Nutrition Care Process Terminology (NCPT)

REFERENCE MANUAL

Standardized Terminology for the Nutrition Care Process

NCPT Version 3.1.0 (released 2023)

eat right. Academy of Nutrition and Dietetics

Nutrition Care Process Terminology (NCPT) Reference Manual: Standardized Terminology for the Nutrition Care Process

ISBN 978-0-88091-282-2

Catalog Number 969226

10 9 8 7 6 5 4 3 2 1

For more information on the Academy of Nutrition and Dietetics, visit www.eatright.org.

Contents

Note: The terminology presented in this *Reference Manual* reflects the current version of the Nutrition Care Process Terminology (NCPT) at the time of publication (version 3.1.0), originally released in 2023 on the electronic Nutrition Care Process Terminology (eNCPT) website, and is subject to change based on continuing development work. For suggested references for each step and term, sign in as a subscriber at nutritioncareprocess.org. Additional resources are available on the Academy's website (eatrightpro.org); sign in as a member and go to eatrightpro.org/practice/nutrition-care-process.

About This Book

The Nutrition Care Process (NCP) is an ongoing and dynamic process designed to improve the consistency and quality of nutrition care and the predictability of nutrition outcomes. It is not intended to standardize nutrition care for clients, but rather to establish a standardized and systematic process for assessing clients across a wide spectrum of health and disease.

The Nutrition Care Process Terminology (NCPT) is an ever-evolving database of assessment, diagnosis, intervention, monitoring, and evaluation terminology that is intended to help practitioners document effectively and efficiently. This process allows for consistent communication both among practitioners and with other health care professionals. It is intended to complement other resources provided by the Academy of Nutrition and Dietetics.

The electronic NCPT (eNCPT) website (nutritioncareprocess.org) is available via subscription from the Academy, but many practitioners and educators also appreciate having a hard copy text available. Although the previous edition of this manual presented an abridged version of the NCPT, this new unabridged edition contains all assessment, diagnostic, intervention, monitoring, and evaluation terminology.

From both a practitioner and educator perspective, this book is a valuable resource. It is also useful to undergraduate and graduate students and dietetic interns. While the NCPT provides the foundation for documentation across all areas of practice in dietetics, it also serves as a valuable educational tool.

For those desiring a more in-depth look at the NCPT, the eNCPT website provides extensive detail and explanation about the complete NCP Terminology for dietetics. Other resources that might be useful include the *eNCPT Clinical Case Studies*, the NCP Scorecard, and the NCP tutorials (nutritioncareprocess.org).

This manual reflects the 2023 version of the NCPT. Some updates include:

- Various revisions and additions to the terminology
- Expanded functional nutrition diagnoses
- Comparative standards in the Assessment/Monitoring and Evaluation domain
- Removal of the alphanumeric NCPT hierarchical codes; symbols are used to represent the domains, classes, subclasses, and terms
- Addition of outlines for each step to highlight the NCPT terminology hierarchy

This book includes the version 3.1.0 of the NCPT released in 2023, which is the same version of the terminology presented on the eNCPT website at the time of publication. Recent changes to the terminology can be found in the Summary of Changes Table on the eNCPT website, which is organized by the steps of the NCP.

Nutrition and dietetics practitioners with decades of experience in both education and practice provided valuable input for this manual, many of whom are currently serving on the eNCPT Board of Editors. We are grateful to each of them for contributing their valuable time, expertise, and input.

Samantha Hutson, PhD, RDN, LDN
Editor-in-Chief, NCPT Board of Editors

Frequently Used Terms and Abbreviations

AI	Adequate Intake
ALT	alanine aminotransferase
AMDR	Acceptable Macronutrient Distribution Range
AST	aspartate aminotransferase
BMI	body mass index
DRI	Dietary Reference Intake
EAR	Estimated Average Requirement
EN	enteral nutrition
GFR	glomerular filtration rate
GI	gastrointestinal
INR	international normalized ratio
LFT	liver function test
MCV	mean corpuscular volume
MNT	medical nutrition therapy
NCP	Nutrition Care Process
PN	parenteral nutrition
RDA	Recommended Dietary Allowance
RDN	Registered Dietitian Nutritionist
RMR	resting metabolic rate
UL	Tolerable Upper Intake Level

Note: Individuals and populations are referred to as clients in association with the NCP. Client also includes supportive individuals (eg, family, caregivers) and structures (eg, social service agencies, faith-based organizations). **Individuals**, **populations**, **supportive individuals**, and **structures** are implied each time a reference is made to client.

The Nutrition Care Process Model

The Nutrition Care Process Model is a graphic visualization that illustrates the steps of the Nutrition Care Process as well as internal and external factors that impact application of the NCP. The central component of the Model is the relationship between the target client or group and the RDN. The innermost of two outer rings represents the skills and abilities of the RDN along with application of evidence-based practice, application of the Academy of Nutrition and Dietetics/Commission on Dietetic Registration Code of Ethics for the Nutrition and Dietetics Profession, and knowledge of the RDN. The outermost ring represents environmental factors such as health care systems, socioeconomics, and practice settings that impact the ability of the target group or client to benefit from RDN services. Screening and referral and outcomes management are also components of the model.

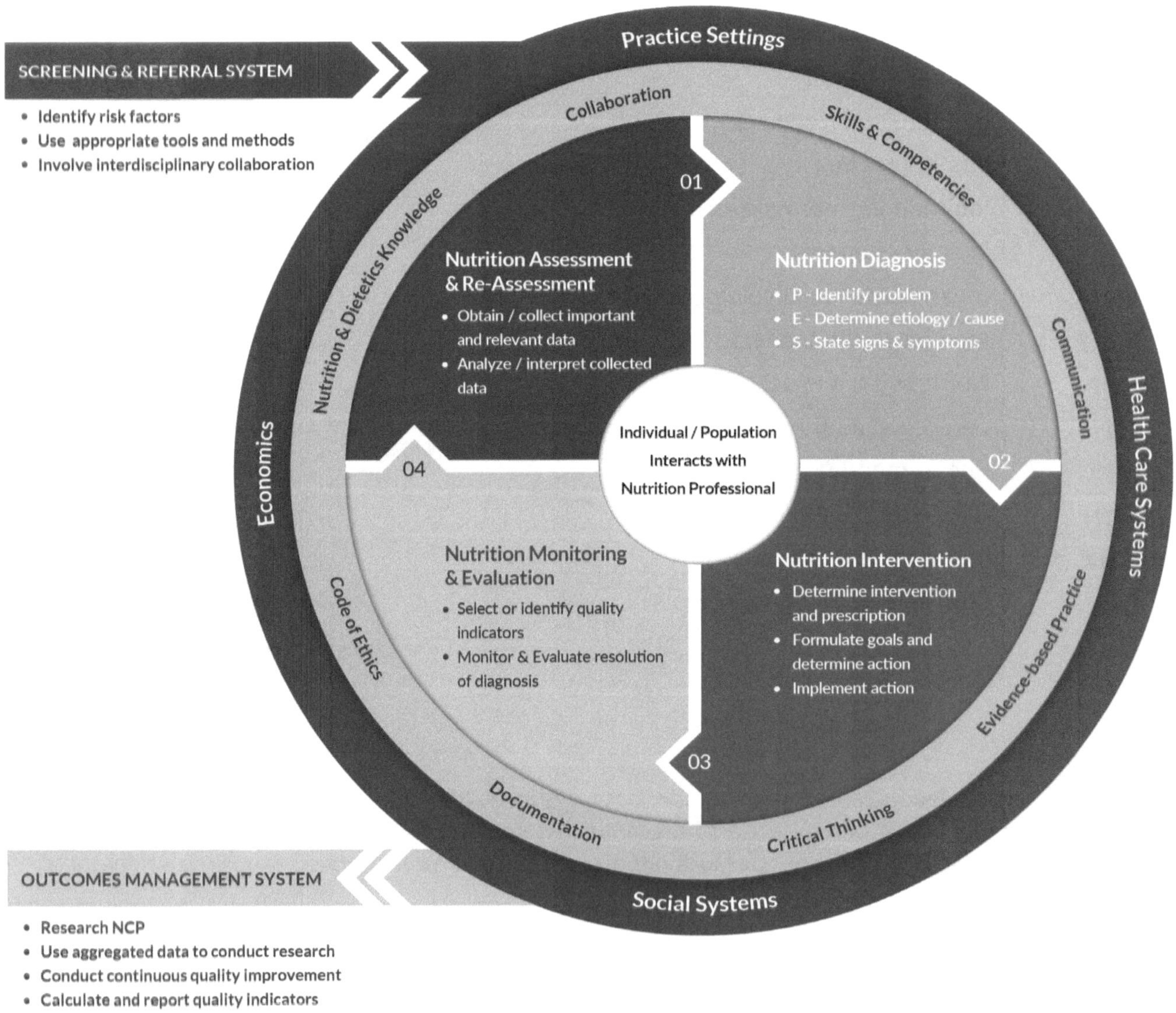

SNAPSHOT
NCP Step 1: Nutrition Assessment

Definition: Nutrition assessment is a systematic approach to collect, interpret, and synthesize relevant data needed to identify nutrition-related problems and their causes. It is an ongoing and dynamic process that involves initial data collection and continual analysis or reassessment of the client's status compared to comparative standards, recommendations, and goals. This contrasts with nutrition monitoring and evaluation where nutrition and dietetics practitioners use the same data to determine changes in client behavior, nutritional status, and the efficacy of nutrition intervention.

Finding nutrition assessment data: For individuals, data can come directly from the client through interview, observation and measurements, a medical record, and the referring health care provider. For population groups, data from surveys, administrative data sets, and epidemiological or research studies are used.

Terminology for Nutrition Assessment is organized in nine domains (categories):

Food/Nutrition Related History	Food and nutrient intake, food and nutrient administration, medication, complementary/alternative medicine use, knowledge/beliefs, food and supplies availability, physical activity, nutrition quality of life
Anthropometric Measurements	Height, weight, body mass index (BMI), growth pattern indices/percentile ranks, and weight history
Biochemical Data, Medical Tests and Procedures	Lab data (eg, electrolytes, glucose) and tests (eg, gastric emptying time, resting metabolic rate)
Nutrition Focused Physical Findings	Physical appearance, muscle and subcutaneous fat wasting, swallow function, appetite, and affect
Client History	Personal history, medical/health/family history treatments and complementary/alternative medicine use, and social history
Assessment, Monitoring and Evaluation Tools	Tools used for health or disease status or risk assessment, reassessment, and monitoring and evaluation
Etiology Category	Categories to communicate the type of nutrition diagnosis etiology
Comparative Standards	What indicator data are compared against
Progress Evaluation	Evaluation of progress toward a nutrition related goal(s) and resolution of a nutrition diagnosis(es)

Use of nutrition assessment data: Nutrition assessment data, or indicators, are compared to reference standards, recommendations, or goals (comparative standards). These norms and standards may be national, institutional, or regulatory. Nutrition assessment findings are then documented in nutrition diagnosis (problem) statements and nutrition intervention goal setting.

Critical Thinking Skills

- Determining important and relevant data to collect
- Determining the need for additional information
- Selecting assessment tools and procedures that match the situation
- Applying assessment tools in valid and reliable ways
- Distinguishing relevant from irrelevant data
- Validating the data

Term selection and organization: The taxonomy or classification system guides the nutrition and dietetics practitioner to logical terminology selection. The terms for Nutrition Assessment and Nutrition Monitoring and Evaluation are combined because the data are the same or related; however, the data purpose and use are distinct in these two steps of the Nutrition Care Process.

For more detailed information about the Nutrition Assessment step, log in as a subscriber to www.nutritioncareprocess.org.

NCP Step 1: Nutrition Assessment

The following is a quick reference outline of the Nutrition Assessment Step. This outline does not include all the terms in this step.

Key: ◆ = NCP Domain; ▲ = NCP Class; ● = NCP Subclass; □ = NCP Term

Key: ◆ = NCP Domain; ▲ = NCP Class; ● = NCP Subclass; ☐ = NCP Term

This is a combined list of Nutrition Assessment and Monitoring and Evaluation terms. All terms can be used for Nutrition Assessment. Client History terms are used for Nutrition Assessment, but not for Nutrition Monitoring and Evaluation. Each term is designated with a five-digit (eg, 99999) Academy unique identifier (ANDUID). This should not be used in nutrition documentation. The ANDUID is for data-tracking purposes in electronic health records.

◆ FOOD/NUTRITION-RELATED HISTORY

Food and nutrient intake, food and nutrient administration, medication and complementary/alternative medicine use, knowledge/beliefs/attitudes, behavior, food and supply availability, physical activity and function, nutrition-related client-centered measures.

▲ Food and Nutrient Intake

Composition and adequacy of food and nutrient intake, meal and snack patterns, current and previous diets and/or food modifications, and eating environment.

● Energy Intake Determination

Ascertaining of the total energy intake from all sources including, food, beverages, breastmilk/formula, supplements, and via enteral and parenteral routes.

	ANDUID
❑ **Energy intake**	**10004**
❑ Estimated energy intake	14219
❑ Total energy estimated intake in 24 hours	11383
❑ Energy estimated intake per kg body weight in 24 hours	14001
❑ Energy estimated intake from oral nutrition in 24 hours	14002
❑ Energy estimated intake from enteral nutrition in 24 hours	14003
❑ Energy estimated intake from parenteral nutrition in 24 hours	14004
❑ Energy estimated intake from intravenous fluids in 24 hours	14005
❑ Measured energy intake	14220
❑ Total energy measured intake in 24 hours	10005
❑ Energy measured intake per kg body weight in 24 hours	14006
❑ Energy measured intake from oral nutrition in 24 hours	14007
❑ Energy measured intake from enteral nutrition in 24 hours	14008
❑ Energy measured intake from parenteral nutrition in 24 hours	14009
❑ Energy measured intake from intravenous fluids in 24 hours	14010

● Food and Beverage Intake Determination

Ascertaining of the type, amount, and pattern of intake of foods and food groups, indices of diet quality, intake of fluids, breastmilk and infant formula

	ANDUID
❑ **Fluid intake**	**10007**
❑ Estimated fluid intake	14011
❑ Total fluid estimated intake in 24 hours	14012
❑ Fluid estimated intake from oral nutrition in 24 hours	11386
❑ Water estimated oral intake in 24 hours	14013
❑ Sugar sweetened beverage estimated oral intake in 24 hours	14014
❑ Beverage with high intensity sweetener estimated oral intake in 24 hours	14015
❑ 100 percent fruit juice estimated oral intake in 24 hours	14016
❑ Liquid mammalian milk product estimated oral intake in 24 hours	14017
❑ Caffeinated beverage estimated oral intake in 24 hours	14018
❑ Nutritionally complete liquid supplement estimated oral intake in 24 hours	14019
❑ Liquid meal replacement estimated oral intake in 24 hours	14020
❑ Fluid estimated intake per kg body weight in 24 hours	14021
❑ Fluid estimated intake from food	10009
❑ Free water estimated intake in 24 hours	14022
❑ Free water estimated intake from breastmilk in 24 hours	14023
❑ Free water estimated intake from infant formula in 24 hours	14024
❑ Free water estimated intake from enteral nutrition in 24 hours	14025
❑ Free water estimated intake from parenteral nutrition in 24 hours	14026
❑ Free water estimated intake from intravenous fluids in 24 hours	14027
❑ Measured fluid intake	14028
❑ Total fluid measured intake in 24 hours	14029

	ANDUID

- ❑ Fluid measured intake from oral nutrition in 24 hours 10008
- ❑ Water measured oral intake in 24 hours 14030
- ❑ Sugar sweetened beverage measured oral intake in 24 hours 14031
- ❑ Beverage with high intensity sweetener measured oral intake in 24 hours 14032
- ❑ 100 percent fruit juice measured oral intake in 24 hours 14033
- ❑ Liquid mammalian milk product measured oral intake in 24 hours 14034
- ❑ Caffeinated beverage measured oral intake in 24 hours 14035
- ❑ Nutritionally complete liquid supplement measured oral intake in 24 hours 14036
- ❑ Liquid meal replacement measured oral intake in 24 hours 14037

❑ Fluid measured intake from food 14038

❑ Fluid measured intake per kg body weight in 24 hours 14039

❑ Free water measured intake in 24 hours 14040
- ❑ Free water measured intake from breastmilk in 24 hours 14041
- ❑ Free water measured intake from infant formula in 24 hours 14042
- ❑ Free water measured intake from enteral nutrition in 24 hours 14043
- ❑ Free water measured intake from parenteral nutrition in 24 hours 14044
- ❑ Free water measured intake from intravenous fluids in 24 hours 14045

❑ Food intake 10011

- ❑ Amount of food 10012
  - ❑ Estimated amount of food 13125
    - ❑ Grain servings estimated in 24 hours 11387
    - ❑ Fruit servings estimated in 24 hours 11389
    - ❑ Vegetable servings estimated in 24 hours 11391
    - ❑ Mammalian milk product servings estimated in 24 hours 11393
    - ❑ Protein food servings estimated in 24 hours 11395
    - ❑ Fat servings estimated in 24 hours 11397
    - ❑ Empty energy servings estimated in 24 hours 11399
    - ❑ Estimated percent of meals eaten in 24 hours 14046
  - ❑ Measured amount of food 13126
    - ❑ Grain servings measured in 24 hours 11388
    - ❑ Fruit servings measured in 24 hours 11390
    - ❑ Vegetable servings measured in 24 hours 11392
    - ❑ Mammalian milk product servings measured in 24 hours 11394
    - ❑ Protein food servings measured in 24 hours 11396
    - ❑ Fat servings measured in 24 hours 11398
    - ❑ Empty energy servings measured in 24 hours 11400
    - ❑ Measured percent of meals eaten in 24 hours 14047
- ❑ Types of food 10013
  - ❑ Fortified food intake 14048
  - ❑ Enriched food intake 14049
  - ❑ Special dietary food intake 14050
  - ❑ Medical food intake 14051
  - ❑ Processed food intake 14052
  - ❑ Quick service food intake 14053
  - ❑ Self prepared food intake 14054
  - ❑ Prepared food intake 14210
- ❑ Meal/snack pattern 10014
  - ❑ Estimated meal and snack pattern 13127
    - ❑ Number of meals estimated in 24 hours 11404
    - ❑ Number of snacks estimated in 24 hours 11402
  - ❑ Measured meal and snack pattern 13128
    - ❑ Number of meals measured in 24 hours 11405
    - ❑ Number of snacks measured in 24 hours 11403
- ❑ Diet quality index 10015
  - ❑ Healthy eating index (HEI) 2015 score 14055
- ❑ Food variety 10016

❑ Breastmilk and infant formula intake 10017

- ❑ Breastmilk intake 10018
  - ❑ Breastmilk feeding attempts in 24 hours 11406
  - ❑ Adequacy of breastmilk intake 11409
  - ❑ Donor breastmilk intake 14056
  - ❑ Mother's expressed breastmilk intake 14057
  - ❑ Estimated breastmilk intake 14058
    - ❑ Breastmilk intake estimated volume in 24 hours 11407
    - ❑ Breastmilk intake estimated volume per kg body weight in 24 hours 14059
  - ❑ Measured breastmilk intake 14060
    - ❑ Breastmilk intake measured volume in 24 hours 11408

Key: ◆ = NCP Domain; ▲ = NCP Class; ● = NCP Subclass; ❑ = NCP Term

ANDUID

- ❑ Breastmilk intake measured volume per kg body weight in 24 hours 14061
- ❑ Infant formula intake 10019
  - ❑ Infant formula feedings in 24 hours 11412
  - ❑ Adequacy of infant formula intake 11413
  - ❑ Infant formula intake composition 14211
  - ❑ Infant formula intake concentration 14062
  - ❑ Estimated infant formula intake 14063
    - ❑ Infant formula intake estimated volume in 24 hours 11410
    - ❑ Infant formula intake estimated volume per kg body weight in 24 hours 14064
  - ❑ Measured infant formula intake 14065
    - ❑ Infant formula intake measured volume in 24 hours 11411
    - ❑ Infant formula intake measured volume per kg body weight in 24 hours 14066

● Enteral and Parenteral Nutrition Intake Determination

Ascertaining of the nutrition support intake from all sources, eg, enteral and parenteral routes.

❑ Enteral nutrition intake **10021**

- ❑ Enteral nutrition formula/solution 10022
  - ❑ Enteral nutrition formula composition 11414
  - ❑ Enteral nutrition formula concentration 11415
  - ❑ Enteral nutrition formula estimated volume in 24 hours 11416
  - ❑ Enteral nutrition formula measured volume in 24 hours 13227
- ❑ Enteral tube feeding flush estimated volume in 24 hours 10023
- ❑ Enteral tube feeding flush measured volume in 24 hours 13228

❑ Parenteral nutrition intake **10024**

- ❑ Parenteral nutrition formula/solution 10025
- ❑ IV fluids 10026

● Bioactive Constituent Intake Determination

Ascertaining of the alcohol, plant stanol and sterol esters, soy protein, psyllium and beta glucan, and caffeine intake from all sources, eg, food, beverages, supplements, and via enteral and parenteral routes.

❑ Alcohol intake **10028**

- ❑ Alcohol intake in one week 14172
- ❑ Alcohol intake in 24 hours 14173
  - ❑ Beer intake in 24 hours 14174
  - ❑ Distilled alcohol intake in 24 hours 14175
  - ❑ Wine intake in 24 hours 14176
  - ❑ Hard cider intake in 24 hours 14177

ANDUID

- ❑ Days per week alcoholic drinks consumed 14188
- ❑ Alcohol intake pattern on drinking days 10031

❑ Bioactive substance intake **10032**

- ❑ Estimated bioactive substance intake 13129
  - ❑ Plant stanol ester estimated intake in 24 hours 11422
  - ❑ Plant sterol ester estimated intake in 24 hours 11424
  - ❑ Soy protein estimated intake in 24 hours 11426
  - ❑ Prebiotic estimated intake 30006
    - ❑ Psyllium estimated intake in 24 hours 11428
    - ❑ Beta glucan estimated intake in 24 hours 11430
- ❑ Measured bioactive substance intake 13130
  - ❑ Plant stanol ester measured intake in 24 hours 11423
  - ❑ Plant sterol ester measured intake in 24 hours 11425
  - ❑ Soy protein measured intake in 24 hours 11427
  - ❑ Prebiotic measured intake 30007
    - ❑ Psyllium measured intake in 24 hours 11429
    - ❑ Beta glucan measured intake in 24 hours 11431
- ❑ Food additive intake 10038
  - ❑ High intensity sweetener additive intake 14067
    - ❑ Excessive high intensity sweetener additive intake 14068
- ❑ Probiotic intake 30008

❑ Caffeine intake **10040**

- ❑ Total caffeine estimated intake in 24 hours 11432
- ❑ Total caffeine measured intake in 24 hours 10041

● Macronutrient Intake Determination

Ascertaining of the fat and cholesterol, protein, carbohydrate, and fiber intake from all sources including food, beverages, supplements, and via enteral and parenteral routes.

❑ Fat intake **11607**

- ❑ Estimated fat intake 13131
  - ❑ Total fat estimated intake in 24 hours 11433
  - ❑ Saturated fat estimated intake in 24 hours 11435
  - ❑ Trans fatty acid estimated intake in 24 hours 11437
  - ❑ Polyunsaturated fat estimated intake in 24 hours 11439
    - ❑ Linoleic acid estimated intake in 24 hours 11602
  - ❑ Monounsaturated fat estimated intake in 24 hours 11441

	ANDUID
❑ Omega 3 fatty acid estimated intake in 24 hours	11443
❑ Alpha linolenic acid estimated intake in 24 hours	11445
❑ Eicosapentaenoic acid estimated intake in 24 hours	11447
❑ Docosahexaenoic acid estimated intake in 24 hours	11449
❑ Essential fatty acid estimated intake in 24 hours	11451
❑ Medium chain triglyceride estimated intake in 24 hours	11453
❑ Fat estimated intake in one meal	14069
❑ Percent saturated fat estimated intake in 24 hours	14070
❑ Fat estimated intake from oral nutrition in 24 hours	13000
❑ Fat estimated intake from enteral nutrition in 24 hours	12014
❑ Fat estimated intake from parenteral nutrition in 24 hours	13001
❑ Fat estimated intake from intravenous fluids in 24 hours	13002
❑ Fat additive estimated intake in 24 hours	14071
❑ Percent fat estimated intake in 24 hours	14216
❑ Measured fat intake	13132
❑ Total fat measured intake in 24 hours	11434
❑ Saturated fat measured intake in 24 hours	11436
❑ Trans fatty acid measured intake in 24 hours	11438
❑ Polyunsaturated fat measured intake in 24 hours	11440
❑ Linoleic acid measured intake in 24 hours	13225
❑ Monounsaturated fat measured intake in 24 hours	11442
❑ Omega 3 fatty acid measured intake in 24 hours	11444
❑ Alpha linolenic acid measured intake in 24 hours	11446
❑ Eicosapentaenoic acid measured intake in 24 hours	11448
❑ Docosahexaenoic acid measured intake in 24 hours	11450
❑ Essential fatty acid measured intake in 24 hours	11452
❑ Medium chain triglyceride measured intake in 24 hours	11454
❑ Fat measured intake in one meal	14072
❑ Percent saturated fat measured intake in 24 hours	14073

	ANDUID
❑ Fat measured intake from oral nutrition in 24 hours	14074
❑ Fat measured intake from enteral nutrition in 24 hours	14075
❑ Fat measured intake from parenteral nutrition in 24 hours	14076
❑ Fat measured intake from intravenous fluids in 24 hours	14077
❑ Fat additive measured intake in 24 hours	14078
❑ Percent fat measured intake in 24 hours	14217
❑ Cholesterol intake	**11608**
❑ Cholesterol estimated intake in 24 hours	11455
❑ Cholesterol measured intake in 24 hours	11456
❑ Protein intake	**10052**
❑ Estimated protein intake	13133
❑ Total protein estimated intake in 24 hours	11457
❑ High biological value protein estimated intake in 24 hours	11459
❑ Casein estimated intake in 24 hours	11461
❑ Whey protein estimated intake in 24 hours	11463
❑ Gluten estimated intake in 24 hours	11465
❑ Protein estimated intake per kg body weight in 24 hours	11467
❑ Natural protein estimated intake in 24 hours	11610
❑ Protein estimated intake in one meal	14079
❑ Percent protein estimated intake in 24 hours	14080
❑ Protein estimated intake from oral nutrition in 24 hours	13003
❑ Protein estimated intake from enteral nutrition in 24 hours	13004
❑ Protein additive estimated intake in 24 hours	14081
❑ Measured protein intake	13134
❑ Total protein measured intake in 24 hours	11458
❑ High biological value protein measured intake in 24 hours	11460
❑ Casein measured intake in 24 hours	11462
❑ Whey protein measured intake in 24 hours	11464
❑ Gluten measured intake in 24 hours	11466
❑ Protein measured intake per kg body weight in 24 hours	11468
❑ Natural protein measured intake in 24 hours	14082
❑ Protein measured intake in one meal	14083
❑ Percent protein measured intake in 24 hours	14212

Key: ◆ = NCP Domain; ▲ = NCP Class; ● = NCP Subclass; ❑ = NCP Term

ANDUID

- ❑ Protein measured intake from oral nutrition in 24 hours 14084
- ❑ Protein measured intake from enteral nutrition in 24 hours 14085
- ❑ Protein additive measured intake in 24 hours 14087

❑ Amino acid intake 11611

- ❑ Estimated amino acid intake 13135
  - ❑ Total amino acid estimated intake in 24 hours 10057
  - ❑ Essential amino acid estimated intake in 24 hours 10058
    - ❑ Histidine estimated intake in 24 hours 11612
    - ❑ Methionine estimated intake in 24 hours 11613
    - ❑ Isoleucine estimated intake in 24 hours 11614
    - ❑ Leucine estimated intake in 24 hours 11615
    - ❑ Lysine estimated intake in 24 hours 11616
    - ❑ Threonine estimated intake in 24 hours 11617
    - ❑ Tryptophan estimated intake in 24 hours 11618
    - ❑ Phenylalanine estimated intake in 24 hours 11619
    - ❑ Valine estimated intake in 24 hours 11620
  - ❑ Nonessential amino acid estimated intake in 24 hours 11621
    - ❑ Arginine estimated intake in 24 hours 11622
    - ❑ Glutamine estimated intake in 24 hours 11623
    - ❑ Homocysteine estimated intake in 24 hours 11624
    - ❑ Tyramine estimated intake in 24 hours 11625
    - ❑ Tyrosine estimated intake in 24 hours 11626
  - ❑ Estimated amino acid intake from enteral nutrition in 24 hours 13005
  - ❑ Estimated amino acid intake from parenteral nutrition in 24 hours 13006
  - ❑ Estimated amino acid intake from intravenous fluids in 24 hours 13007
- ❑ Measured amino acid intake 13226
  - ❑ Total amino acid measured intake in 24 hours 13137
  - ❑ Essential amino acid measured intake in 24 hours 13138
    - ❑ Histidine measured intake in 24 hours 13139
    - ❑ Methionine measured intake in 24 hours 13140
    - ❑ Isoleucine measured intake in 24 hours 13141
    - ❑ Leucine measured intake in 24 hours 13142
    - ❑ Lysine measured intake in 24 hours 13143
    - ❑ Threonine measured intake in 24 hours 13144
    - ❑ Tryptophan measured intake in 24 hours 13145
    - ❑ Phenylalanine measured intake in 24 hours 13146
    - ❑ Valine measured intake in 24 hours 13147
  - ❑ Nonessential amino acid measured intake in 24 hours 13148
    - ❑ Arginine measured intake in 24 hours 13136
    - ❑ Glutamine measured intake in 24 hours 13149
    - ❑ Homocysteine measured intake in 24 hours 13150
    - ❑ Tyramine measured intake in 24 hours 13151
    - ❑ Tyrosine measured intake in 24 hours 13152
  - ❑ Measured amino acid intake from enteral nutrition in 24 hours 30009
  - ❑ Measured amino acid intake from parenteral nutrition in 24 hours 30010
  - ❑ Measured amino acid intake from intravenous fluids in 24 hours 30011

❑ Carbohydrate intake 10059

- ❑ Estimated carbohydrate intake 13153
  - ❑ Total carbohydrate estimated intake in 24 hours 10060
  - ❑ Complex carbohydrate estimated intake in 24 hours 11627
  - ❑ Simple carbohydrate estimated intake in 24 hours 11628
  - ❑ Galactose estimated intake in 24 hours 11629
  - ❑ Lactose estimated intake in 24 hours 11630
  - ❑ Fructose estimated intake in 24 hours 11631
  - ❑ Carbohydrate estimated intake per kg body weight in 24 hours 14088
  - ❑ Carbohydrate estimated intake in one meal 14089
  - ❑ Percent carbohydrate estimated intake in 24 hours 14090
  - ❑ Carbohydrate estimated intake from oral nutrition in 24 hours 12143

	ANDUID
❑ Carbohydrate estimated intake from enteral nutrition in 24 hours	12011
❑ Carbohydrate estimated intake from parenteral nutrition in 24 hours	11180
❑ Carbohydrate estimated intake from intravenous fluids in 24 hours	11240
❑ Carbohydrate additive estimated intake in 24 hours	14091
❑ Estimated daily glycemic index value	12013
❑ Estimated daily glycemic load	12142
❑ Insulin to carbohydrate ratio	10066
❑ Measured carbohydrate intake	13154
❑ Total carbohydrate measured intake in 24 hours	13155
❑ Complex carbohydrate measured intake in 24 hours	13156
❑ Simple carbohydrate measured intake in 24 hours	13157
❑ Galactose measured intake in 24 hours	13158
❑ Lactose measured intake in 24 hours	13159
❑ Fructose measured intake in 24 hours	13160
❑ Carbohydrate measured intake per kg body weight in 24 hours	14092
❑ Carbohydrate measured intake in one meal	14093
❑ Percent carbohydrate measured intake in 24 hours	14094
❑ Carbohydrate measured intake from oral nutrition in 24 hours	14095
❑ Carbohydrate measured intake from enteral nutrition in 24 hours	14096
❑ Carbohydrate measured intake from parenteral nutrition in 24 hours	14097
❑ Carbohydrate measured intake from intravenous fluids in 24 hours	14098
❑ Carbohydrate additive measured intake in 24 hours	14099
❑ Fiber intake	**10067**
❑ Estimated fiber intake	13161
❑ Total fiber estimated intake in 24 hours	10068
❑ Soluble fiber estimated intake in 24 hours	10069
❑ Insoluble fiber estimated intake in 24 hours	10070
❑ Fiber estimated intake from oral nutrition in 24 hours	14213
❑ Fiber estimated intake from enteral nutrition in 24 hours	14100
❑ Fiber additive estimated intake in 24 hours	14214
❑ Measured fiber intake	11519

	ANDUID
❑ Total fiber measured intake in 24 hours	13162
❑ Soluble fiber measured intake in 24 hours	13163
❑ Insoluble fiber measured intake in 24 hours	13164
❑ Fiber measured intake from oral nutrition in 24 hours	14101
❑ Fiber measured intake from enteral nutrition in 24 hours	14102
❑ Fiber additive measured intake in 24 hours	14103

● Micronutrient Intake Determination

Ascertaining of the vitamin and mineral intake from all sources, including food, beverages, supplements, and via enteral and parenteral routes.

❑ Vitamin intake	**10072**
❑ Estimated vitamin intake	13165
❑ Vitamin A estimated intake in 24 hours	10073
❑ Vitamin C estimated intake in 24 hours	10074
❑ Vitamin D estimated intake in 24 hours	10075
❑ Vitamin E estimated intake in 24 hours	10076
❑ Vitamin K estimated intake in 24 hours	10077
❑ Thiamin estimated intake in 24 hours	10078
❑ Riboflavin estimated intake in 24 hours	10079
❑ Niacin estimated intake in 24 hours	10080
❑ Folate estimated intake in 24 hours	10081
❑ Vitamin B6 estimated intake in 24 hours	10082
❑ Vitamin B12 estimated intake in 24 hours	10083
❑ Pantothenic acid estimated intake in 24 hours	10084
❑ Biotin estimated intake in 24 hours	10085
❑ Multivitamin estimated intake in 24 hours	10086
❑ Measured vitamin intake	13167
❑ Vitamin A measured intake in 24 hours	13168
❑ Vitamin C measured intake in 24 hours	13169
❑ Vitamin D measured intake in 24 hours	13170
❑ Vitamin E measured intake in 24 hours	13171
❑ Vitamin K measured intake in 24 hours	13172
❑ Thiamin measured intake in 24 hours	13173
❑ Riboflavin measured intake in 24 hours	13174
❑ Niacin measured intake in 24 hours	13175
❑ Folate measured intake in 24 hours	13176
❑ Vitamin B6 measured intake in 24 hours	13177
❑ Vitamin B12 measured intake in 24 hours	13178
❑ Pantothenic acid measured intake in 24 hours	13179
❑ Biotin measured intake in 24 hours	13180

Key: ◆ = NCP Domain; ▲ = NCP Class; ● = NCP Subclass; ❑ = NCP Term

	ANDUID
❑ Multivitamin measured intake in 24 hours	13181
❑ Mineral/element intake	**10088**
❑ Estimated mineral intake	13182
❑ Calcium estimated intake in 24 hours	10089
❑ Chloride estimated intake in 24 hours	10090
❑ Iron estimated intake in 24 hours	10091
❑ Magnesium estimated intake in 24 hours	10092
❑ Potassium estimated intake in 24 hours	10093
❑ Phosphorus estimated intake in 24 hours	10094
❑ Sodium estimated intake in 24 hours	10095
❑ Zinc estimated intake in 24 hours	10096
❑ Sulfate estimated intake in 24 hours	10097
❑ Fluoride estimated intake in 24 hours	10098
❑ Copper estimated intake in 24 hours	10099
❑ Iodine estimated intake in 24 hours	10100
❑ Selenium estimated intake in 24 hours	10101
❑ Manganese estimated intake in 24 hours	10102
❑ Chromium estimated intake in 24 hours	10103
❑ Molybdenum estimated intake in 24 hours	10104
❑ Boron estimated intake in 24 hours	10105
❑ Cobalt estimated intake in 24 hours	10106
❑ Multimineral estimated intake in 24 hours	10107
❑ Multitrace element estimated intake in 24 hours	10108
❑ Measured mineral intake	13183
❑ Calcium measured intake in 24 hours	13184
❑ Chloride measured intake in 24 hours	13185
❑ Iron measured intake in 24 hours	13186
❑ Magnesium measured intake in 24 hours	13187
❑ Potassium measured intake in 24 hours	13188
❑ Phosphorus measured intake in 24 hours	13189
❑ Sodium measured intake in 24 hours	13190
❑ Zinc measured intake in 24 hours	13191
❑ Sulfate measured intake in 24 hours	13192
❑ Fluoride measured intake in 24 hours	13193
❑ Copper measured intake in 24 hours	13194
❑ Iodine measured intake in 24 hours	13195
❑ Selenium measured intake in 24 hours	13196
❑ Manganese measured intake in 24 hours	13197
❑ Chromium measured intake in 24 hours	13198
❑ Molybdenum measured intake in 24 hours	13199

	ANDUID
❑ Boron measured intake in 24 hours	13200
❑ Cobalt measured intake in 24 hours	13201
❑ Multimineral measured intake in 24 hours	13202
❑ Multitrace element measured intake in 24 hours	13203

● Food and Nutrition Component Intake Determination

Ascertaining of the intake of substances for modifying the composition of oral or enteral nutrition intake.

❑ Consistency modifier intake	**14301**
❑ Estimated consistency modifier intake	14104
❑ Thickener additive estimated intake in 24 hours	14105
❑ Measured consistency modifier intake	14106
❑ Thickener additive measured intake in 24 hours	14107

▲ Food and Nutrient Administration

Current and previous diets and/or food modifications, eating environment, and enteral and parenteral nutrition administration.

● Diet History

Description of food and drink regularly provided or consumed, past diets followed or prescribed and counseling received, and the eating environment.

❑ Diet order	**10112**
❑ General healthful diet order	10113
❑ Modified diet order	10114
❑ Enteral nutrition order	10115
❑ Parenteral nutrition order	10116
❑ Diet experience	**10117**
❑ Previously prescribed diets	10118
❑ Previous diet/nutrition education/counseling	10119
❑ Self selected diet/s followed	10120
❑ Dieting attempts	10121
❑ Food allergies	10805
❑ Food intolerance	10806
❑ Eating environment	**10122**
❑ Location	10123
❑ Atmosphere	10124
❑ Caregiver/companion	10125
❑ Appropriate breastfeeding accommodations/facility	10126
❑ Eats alone	10127
❑ Enteral and parenteral nutrition administration	**10128**
Enteral nutrition administration assessment	30012

	ANDUID
❑ Method of enteral nutrition feeding administration	30013
❑ Orogastric enteral nutrition feeding administration	30014
❑ Oroenteric enteral nutrition feeding administration	30015
❑ Nasogastric enteral nutrition feeding administration	30017
❑ Nasoduodenal enteral nutrition feeding administration	30016
❑ Nasojejunal enteral nutrition feeding administration	30018
❑ Gastrostomy enteral nutrition feeding administration	30019
❑ Jejunostomy enteral nutrition feeding administration	30020
❑ Continuous enteral nutrition feeding	30024
❑ Bolus enteral nutrition feeding	30025
❑ Intermittent enteral nutrition feeding	30026
❑ Enteral nutrition feeding access device patency status	30027
❑ Body position for enteral nutrition administration	10804
❑ Supine body position for enteral nutrition administration	30028
❑ Prone body position for enteral nutrition administration	30029
❑ Degree elevation of head of bed for enteral nutrition administration	30030
❑ Parenteral nutrition administration assessment	30031
❑ Method of parenteral nutrition administration	30032
❑ Peripheral venous parenteral nutrition administration	30033
❑ Central venous parenteral nutrition administration	30034
❑ Intradialytic parenteral nutrition administration	30035
❑ Intraperitoneal parenteral nutrition administration	30036
❑ Continuous parenteral nutrition administration	30037
❑ Cyclic parenteral nutrition administration	30038
❑ Parenteral nutrition access device patency status	30039
❑ Fasting determination	**11632**
❑ Reported fasting pattern in one calendar day	11633
❑ Reported fasting pattern in one calendar week	11634

	ANDUID
❑ Reported fasting pattern in one calendar month	11635
❑ Reported fasting pattern in one calendar year	11636
❑ Reported fasting tolerance	11637

▲ Medication and Complementary/Alternative Medicine Use

Prescription and over the counter medications, including herbal preparations and complementary/alternative medicine products used.

● Medications	**10797**
❑ Prescription medication use	10820
❑ Insulin sensitivity factor	11241
❑ Over the counter (OTC) medication use	10134
❑ Misuse of medication	10135
● Complementary/Alternative Medicine	**10136**
❑ Nutrition related complementary/ alternative medicine use	10137

▲ Knowledge Belief Attitude Determination

Ascertaining of the client's understanding of nutrition-related concepts, conviction of the truth and feelings/ emotions toward some nutrition-related statement or phenomenon, and readiness to change nutrition-related behaviors.

● Food and nutrition knowledge	**10141**
❑ Nutrition knowledge of community	13204
❑ Nutrition knowledge of supportive individuals	13205
❑ Nutrition knowledge of individual client	13206
● Food and nutrition skill	**14000**
❑ Nutrition skill of the community	13207
❑ Nutrition skill of supportive individuals	13208
❑ Nutrition skill of individual client	13209
● Belief and attitude determination	**10144**
❑ Nutrition priority of individual client	14508
❑ Nutrition priority of client's supportive individuals	14509
❑ Nutrition priority of client's supportive structures	14510
❑ Nutrition priority of client's stakeholders	14511
❑ Conflict with individual client's value system	14512
❑ Conflict with client's supportive individuals' value system	14513
❑ Conflict with client's supportive structures' value system	14514
❑ Conflict with client's stakeholders' value system	14515
❑ Behavioral beliefs	14516

Key: ◆ = NCP Domain; ▲ = NCP Class; ● = NCP Subclass; ❑ = NCP Term

	ANDUID
❑ Perceived susceptibility to nutrition related health problems score	14517
❑ Perceived severity of risk to health score	14518
❑ Perceived benefit of nutrition related change score	14519
❑ Likelihood of performing nutrition related behavior score	14520
❑ Perceived control over nutrition related behavior score	14521
❑ Nutrition self efficacy score	14522
❑ Perceived barrier to nutrition related behavior score	14523
❑ Readiness to change nutrition related behavior stage	10151
❑ Precontemplation stage for readiness to change	14524
❑ Contemplation stage for readiness to change	14525
❑ Preparation stage for readiness to change	14526
❑ Action stage for readiness to change	14527
❑ Maintenance stage for readiness to change	14528
❑ Relapse stage for readiness to change	14529
❑ Readiness to change nutrition related behavior score	14590
❑ Negative emotions about food and nutrition	14530
❑ Positive emotions about food and nutrition	14531
❑ Unrealistic nutrition related goals	10154
❑ Unscientific nutrition belief	14532
❑ Body image disturbance	10146
❑ Preoccupation with food	10149
❑ Preoccupation with body weight	10150
❑ Preoccupation with body shape	14533
❑ Negative nutrition self talk	14534
❑ Positive nutrition self talk	14535
❑ Preferences for food	10156
❑ Preferences for beverages	14537
❑ Craving for nonfood item	30040

▲ Behavior Determination

Ascertaining of the client activities and actions, which influence achievement of nutrition related goals.

● Adherence behavior	**10159**
❑ Self reported nutrition adherence score	10160
❑ Nutrition encounter ratio	14215
❑ Ability to recall nutrition goals	10162
❑ Nutrition self monitoring at agreed upon rate	10163
❑ Nutrition self management as agreed upon	10164
● Avoidance behavior	**10165**
❑ Avoidance	10166
❑ Restrictive eating	10167
❑ Cause of avoidance behavior	10168
● Binge eating and purging behavior	**10169**
❑ Binge eating behavior	10170
❑ Self induced purging behavior	10171
❑ Number of binge eating episodes per week	30041
❑ Number of self induced purging episodes per week	30042
● Eating behavior	**10172**
❑ Duration of typical eating occasion	10173
❑ Percentage of typical eating occasion spent consuming food	10174
❑ Refusing food	10176
❑ Fatigue during eating	10179
❑ Readiness to consume new food	10180
❑ Aversion to particular food	30043
❑ Sensory aversion to particular food	10182
❑ Aversion to particular beverage	30044
❑ Distracted during eating	30045
● Social network behavior	**10183**
❑ Ability to build and utilize social network	10184

▲ Factors Affecting Access to Food and Food/Nutrition Related Supplies

Factors that affect intake and availability of a sufficient quantity of safe, healthful food as well as food/nutrition-related supplies.

● Food and nutrition program participation	**10186**
❑ Eligibility for government nutrition programs	10187
❑ Enrollment in government nutrition programs	14538
❑ Eligibility for community nutrition programs	10189
❑ Enrollment in community nutrition programs	14539
❑ Awareness of programs offering food support and nutrition intervention	14540
● Safe food availability	**10191**
❑ Availability of shopping facilities	10192
❑ Ability to procure safe food	10800
❑ Access to food preparation equipment	14541
❑ Availability of food refrigeration	14542
❑ Ability to store food safely	14543
❑ Ability to identify safe food	10801
❑ Individual client food security level	14544
❑ Household food security level	14545

	ANDUID
❑ Situational food insecurity	14546
❑ Chronic food insecurity	14547
● Safe water availability	**10197**
❑ Availability of potable water	10198
❑ Ability to decontaminate water	14548
❑ Awareness of public health water alert	14549
● Food and nutrition related supplies availability	**10200**
❑ Access to food and nutrition related supplies	10201
❑ Access to assistive eating devices	10202
❑ Access to assistive food preparation devices	10203
● Food and nutrition sanitation	**14550**
❑ Availability of suitable sanitation facilities	14551
❑ Ability to wash hands with soap and water	14552

▲ Physical Activity and Function

Physical activity, cognitive and physical ability to engage in specific tasks, eg, breastfeeding and self-feeding.

	ANDUID
● Breastfeeding assessment	**10205**
❑ Initiation of breastfeeding	10206
❑ Start breastfeeding	14108
❑ Stop breastfeeding	14109
❑ Breastfeeding approach	14110
❑ Exclusive breastfeeding	10208
❑ Predominant breastfeeding	14111
❑ Partial breastfeeding	14112
❑ Breastfeeding difficulties	10209
❑ Infant able to latch on to nipple for feeding	14113
❑ Infant unable to latch on to nipple for feeding	14114
❑ Difficulty latching onto nipple for feeding	14115
❑ Abscess of breast tissue with lactating capability	14116
❑ Cracked nipple associated with lactation	14117
❑ Infection of nipple associated with lactation	14118
❑ Non purulent mastitis associated with lactation	14119
❑ Retracted nipple associated with lactation	14120
❑ Inversion of nipple associated with lactation	14121
❑ Breast tissue with lactating capability engorged	14122
❑ Previous surgery on breast tissue with lactating capability	14123
❑ Abnormality of breast tissue with lactating capability	14124
❑ Inadequate flow of breastmilk	14125
❑ Finding related to infant's ability to suck	14126
❑ Infant able to suck	14127
❑ Infant unable to suck	14128
❑ Difficulty sucking	14129
● Nutrition related activities of daily living and instrumental activities of daily living	**10210**
❑ Ability to perform shopping activities	30046
❑ Ability to plan meals	30047
❑ Ability to prepare food for eating	30048
❑ Ability to prepare meal	30049
❑ Ability to self feed	10212
❑ Ability to position self in relation to food	10213
❑ Feeding assisted	10214
❑ Ability to use cutlery to feed self	30050
❑ Ability to use adaptive eating device for self feeding	10215
❑ Ability to self administer enteral nutrition feeding	30051
❑ Ability to self administer parenteral nutrition	30052
❑ Ability to remember to eat	10139
❑ Ability to remember to infuse enteral nutrition	30053
❑ Ability to remember to infuse parenteral nutrition	30054
❑ Nutrition related activities of daily living (ADL) score	10220
❑ Nutrition related instrumental activities of daily living (IADL) score	10221
❑ Ability to open and close containers	30055
● Physical activity	**10222**
❑ Physical activity history	10223
❑ Consistency	10224
❑ Frequency	10225
❑ Duration	10226
❑ Intensity	10227
❑ Type of physical activity	10228
❑ Strength	10229
❑ Handgrip strength	11680
❑ TV/screen time	10230
❑ Other sedentary activity time	10231
❑ Involuntary physical movement	10232
❑ Non exercise activity thermogenesis	10233
● Factors affecting access to physical activity	**10821**
❑ Perceived neighborhood safety	10822
❑ Perceived walkability of neighborhood	10823
❑ Perceived proximity to parks	10824
❑ Access to physical activity facility	10825

Key: ◆ = NCP Domain; ▲ = NCP Class; ● = NCP Subclass; ❑ = NCP Term

▲ Nutrition Related Client Centered Measures

Client's perception of their nutrition intervention and its impact on life.

	ANDUID
● **Food and/or nutrition quality of life**	**10235**
❑ Food and/or nutrition quality of life response	10236
❑ Food and/or nutrition related concern	30056
❑ Client reported experience measure	30057
❑ Client reported outcome measure	30058

◆ ANTHROPOMETRIC MEASUREMENTS

Body height, body weight, body frame, body weight change, body mass, growth pattern indices, and body compartment estimates.

▲ Nutrition Focused Anthropometric Measurements

Anthropometric indicators that may be important for determining nutrition status.

	ANDUID
● **Body composition/growth/weight history**	**10238**
❑ Body height	10239
❑ Measured body height	11377
❑ Measured body length	12015
❑ Birth length	12016
❑ Preamputation measured body height	12017
❑ Preamputation estimated body height	12018
❑ Estimated body height	12019
❑ Stated body height	12020
❑ Measured peak adult body height	12021
❑ Stated peak adult body height	12022
❑ Knee height measure	12023
❑ Tibia length measure	12024
❑ Arm span measure	12025
❑ Arm demispan measure	12026
❑ Arm halfspan measure	12027
❑ Height measurement device	12028
❑ Body weight	10240
❑ Measured body weight	12029
❑ Stated body weight	12030
❑ Stated peak body weight	12031
❑ Measured peak body weight	12032
❑ Usual stated body weight (UBW)	12033
❑ Usual body weight (UBW) percentage	12034
❑ Birth weight	12035
❑ Stated prepregnancy body weight	12036
❑ Dosing body weight	12037
❑ Estimated dry body weight	12038
❑ Preamputation measured body weight	12039
❑ Preamputation estimated body weight	12040
❑ Postamputation measured body weight	12041
❑ Postamputation estimated body weight	12042
❑ Predialysis body weight	12043
❑ Postdialysis body weight	12044
❑ Body frame	10241
❑ Body frame size	12045
❑ Wrist joint circumference	12046
❑ Body weight change	10242
❑ Body weight gain	12047
❑ Body weight loss	12048
❑ Body weight change percentage	12049
❑ Measured interdialytic body weight gain	12050
❑ Measured interdialytic body weight loss	12051
❑ Measured gestational body weight gain	12052
❑ Measured gestational body weight loss	12053
❑ Body weight change intent	12054
❑ Body mass	10243
❑ Body mass index (BMI)	12055
❑ Body mass index prime ratio (BMI prime)	12056
❑ Appendicular skeletal muscle mass	30060
❑ Appendicular skeletal muscle mass index	30061
❑ Fat free mass	30062
❑ Fat free mass index	30063
❑ Skeletal muscle mass	30064
❑ Skeletal muscle mass index	30065
❑ Lean soft tissue mass	30066
❑ Method for assessing muscle mass	30067
❑ Growth pattern indices	10244
❑ Body mass index (BMI) for age percentile	12057
❑ Body mass index (BMI) for age z score	12058
❑ Head occipital frontal circumference	12059
❑ Birth head occipital frontal circumference	12060
❑ Head occipital frontal circumference for age percentile	12061
❑ Head occipital frontal circumference for age z score	12062
❑ Body length for age percentile	12063
❑ Body length for age z score	12064
❑ Body stature for age percentile	12065
❑ Body stature for age z score	12066
❑ Body weight for length percentile	12067
❑ Body weight for length z score	12068
❑ Body weight for age percentile	12069
❑ Body weight for age z score	12070
❑ Body weight for stature percentile	12071
❑ Body weight for stature z score	12072
❑ Mid parental body height comparator	12073
❑ Body compartment estimates	10245
❑ Body fat percentage	12074
❑ Body fat percentage technique	12075
❑ Body surface area	12076
❑ Calculated body surface area	12077

	ANDUID
❑ Bone maturation age	12078
❑ Bone mineral density t score	12079
❑ Bone mineral density z score	12080
❑ Bone mineral density technique	12081
❑ Mid arm muscle circumference	12082
❑ Mid arm muscle circumference percentile	12083
❑ Triceps skinfold thickness	12084
❑ Triceps skinfold percentile	12085
❑ Triceps skinfold z score	12086
❑ Waist circumference	12087
❑ Waist circumference narrowest point	12088
❑ Waist circumference iliac crest	12089
❑ Hip circumference	12090
❑ Waist to hip ratio	12091
❑ Mid upper arm circumference	12092
❑ Mid upper arm circumference left arm	12093
❑ Mid upper arm circumference z score	12094
❑ Waist circumference to body height ratio	30068
❑ Left calf circumference	30069
❑ Right calf circumference	30070
❑ Lumbar muscle cross section area	30071
❑ Muscle thickness	30072
❑ Thigh circumference	30073

◆ BIOCHEMICAL DATA, MEDICAL TESTS AND PROCEDURES

Laboratory data, (eg, electrolytes, glucose, and lipid panel) and tests (eg, gastric emptying time, resting metabolic rate).

▲ Nutrition Focused Biochemical Data, Tests, and Procedures

Laboratory data and tests that may be important for determining nutrition status.

	ANDUID
● Acid base balance	**10247**
❑ Arterial pH	10248
❑ Arterial bicarbonate	10249
❑ Partial pressure of carbon dioxide in arterial blood (PaCO2)	10250
❑ Partial pressure of oxygen in arterial blood (PaO2)	10251
❑ Venous pH	10252
❑ Venous bicarbonate	10253
● Electrolyte and renal profile	**10254**
❑ BUN	10255
❑ Creatinine	10256
❑ BUN:creatinine ratio	10257
❑ Glomerular filtration rate	10258
❑ Sodium	10259
❑ Chloride	10260
❑ Potassium	10261
❑ Magnesium	10262
❑ Calcium, serum	10263
❑ Calcium, ionized	10264
❑ Phosphorus	10265
❑ Serum osmolality	10266
❑ Parathyroid hormone	10267
● Essential fatty acid profile	**10268**
❑ Triene:tetraene ratio	10269
● Gastrointestinal profile	**10270**
❑ Alkaline phosphatase	10271
❑ Alanine aminotransferase (ALT)	10272
❑ Aspartate aminotransferase (AST)	10273
❑ Gamma glutamyl transferase (GGT)	10274
❑ Gastric residual volume	10275
❑ Bilirubin, total	10276
❑ Ammonia, serum	10277
❑ Toxicology report, including alcohol	10278
❑ Prothrombin time (PT)	10279
❑ Partial thromboplastin time (PTT)	10280
❑ INR ratio	10281
❑ Amylase	10283
❑ Lipase	10284
❑ Fecal fat, 24 hour	11242
❑ Fecal fat, 72 hour	11243
❑ Fecal fat, qualitative	11244
❑ Fecal calprotectin	11245
❑ Fecal lactoferrin	11246
❑ Pancreatic elastase	11150
❑ 5'nucleotidase	11247
❑ D xylose	10286
❑ Lactulose hydrogen breath test	11248
❑ Lactose hydrogen breath test	11249
❑ Fructose hydrogen breath test	11250
❑ Glucose hydrogen breath test	11251
❑ Urea hydrogen breath test	11252
❑ Intestinal biopsy	10288
❑ Stool culture	10289
❑ Gastric emptying time	10290
❑ Small bowel transit time	10291
❑ Abdominal X ray	11253
❑ Abdominal CT (computed tomography)	11254
❑ Abdominal ultrasound	11255
❑ Endoscopic ultrasound	11256
❑ Pelvic CT (computed tomography)	11257
❑ Modified barium swallow	11258
❑ Barium swallow	11259
❑ Esophagogastroduodenoscopy	11260
❑ Endoscopic retrograde cholangiopancreatography (ERCP)	11261
❑ Capsule endoscopy	11262

Key: ◆ = NCP Domain; ▲ = NCP Class; ● = NCP Subclass; ☐ = NCP Term

	ANDUID
❑ Esophageal manometry	11263
❑ Esophageal pH test	11264
❑ Gastroesophageal reflux monitoring	11265
❑ Gastrointestinal sphincter monitoring	11266
❑ Urate	11638
● **Glucose/endocrine profile**	**10294**
❑ Glucose, fasting	10295
❑ Glucose, casual	10296
❑ Hemoglobin A1c (HgbA1c)	10297
❑ Preprandial capillary plasma glucose	10298
❑ Peak postprandial capillary plasma glucose	10299
❑ Glucose tolerance test	10300
❑ Cortisol level	10301
❑ IGF binding protein	10302
❑ Thyroid stimulating hormone	11639
❑ Thyroxine test	11640
❑ Triiodothyronine	11641
❑ Adrenocorticotropic hormone	11642
❑ Follicle stimulating hormone	11643
❑ Growth hormone	11644
❑ Luteinizing hormone	11645
● **Inflammatory profile**	**10304**
❑ C reactive protein	10305
● **Lipid profile**	**10306**
❑ Cholesterol, serum	10307
❑ Cholesterol, HDL	10308
❑ Cholesterol, LDL	10309
❑ Cholesterol, non HDL	10310
❑ Total cholesterol:HDL cholesterol ratio	10311
❑ LDL:HDL ratio	10312
❑ Triglycerides, serum	10313
● **Metabolic rate profile**	**10314**
❑ Resting metabolic rate, measured	10315
❑ Respiratory quotient, measured	10316
● **Mineral profile**	**10317**
❑ Copper, serum or plasma	10318
❑ Iodine, urinary excretion	10319
❑ Zinc, serum or plasma	10320
❑ Boron, serum or plasma	10841
❑ Chromium, serum or urinary	10842
❑ Fluoride, plasma	10843
❑ Manganese, urinary, blood, plasma	10844
❑ Molybdenum, serum	10845
❑ Selenium, serum or urinary	10846
● **Nutritional anemia profile**	**10322**
❑ Hemoglobin	10323
❑ Hematocrit	10324
❑ Mean corpuscular volume	10325
❑ Red blood cell folate	10326

	ANDUID
❑ Red cell distribution width	10327
❑ B12, serum	10328
❑ Methylmalonic acid, serum	10329
❑ Folate, serum	10330
❑ Homocysteine, serum	10331
❑ Ferritin, serum	10332
❑ Iron, serum	10333
❑ Total iron binding capacity	10334
❑ Transferrin saturation	10335
● **Protein profile**	**10336**
❑ Albumin	10337
❑ Prealbumin	10338
❑ Transferrin	10339
❑ Phenylalanine, plasma	10340
❑ Tyrosine, plasma	10341
❑ Amino acid panel	10342
❑ Phenylalanine, dried blood spot	11151
❑ Tyrosine, dried blood spot	11152
❑ Phenylalanine:tyrosine ratio	11153
❑ Hydroxyproline	11154
❑ Threonine	11155
❑ Serine	11156
❑ Asparagine	11157
❑ Glutamate	11158
❑ Glutamine	11159
❑ Proline	11160
❑ Glycine	11161
❑ Alanine	11162
❑ Citrulline	11163
❑ Valine	11164
❑ Cysteine	11165
❑ Methionine	11166
❑ Isoleucine	11167
❑ Leucine	11168
❑ Ornithine	11169
❑ Lysine	11170
❑ Histidine	11171
❑ Arginine	11172
❑ Lysine:arginine ratio	11173
❑ Tryptophan	11174
❑ Plasma organic acid panel	11175
❑ Organic acids/creatinine	11176
❑ 3 hydroxybutyrate	11181
❑ 3 hydroxyisovalerate	11182
❑ Acetoacetate	11183
❑ Ethylmalonate	11184
❑ Succinate	11185
❑ Fumarate	11186
❑ Glutarate	11187
❑ 3 methylglutarate	11188
❑ Adipate	11189

	ANDUID
❑ 2 hydroxyglutarate	11190
❑ 3 hydroxyphenylacetate	11191
❑ 2 ketoglutarate	11192
❑ Citrate	11193
❑ Propionate	11194
❑ Methylcitrate	11195
❑ 3 hydroxy propionate	11196
❑ Beta hydroxy butyrate	11197
❑ Creatine kinase	11198
❑ Troponin I. cardiac	11199
❑ Troponin T. cardiac	11200
❑ B type natriuretic peptide	11201
❑ Succinylacetone	11202
❑ Total serum immunoglobulin A	11267
❑ Tissue transglutaminase antibodies (IgA)	11268
❑ Tissue transglutaminase antibodies (IgG)	11269
❑ Deamidated gliadin peptide antibodies (IgG)	11270
❑ Endomysial antibodies	11271
❑ Carbohydrate deficient transferrin	10847

● Urine profile **10344**

❑ Urine color	10345
❑ Urine osmolality	10346
❑ Urine specific gravity	10347
❑ Urine volume	10349
❑ Urine calcium, 24 hour	11272
❑ Urine d xylose	11273
❑ Urine glucose	11203
❑ Urine ketones	11204
❑ Urine sodium	11205
❑ Urine microalbumin	11206
❑ Urine protein, random	11207
❑ Urine protein, 24 hour	11208
❑ Urine uric acid, random	11209
❑ Urine uric acid, 24 hour	11210
❑ Urine organic acid panel	11211
❑ Urine glutarate	11212
❑ Urine methylmalonate	11213
❑ Urine acylglycines/creatinine	11214
❑ Urine argininosuccinate	11215
❑ Urine succinylacetone/creatinine	11216
❑ Urine orotate	11217
❑ Urine orotate/creatinine	11218
❑ Urine 2 hydroxyisovalerate	11219
❑ Urine 2 oxoisovalerate	11220
❑ Urine galactitol	11221
❑ Urine reducing substances	11222
❑ Urine porphyrins	11274
❑ Urine creatinine, 24 hour	14189
❑ Urine citrate, 24 hours	14190
❑ Urine phosphorus, 24 hour	14191
❑ Urine pH, random	14192

	ANDUID
❑ Urine pH, 24 hour	14193
❑ Urine sodium, 24 hour	14194
❑ Urine urea nitrogen, 24 hour	14195
❑ Urine oxalate, 24 hour	14196
❑ Urine chloride, 24 hour	14197
❑ Urine ammonium, 24 hour	14198
❑ Urine magnesium, 24 hour	14199
❑ Urine potassium, 24 hour	14200
❑ Urine sulfate, 24 hour	14201
❑ Urine cystine, 24 hour	14202
❑ Calcium oxalate supersaturation in 24 hour urine	14203
❑ Calcium phosphate supersaturation in 24 hour urine	14204
❑ Brushite supersaturation in 24 hour urine	14205
❑ Uric acid supersaturation in 24 hour urine	14218

● Vitamin profile **10350**

❑ Vitamin A, serum or plasma retinol	10351
❑ Vitamin C, plasma or serum	10352
❑ Vitamin D, 25 hydroxy	10353
❑ Vitamin E, plasma alpha tocopherol	10354
❑ Thiamin, activity coefficient for erythrocyte transketolase activity	10355
❑ Riboflavin, activity coefficient for erythrocyte glutathione reductase activity	10356
❑ Niacin, urinary N'methyl nicotinamide concentration	10357
❑ Vitamin B6, plasma or serum pyridoxal 5'phosphate concentration	10358
❑ Pantothenic acid, urinary pantothenate excretion, plasma	10850
❑ Biotin, urinary 3 hydroxyisovaleric acid excretion	11275
❑ Biotin, lymphocyte propionyl CoA carboxylase in pregnancy, serum	11276
❑ Biotinidase	11223
❑ Protein induced by vitamin K absence or antagonist II	11224

● Carbohydrate metabolism profile **11225**

❑ Galactose 1 phosphate in red blood cell	11226
❑ Galactose 1 phosphate uridyl transferase	11227
❑ Fructose	11228
❑ Lactate	11177
❑ Pyruvate	11178
❑ Lactate:pyruvate ratio	11179

● Fatty acid profile **11229**

❑ Acylcarnitine panel	11230
❑ Acylcarnitine, plasma	11231
❑ Free carnitine	11232

Key: ◆ = NCP Domain; ▲ = NCP Class; ● = NCP Subclass; ☐ = NCP Term

ANDUID

- ❑ Total carnitine 11233
- ❑ Free carnitine:total carnitine 11234
- ❑ Fatty acid panel mitochondrial C8 to C18 11235
- ❑ Fatty acid panel essential C12 to C22 11236
- ❑ Fatty acid panel peroxisomal C22 to C26 11237
- ❑ MCAD enzyme assay in fibroblasts or other tissues 11238
- ❑ Fatty acid beta oxidation in fibroblasts 11239

◆ PHYSICAL EXAM FINDINGS

Findings from a physical exam, interview, or the health record.

▲ Nutrition Focused Physical Exam

Physical exam, interview, or health record findings that may be important for determining nutrition status.

● Nutrition focused physical findings 10361

- ❑ Overall finding 10362
    - ❑ Asthenia 30077
    - ❑ Buffalo hump 11647
    - ❑ Cachexia 11648
    - ❑ Cushingoid appearance 11649
    - ❑ Ectomorph 11650
    - ❑ Endomorph 11651
    - ❑ Lethargic 11652
    - ❑ Mesomorph 11653
    - ❑ Neglect of personal hygiene 11654
    - ❑ Obese 11655
    - ❑ Short stature for age 11656
    - ❑ Tall stature 11657
    - ❑ Body language that may suggest discomfort with interaction 14553
- ❑ Adipose finding 11658
    - ❑ Atrophy of orbital fat 11659
    - ❑ Excess subcutaneous fat 11660
    - ❑ Loss of subcutaneous fat 11661
    - ❑ Central adiposity 11662
    - ❑ Loss of subcutaneous triceps fat 12095
    - ❑ Loss of subcutaneous biceps fat 12096
    - ❑ Loss of subcutaneous fat overlying the ribs 12097
    - ❑ Lipodystrophy 14554
- ❑ Bone finding 11663
    - ❑ Bow legs 11664
    - ❑ Frontal bossing 11665
    - ❑ Harrison's sulcus 11666
    - ❑ Rachitic rosary 11667
    - ❑ Rickets 11668
    - ❑ Scoliosis 11669
    - ❑ Acromion abnormal prominence 12098
    - ❑ Bone widening at ends 12099
    - ❑ Clavicle abnormal prominence 12100
    - ❑ Rib abnormal prominence 12101

ANDUID

    - ❑ Scapula abnormal prominence 12102
    - ❑ Spine abnormal prominence 12103
    - ❑ Iliac crest abnormal prominence 12104
    - ❑ Patella abnormal prominence 12105
    - ❑ Lordosis 14556
- ❑ Cardiovascular pulmonary system finding 10364
    - ❑ Absent breath sounds 11670
    - ❑ Bradycardia 11671
    - ❑ Bradypnea 11672
    - ❑ Decreased breath sounds 11673
    - ❑ Dyspnea 11674
    - ❑ Increased breath sounds 11675
    - ❑ Normal breath sounds 11676
    - ❑ Tachypnea 11677
    - ❑ Tachycardia 11678
    - ❑ Respiratory crackles 11679
    - ❑ Decreased functional residual capacity 30074
    - ❑ Diaphragmatic weakness 30075
- ❑ Digestive system finding 11682
    - ❑ Abdominal bloating 11684
    - ❑ Abdominal cramping 11685
    - ❑ Abdominal distension 11686
    - ❑ Abdominal pain 11687
    - ❑ Absence of bowel sounds 11688
    - ❑ Anorexia 11689
    - ❑ Ascites 11690
    - ❑ Bulky stool 11691
    - ❑ Constipation 11692
    - ❑ Decrease in appetite 11693
    - ❑ Diarrhea 11694
    - ❑ Early satiety 11695
    - ❑ Epigastric pain 11696
    - ❑ Excessive appetite 11697
    - ❑ Excessive belching 11698
    - ❑ Excessive flatus 11699
    - ❑ Fatty stool 11700
    - ❑ Heartburn 11701
    - ❑ Hyperactive bowel sounds 11702
    - ❑ Hypoactive bowel sounds 11703
    - ❑ Increased appetite 11704
    - ❑ Liquid stool 11705
    - ❑ Loose stool 11706
    - ❑ Nausea 11707
    - ❑ Normal bowel sounds 11708
    - ❑ Retching 11709
    - ❑ Vomiting 11710
    - ❑ Gastrointestinal drainage volume 12106
    - ❑ Gastric drainage volume 12107
    - ❑ Bile duct fluid drainage volume 12108
    - ❑ Pancreatic fluid drainage volume 12109
    - ❑ Chylous fluid drainage volume 12110
    - ❑ Wound drainage volume 12111

ANDUID

  - ❑ Intestinal fistula output volume 12112
  - ❑ Normal stool 14557
- ❑ Edema finding 11711
  - ❑ +1 pitting edema 11712
  - ❑ +2 pitting edema 11713
  - ❑ +3 pitting edema 11714
  - ❑ +4 pitting edema 11715
  - ❑ Anasarca 11716
  - ❑ Ankle edema 11717
  - ❑ Edema of calf 11718
  - ❑ Edema of eyelid 11719
  - ❑ Edema of foot 11720
  - ❑ Edema of hand 11721
  - ❑ Edema of scrotum 11722
  - ❑ Edema of thigh 11723
  - ❑ Edema of vulva 11724
  - ❑ Mucosal edema 11725
  - ❑ Sacral edema 11726
- ❑ Extremity finding 11727
  - ❑ Amputated foot 11728
  - ❑ Amputated hand 11729
  - ❑ Amputated leg 11730
  - ❑ Athetoid movement 11731
  - ❑ Decreased range of ankle movement 11732
  - ❑ Decreased range of cervical spine movement 11733
  - ❑ Decreased range of elbow movement 11734
  - ❑ Decreased range of finger movement 11735
  - ❑ Decreased range of foot movement 11736
  - ❑ Decreased range of hip movement 11737
  - ❑ Decreased range of knee movement 11738
  - ❑ Decreased range of lumbar spine movement 11739
  - ❑ Decreased range of shoulder movement 11740
  - ❑ Decreased range of subtalar movement 11741
  - ❑ Decreased range of thumb movement 11742
  - ❑ Decreased range of toe movement 11743
  - ❑ Decreased range of thoracic spine movement 11744
  - ❑ Decreased range of wrist movement 11745
  - ❑ Hypertonia 11746
  - ❑ Hypotonia 11747
  - ❑ Joint arthralgia 11748
  - ❑ Lower limb spasticity 11749
  - ❑ Peripheral cyanosis 11750
  - ❑ Spasticity 11751
  - ❑ Tetany 11752
  - ❑ Upper limb spasticity 11753
  - ❑ Talipes planus 14558
- ❑ Eye finding 11754
  - ❑ Abnormal vision 11755
  - ❑ Angular blepharitis 11756

ANDUID

  - ❑ Bitot's spots 11757
  - ❑ Circles under eyes 11758
  - ❑ Corneal arcus 11759
  - ❑ Conjunctival discoloration 11760
  - ❑ Conjunctival hemorrhage 11761
  - ❑ Conjunctival keratinization 11762
  - ❑ Excessive tear production 11763
  - ❑ Keratomalacia 11764
  - ❑ Jaundiced sclera 11765
  - ❑ Night blindness 11766
  - ❑ Ophthalmoplegia 11767
  - ❑ Sunken eyes 11768
  - ❑ Xerophthalmia 11769
  - ❑ Xanthelasma 11770
  - ❑ Pale conjunctiva 12113
- ❑ Genitourinary system finding (9) 11771
  - ❑ Amenorrhea 11772
  - ❑ Anuria 11773
  - ❑ Delay in sexual development and/or puberty 11774
  - ❑ Menorrhagia 11775
  - ❑ Oliguria 11776
  - ❑ Polyuria 11777
- ❑ Hair finding 11778
  - ❑ Abnormal keratinization of hair follicle 11779
  - ❑ Alopecia 11780
  - ❑ Brittle hair 11781
  - ❑ Corkscrew hairs 11782
  - ❑ Dry hair 11783
  - ❑ Fine hair 11784
  - ❑ Follicular hyperkeratosis 11785
  - ❑ Hair changes due to malnutrition 11786
  - ❑ Hair lacks luster 11787
  - ❑ Hypertrichosis 11788
  - ❑ Increased loss of hair 11789
  - ❑ Nutritional hair color change 11790
  - ❑ White hair 11791
  - ❑ Easily pluckable hair 12114
  - ❑ Lanugo hair formation 12115
- ❑ Head finding 11792
  - ❑ Altered olfactory sense 11793
  - ❑ Anosmia 11794
  - ❑ Bulging fontanelle 11795
  - ❑ Epistaxis 11796
  - ❑ Headache 11797
  - ❑ Hyposmia 11798
  - ❑ Macrocephaly 11799
  - ❑ Microcephaly 11800
  - ❑ Nasal mucosa dry 11801
  - ❑ Sunken fontanelle 11802
- ❑ Hand and nail finding 11803
  - ❑ Beau's lines 11804

Key: ◆ = NCP Domain; ▲ = NCP Class; ● = NCP Subclass; ☐ = NCP Term

	ANDUID
❑ Clubbing of nail	11805
❑ Flaking of nails	11806
❑ Koilonychia	11807
❑ Leukonychia	11808
❑ Longitudinal grooving of nails	11809
❑ Muehrcke's lines	11810
❑ Nail changes	11811
❑ Palmar erythema	11812
❑ Ridged nails	11813
❑ Splits in nails	11814
❑ Thin nails	11815
❑ Trachyonychia	11816
❑ Splinter hemorrhage under nail	11817
❑ White flecks in nails	11818
❑ Blue nail bed	12116
❑ Pale nail bed	12117
❑ Russell's sign	12118
❑ Mouth finding	11819
❑ Ageusia	11820
❑ Angular stomatitis	11821
❑ Aphthous ulcer of mouth	11822
❑ Aptyalism	11823
❑ Blue lips	11824
❑ Blue line on gingiva	11825
❑ Candidiasis of the mouth	11826
❑ Cheilosis	11827
❑ Cheilitis	11828
❑ Cleft palate	11829
❑ Cracked lips	11830
❑ Drooling	11831
❑ Dry mucous membranes	11832
❑ Dysgeusia	11833
❑ Excessive salivation	11834
❑ Excessive thirst	11835
❑ Gingival hypertrophy	11836
❑ Gingivitis	11837
❑ Halitosis	11838
❑ Hemorrhagic gingivitis	11839
❑ Hypogeusia	11840
❑ Ketotic breath	11841
❑ Micrognathia	11842
❑ Swollen gums	11843
❑ Oral candidiasis	11844
❑ Oral lesion	11845
❑ Parotid swelling	11846
❑ Poor oral hygiene	11847
❑ Retains food in mouth	11848
❑ Stomatitis	11849
❑ Uremic breath	11850
❑ Pale gums	12119
❑ Cleft lip	14559
❑ Muscle finding	11851

	ANDUID
❑ Muscle atrophy	11852
❑ Muscle contracture	11853
❑ Muscle cramp	11854
❑ Muscle pain	11855
❑ Muscle weakness	11856
❑ Quadriceps muscle atrophy	11857
❑ Deltoid muscle atrophy	12120
❑ Gastrocnemius muscle atrophy	12121
❑ Gluteal muscle atrophy	12122
❑ Interosseous hand muscle atrophy	12123
❑ Pectoral muscle atrophy	12124
❑ Temporalis muscle atrophy	12125
❑ Trapezius muscle atrophy	12126
❑ Latissimus dorsi muscle atrophy	12150
❑ Abnormal muscle function	30078
❑ Loss of muscle function	30079
❑ Low muscle function	30080
❑ Loss of physical performance	30081
❑ Skeletal muscle problem	30082
❑ Skeletal muscle power problem	30083
❑ Neck finding	11858
❑ Goiter	11859
❑ Nerve, cognition, and feeling finding	10368
❑ Abnormal gait	11860
❑ Absent reflex	11861
❑ Asterixis	11862
❑ Ataxia	11863
❑ Clouded consciousness	11864
❑ Cranial nerve finding	11865
❑ Decreased vibratory sense	11866
❑ Delirious	11867
❑ Dementia	11868
❑ Depressed mood	11869
❑ Disoriented	11870
❑ Dizziness	11871
❑ Feels cold	11872
❑ Flat affect	11873
❑ Hyperreflexia	11874
❑ Hyporeflexia	11875
❑ Inappropriate affect	11876
❑ Many seizures a day	11877
❑ Numbness of foot	11878
❑ Numbness of hand	11879
❑ Peripheral nerve disease	11880
❑ Tremor of outstretched hand	11881
❑ Tingling of foot	11882
❑ Tingling of hand	11883
❑ Skin finding	10369
❑ Acanthosis nigricans	11884
❑ Calcinosis	11885
❑ Carotenemia	11886
❑ Cutaneous xanthoma	11887

	ANDUID
❑ Decreased skin turgor	11888
❑ Dermatitis	11889
❑ Diaper rash	11890
❑ Dry skin	11891
❑ Ecchymosis	11892
❑ Erythema	11893
❑ Eczema	11894
❑ Flushing	11895
❑ Hirsutism	11896
❑ Hyperpigmentation of skin	11897
❑ Impaired skin integrity	11898
❑ Jaundice	11899
❑ Keratinization of skin	11900
❑ Pale complexion	11901
❑ Peeling skin	11902
❑ Petechiae	11903
❑ Impaired wound healing	11904
❑ Pressure injury of ankles	11905
❑ Pressure injury of back	11906
❑ Pressure injury of breast	11907
❑ Pressure injury of buttock	11908
❑ Pressure injury of dorsum of foot	11909
❑ Pressure injury of elbow	11910
❑ Pressure injury of head	11911
❑ Pressure injury of heel	11912
❑ Pressure injury of hip	11913
❑ Pressure injury of knee	11914
❑ Pressure injury of natal cleft	11915
❑ Pressure injury of shoulder	11916
❑ Pressure injury stage 1	11917
❑ Pressure injury stage 2	11918
❑ Pressure injury stage 3	11919
❑ Pressure injury stage 4	11920
❑ Pruritus of the skin	11921
❑ Psoriasis	11922
❑ Scaling skin	11923
❑ Seborrheic dermatitis	11924
❑ Skin rash	11925
❑ Venous stasis ulcer of leg	11926
❑ Yellow skin	11927
❑ Perifollicular hemorrhages	12127
❑ Pressure injury of the coccyx	12128
❑ Pressure injury of the sacrum	12129
❑ Vesiculobullous rash	12130
❑ Acne	14560
❑ Intertrigo	14561
❑ Excess panniculus of abdomen	14562
❑ Skin striae	14563
❑ Teeth finding	10928
❑ Baby bottle tooth decay	11929
❑ Broken denture	11930
❑ Broken teeth	11931

	ANDUID
❑ Dental caries	11932
❑ Dental fluorosis	11933
❑ Dental plaque	11934
❑ Denture loose	11935
❑ Denture lost	11936
❑ Denture present	11937
❑ Edentulous	11938
❑ Erosion of teeth	11939
❑ Impaired dentition	11940
❑ Ill fitting denture	11941
❑ Mottling of enamel	11942
❑ Partially edentulous mandible	11943
❑ Partially edentulous maxilla	11944
❑ Rampant dental caries	11945
❑ Throat and swallowing finding	11946
❑ Choking during swallowing	11947
❑ Cough	11948
❑ Dysphagia	11949
❑ Esophageal lesion	11950
❑ Food sticks on swallowing	11951
❑ Gagging	11952
❑ Hoarse voice	11953
❑ Hypoactive gag reflex	11954
❑ Odynophagia	11955
❑ Swallow impairment	11956
❑ Suck swallow incoordination	11957
❑ Tongue finding	11958
❑ Atrophy of tongue papillae	11959
❑ Beefy red tongue	11960
❑ Difficulty moving tongue	11961
❑ Dry tongue	11962
❑ Glossitis	11963
❑ Glossodynia	11964
❑ Hypertrophy of tongue papillae	11965
❑ Lesion of the tongue	11966
❑ Strawberry tongue	11967
❑ Macroglossia	11968
❑ Short frenulum of tongue	11969
❑ Split frenulum of tongue	11970
❑ Blue tongue	12131
❑ Cracked tongue	12132
❑ Magenta tongue	12133
❑ Pale tongue	12134
❑ Vital signs	10370
❑ Blood pressure, systolic	14206
❑ Blood pressure, diastolic	14207
❑ Blood pressure, systolic, reported	14208
❑ Blood pressure, diastolic, reported	14209
❑ Heart rate	12139
❑ Jugular venous pressure	12140
❑ Mean arterial pressure	12138
❑ Pulse rate	12141

Key: ◆ = NCP Domain; ▲ = NCP Class; ● = NCP Subclass; ❑ = NCP Term

	ANDUID
❑ Respiratory rate	12137
❑ Body temperature	12136

◆ CLIENT HISTORY

Current and past information related to personal, health, family, and social history. Client History terms are used for Nutrition Assessment, but not for Nutrition Monitoring and Evaluation.

▲ Personal History

General client information such as age, gender, sex, race, ethnicity, language, education, and role in family.

● Personal data	**10373**
❑ Age	10374
❑ Corrected age	30084
❑ Gender	10375
❑ Sex	11138
❑ Race	11139
❑ Ethnicity	11140
❑ Language	10377
❑ Literacy factors	10378
❑ Education	10379
❑ Role in family	10380
❑ Tobacco use	10381
❑ Physical ability difference	10382
❑ Mobility	10383

▲ Client and/or Family Health History

Client and/or family health history that may have a nutritional impact.

	ANDUID
● Individual client and/or family nutrition-related health history	**10385**
❑ Individual client nutrition related health history	30085
❑ Cancer history	14612
❑ Cardiovascular disease history	10387
❑ Endocrine disease history	10388
❑ Excretory disease history	10389
❑ Gastrointestinal disease history	10390
❑ Gynecological history	10391
❑ Hematologic disease history	10392
❑ Immune disease history	10393
❑ Integumentary disease history	10394
❑ Musculoskeletal disease history	10395
❑ Neurological disease history	10396
❑ Psychological disease history	10397
❑ Respiratory disease history	10398
❑ Metabolic disease history	14613
❑ Family nutrition related health history	14594
❑ Family history of cancer	14595
❑ Family history of cardiovascular disease	14596
❑ Family history of endocrine disease	14597
❑ Family history of excretory disease	14698
❑ Family history of gastrointestinal disease	14599
❑ Family history of gynecological disorder	14600
❑ Family history of hematologic disease	14601
❑ Family history of immune disease	14602
❑ Family history of integumentary disease	14063
❑ Family history of musculoskeletal disease	14604
❑ Family history of neurological disease	14605
❑ Family history of psychological disease	14066
❑ Family history of respiratory disease	14067
❑ Family history of metabolic disease	14608
● Treatments/therapy	**10400**

Documented medical or surgical treatments that may impact nutritional status of the client

❑ Medical treatment/therapy	10401
❑ Surgical treatment	10402
❑ Palliative/end of life care	10404

▲ Social Context

The social factors, forces, and/or environment that may impact client health.

● Social history	**10406**
❑ Socioeconomic factors	10407
❑ Living/housing situation	10408
❑ Domestic issues	10409
❑ Social and medical support	10410
❑ Geographic location of home	10411
❑ Occupation	10412
❑ Religion	10413
❑ History of recent crisis	10414
❑ Daily stress level	10415

◆ ASSESSMENT, MONITORING AND EVALUATION TOOLS

Tools used for health or disease status or risk assessment, reassessment, and monitoring and evaluation.

▲ Nutrition assessment, monitoring and evaluation tool ratings	**14303**
❑ Subjective global assessment (SGA) rating	14132
❑ Subjective global assessment (SGA) score	82159
❑ The scored patient generated subjective global assessment (PG-SGA) rating	14133
❑ The scored patient generated subjective global assessment (PG-SGA) score	14134
❑ Mini nutritional assessment long form (MNA-LF) rating	14135
❑ Mini nutritional assessment long form (MNA-LF) score	82160

Key: ◆ = NCP Domain; ▲ = NCP Class; ● = NCP Subclass; ❑ = NCP Term

	ANDUID
❑ Subjective global nutritional assessment (SGNA) for children rating	14564
❑ Subjective global nutritional assessment (SGNA) for children score	82161
▲ Household food security assessment tool scores	**14304**
❑ US household food security module: six item short form raw score	14137
❑ US household food security module: six item short form scale score	14138
❑ Food insecurity experience scale (FIES) raw score	14139
▲ Food variety assessment tool scores	**14305**
❑ Minimum dietary diversity for women (MDD-W) indicator score	14141
▲ Dysphagia assessment, monitoring and evaluation tool scores	**30086**
❑ International Dysphagia Diet Standardisation Initiative Framework drinks level	30087
❑ International Dysphagia Diet Standardisation Initiative Framework food level	30088
❑ International Dysphagia Diet Standardisation Initiative Functional Diet Scale score	30089

◆ ETIOLOGY CATEGORY

Categories to communicate the type of nutrition diagnosis etiology.

▲ Nutrition Diagnosis Etiology Category Identification	**14566**
❑ Beliefs attitudes etiology	14567
❑ Cultural etiology	14568
❑ Knowledge etiology	14569
❑ Physical function etiology	14570
❑ Physiologic metabolic etiology	14571
❑ Psychological etiology	14572
❑ Social personal etiology	14573
❑ Treatment etiology	14574
❑ Access etiology	14575
❑ Behavior etiology	14576

◆ COMPARATIVE STANDARDS

What indicator data are compared against.

	ANDUID
▲ Energy Needs	
● Estimated energy needs	**10418**
❑ Total energy estimated needs in 24 hours	12205
❑ Method for estimating 24 hour energy needs	10420
❑ Energy estimated needs per kg body weight in 24 hours	13008
▲ Macronutrient Needs	
● Estimated fat needs	**10422**
❑ Total fat estimated needs in 24 hours	12206
❑ Fat estimated needs per kg body weight in 24 hours	13010
❑ Method for estimating 24 hour fat needs	10425
❑ Proportion of energy needs from fat in 24 hours	13009
● Estimated protein needs	**10426**
❑ Total protein estimated needs in 24 hours	12207
❑ Protein estimated needs per kg body weight in 24 hours	13011
❑ Method for estimating 24 hour protein needs	10429
❑ Proportion of energy needs from protein in 24 hours	13012
● Estimated carbohydrate needs	**10430**
❑ Total carbohydrate estimated needs in 24 hours	12208
❑ Carbohydrate estimated needs per kg body weight in 24 hours	13013
❑ Method for estimating 24 hour carbohydrate needs	10433
❑ Proportion of energy needs from carbohydrate in 24 hours	13014
● Estimated fiber needs	**10434**
❑ Total fiber estimated needs in 24 hours	12209
❑ Method for estimating 24 hour fiber needs	10437
▲ Fluid Needs	
● Estimated fluid needs	**10439**
❑ Total fluid estimated needs in 24 hours	10440
❑ Method for estimating 24 hour fluid needs	10441
▲ Micronutrient Needs	
● Estimated vitamin needs	**10443**
❑ Estimated vitamin A needs in 24 hours	10444
❑ Estimated vitamin C needs in 24 hours	10445
❑ Estimated vitamin D needs in 24 hours	10446
❑ Estimated vitamin E needs in 24 hours	10447
❑ Estimated vitamin K needs in 24 hours	10448
❑ Estimated thiamin needs in 24 hours	10449
❑ Estimated riboflavin needs in 24 hours	10450
❑ Estimated niacin needs in 24 hours	10451
❑ Estimated folate needs in 24 hours	10452
❑ Estimated vitamin B6 needs in 24 hours	10453
❑ Estimated vitamin B12 needs in 24 hours	10454
❑ Estimated pantothenic acid needs in 24 hours	10455
❑ Estimated biotin needs in 24 hours	10456
❑ Method for estimating 24 hour vitamin needs	10458

Key: ◆ = NCP Domain; ▲ = NCP Class; ● = NCP Subclass; ❑ = NCP Term

	ANDUID
● **Estimated mineral needs**	**10459**
❑ Estimated calcium needs in 24 hours	10460
❑ Estimated chloride needs in 24 hours	10461
❑ Estimated iron needs in 24 hours	10462
❑ Estimated magnesium needs in 24 hours	10463
❑ Estimated potassium needs in 24 hours	10464
❑ Estimated phosphorus needs in 24 hours	10465
❑ Estimated sodium needs in 24 hours	10466
❑ Estimated zinc needs in 24 hours	10467
❑ Estimated sulfate needs in 24 hours	10469
❑ Estimated fluoride needs in 24 hours	10470
❑ Estimated copper needs in 24 hours	10471
❑ Estimated iodine needs in 24 hours	10473
❑ Estimated selenium needs in 24 hours	10474
❑ Estimated manganese needs in 24 hours	10475
❑ Estimated chromium needs in 24 hours	10476
❑ Estimated molybdenum needs in 24 hours	10477
❑ Estimated boron needs in 24 hours	10478
❑ Estimated cobalt needs in 24 hours	10479
❑ Method for estimating 24 hour mineral needs	10480
▲ **Weight and Growth Recommendation**	
● **Recommended body weight/body mass index/growth**	**10482**
❑ Ideal/reference body weight (IBW)	10483
❑ Recommended body mass index (BMI)	10484
❑ Goal body weight	12144

	ANDUID
❑ Goal body weight gain in 24 hours	12145
❑ Goal body weight for length z score	12146
❑ Goal mid upper arm circumference z score	12147
❑ Goal body mass index (BMI) for age z score	12148
❑ Percent median body mass index (BMI)	12149

◆ PROGRESS EVALUATION

Evaluation of progress toward a nutrition related goal(s) and resolution of a nutrition diagnosis(es).

▲ **Intervention goal status**	**14578**
❑ New goal identified	14579
❑ Goal achieved	14580
❑ Goal discontinued	14581
❑ Goal not achieved	14582
❑ Some progress toward goal	14583
❑ Some digression away from goal	14584
▲ **Nutrition diagnosis status**	**14585**
❑ New nutrition diagnosis	14586
❑ Active nutrition diagnosis	14587
❑ Resolved nutrition diagnosis	14588
❑ Discontinued nutrition diagnosis	14589

Energy Intake

Definition

Amount of energy intake from all sources including food, beverages, breastmilk/formula, supplements, and via enteral and parenteral routes.

Note: Whenever possible, nutrient intake data should be considered in combination with clinical, biochemical, anthropometric information, medical diagnosis, clinical status, and/or other factors to provide a valid assessment of nutritional status based on a totality of the evidence. (Institute of Medicine. *Dietary Reference Intakes: Applications in Dietary Assessment.* National Academies Press; 2000.)

Nutrition Assessment and Monitoring and Evaluation

Indicators

Estimated energy intake

- Total energy estimated intake in 24 hours (calories, kcal or kJ/day)—defined as the approximate intake in one day of all energy
- Energy estimated intake per kg body weight in 24 hours (calories, kcal, or kJ/kg/day)—defined as the approximate intake per kg of body weight in one day of all energy
- Energy estimated intake from oral nutrition in 24 hours (calories, kcal, or kJ/day)—defined as the estimated intake of energy in one day derived from oral intake
- Energy estimated intake from enteral nutrition in 24 hours (calories, kcal, or kJ/day)—defined as the estimated intake of energy in one day derived from enteral nutrition infusion
- Energy estimated intake from parenteral nutrition in 24 hours (calories, kcal, or kJ/day)—defined as the estimated intake of energy in one day derived from parenteral nutrition infusion
- Energy estimated intake from intravenous (IV) fluids in 24 hours (calories, kcal, or kJ/day)—defined as the estimated intake of energy in one day derived from IV fluid infusion

Measured energy intake

- Total energy measured intake in 24 hours (calories, kcal, or kJ/day)—defined as the known quantity of intake in one day of all energy
- Energy measured intake per kg body weight in 24 hours (calories, kcal, or kJ/kg/day)—defined as the known quantity of intake per kg of body weight in one day of all energy
- Energy measured intake from oral nutrition in 24 hours (calories, kcal, or kJ/day)—defined as the known quantity of energy in one day derived from oral intake
- Energy measured intake from enteral nutrition in 24 hours (calories, kcal, or kJ/day)—defined as the known quantity of energy in one day derived from enteral nutrition infusion
- Energy measured intake from parenteral nutrition in 24 hours (calories, kcal, or kJ/day)—defined as the known quantity of energy in one day derived from parenteral nutrition infusion
- Energy measured intake from IV fluids in 24 hours (calories, kcal, or kJ/day)—defined as the known quantity of energy in one day derived from IV fluid infusion

Note: Weight and weight change can be found on the Body Composition/Growth/Weight History reference sheet on page 129.

In almost all nutrition settings, food and nutrient intakes are estimates; therefore, estimated intake terms should be used. The exception is research settings where exact measurement of intake is done. Then, measured intake terms are appropriate.

Energy Intake

Examples of the measurement methods or data sources for these outcome indicators: Food intake records, 24-hour recalls, 3- to 5-day food diary, food frequency questionnaire, caretaker intake records, menu analysis, intake and output records

Typically used with the following domains of nutrition interventions: Food and/or nutrient delivery, nutrition education, nutrition counseling, coordination of nutrition care by nutrition professional

Typically used to determine and to monitor and evaluate change in the following nutrition diagnoses: Inadequate energy intake, excessive energy intake, malnutrition (undernutrition), inadequate protein energy intake, underweight, unintended weight loss, overweight/obesity, unintended weight gain, swallowing difficulty, breastfeeding difficulty, altered gastrointestinal function, limited adherence to nutrition related recommendations

Note: Judgment must be used to select indicators and determine the appropriate measurement techniques and reference standards for a given client population and setting. Once identified, these indicators, measurement techniques, and reference standards should be identified in policies and procedures or other documents for use in client records, quality or performance improvement, or in formal research projects.

Client Example(s)

Example of one of the nutrition care indicators (includes sample initial and reassessment of documentation for one of the indicators)

Indicator(s) Selected

Total energy estimated intake in 24 hours (kcal/day)

Criteria for Evaluation

Comparison to reference standard, recommendation, or goal:

1. Reference standard: Food diary indicates that client consumes approximately 2,600 calories/kcal (11,000 kJ) per day. 145% of estimated energy needs per day.
2. Recommendation: Client's recommended calorie intake level is 1,800 to 2,000 calories/kcal (7,500 to 8,400 kJ) per day.
3. Goal: Client's goal calorie intake level is 1,800 calories/kcal (7,500 kJ) per day.

Sample Nutrition Assessment and Monitoring and Evaluation Documentation	
Initial encounter	Based on client food diary, client's total energy estimated intake in 24 hours averages approximately 2,600 calories/kcal (11,000 kJ) per day, 145% of recommended level of 1,800 calories/kcal (7,500 kJ) per day. Client's goal is 1,800 calories/kcal (7,500 kJ) per day. Will evaluate calorie intake at next encounter in 2 weeks.
Reassessment after nutrition intervention	Significant progress toward meeting goal. Based on client's food diary, client consuming approximately 2,100 calories/kcal (9,000 kJ) per day, 117% of goal level of 1,800 calories/kcal (7,500 kJ) per day. Will evaluate energy intake at next encounter in 2 weeks.

Fluid Intake

Definition

Amount of fluid consumed from all sources including food, beverages, breastmilk, infant formula, supplements, and via enteral and parenteral routes.

Note: Whenever possible, nutrient intake data should be considered in combination with clinical, biochemical, and anthropometric information, medical diagnosis, clinical status, and/or other factors to provide a valid assessment of nutritional status based on a totality of the evidence. (Institute of Medicine. *Dietary Reference Intakes: Applications in Dietary Assessment.* National Academies Press; 2000.)

Nutrition Assessment and Monitoring and Evaluation

Indicators

Estimated fluid intake

- Total fluid estimated intake in 24 hours (mL/day)—defined as the approximate intake in one day of fluid from all sources
- Fluid estimated intake from oral nutrition in 24 hours (mL/day)—defined as the approximate intake in one day of fluid from oral intake
- Water estimated oral intake in 24 hours (mL/day)—defined as the approximate intake in one day of water
- Sugar sweetened beverage estimated oral intake in 24 hours (mL/day)—defined as the approximate intake in one day of sugar sweetened beverages
- Beverage with high intensity sweetener estimated oral intake in 24 hours (mL/day)—defined as the approximate intake in one day of high intensity, nonnutritive and nutritive, sweetened beverages that contain nutritive and nonnutritive sugar substitutes
- 100 percent fruit juice estimated oral intake in 24 hours (mL/day)—defined as the approximate intake in one day of 100% fruit juice
- Liquid mammalian milk product estimated oral intake in 24 hours (mL/day)—defined as the approximate intake in one day of mammalian milk beverages
- Caffeinated beverage estimated oral intake in 24 hours (mL/day)—defined as the approximate intake in one day of caffeinated beverages
- Nutritionally complete liquid supplement estimated oral intake in 24 hours (mL/day)—defined as the approximate intake in one day of liquid oral enteral nutrition supplements
- Liquid meal replacement estimated oral intake in 24 hours (mL/day)—defined as the approximate intake in one day of liquid meal replacement
- Fluid estimated intake per kg body weight in 24 hours (mL/kg/day)—defined as the approximate intake per kg of body weight in one day of fluid from all sources
- Fluid estimated intake from food in 24 hours (mL/day)—defined as the approximate intake in one day of fluid from food intake
- Free water estimated intake in 24 hours (mL/day)—defined as the approximate intake in one day of free water from all sources
- Free water estimated intake from breastmilk in 24 hours (mL/day)—defined as the approximate intake in one day of free water derived from breastmilk
- Free water estimated intake from infant formula in 24 hours (mL/day)—defined as the approximate intake in one day of free water derived from infant formula

Fluid Intake

- Free water estimated intake from enteral nutrition in 24 hours (mL/day)—defined as the approximate intake of free water per day derived from enteral nutrition infusion
- Free water estimated intake from parenteral nutrition in 24 hours (mL/day)—defined as the approximate intake of free water per day derived from parenteral nutrition infusion
- Free water estimated intake from intravenous fluids in 24 hours (mL/day)—defined as the approximate intake of free water per day derived from intravenous fluid (IV) infusion

Measured fluid intake

- Total fluid measured intake in 24 hours (mL/day)—defined as the known quantity of intake in one day of fluid from all sources
- Fluid measured intake from oral nutrition in 24 hours (mL/day)—defined as the known quantity of intake in one day of fluid from oral intake
- Water measured oral intake in 24 hours (mL/day)—defined as the known quantity of intake in one day of water
- Sugar sweetened beverage measured oral intake in 24 hours (mL/day)—defined as the known quantity of intake in one day of sugar sweetened beverages
- Beverage with high intensity sweetener measured oral intake in 24 hours (mL/day)—defined as the known quantity of intake in one day of high intensity sweetened beverages that contain nutritive and nonnutritive sugar substitutes
- 100 percent fruit juice measured oral intake in 24 hours (mL/day)—defined as the known quantity of intake in one day of 100% fruit juice
- Liquid mammalian milk product measured oral intake in 24 hours (mL/day)—defined as the known quantity of intake in one day of mammalian milk beverages
- Caffeinated beverage measured oral intake in 24 hours (mL/day)—defined as the known quantity of intake in one day of caffeinated beverages
- Nutritionally complete liquid supplement measured oral intake in 24 hours (mL/day)—defined as the known quantity of intake in one day of nutrition supplements
- Liquid meal replacement measured oral intake in 24 hours (mL/day)—defined as the known quantity of intake in one day of a liquid that can replace a meal
- Fluid measured intake from food in 24 hours (mL/day)—defined as the known quantity of intake in one day of fluid from food intake
- Fluid measured intake per kg body weight in 24 hours (mL/kg/day)—defined as the known quantity of intake per kg of body weight in one day of fluid from all sources
- Free water measured intake in 24 hours—defined as the known quantity of intake from all sources
- Free water measured intake from breastmilk in 24 hours (mL/day)—defined as the known quantity of intake in one day of free water derived from breastmilk
- Free water measured intake from infant formula in 24 hours (mL/day)—defined as the known quantity of intake in one day of free water derived from infant formula
- Free water measured intake from enteral nutrition in 24 hours (mL/day)—defined as the known quantity of intake of free water per day derived from enteral nutrition infusion
- Free water measured intake from parenteral nutrition in 24 hours (mL/day)—defined as the known quantity of intake of free water per day derived from parenteral nutrition infusion
- Free water measured intake from intravenous fluids in 24 hours (mL/day)—defined as the known quantity of intake of free water per day derived from intravenous fluid (IV) infusion

Fluid Intake

Note: Alcohol intake is recorded on the Alcohol Intake reference sheet on page 46. Total volumes of breastmilk and infant formula can be found on the Breastmilk and Infant Formula Intake reference sheet on page 39. Total volume of enteral nutrition can be found on the Enteral Nutrition Intake reference sheet on page 42. Total volume of parenteral nutrition can be found on the Parenteral Nutrition Intake reference sheet on page 44. Biochemical measures of hydration status can be found on the Electrolyte and Renal Profile and Urine Profile reference sheets on pages 135 and 154, respectively.

In almost all nutrition settings, food and nutrient intakes are estimates; therefore, estimated intake terms should be used. The exception is research settings where exact measurement of intake is done. Then, measured intake terms are appropriate.

Examples of the measurement methods or data sources for these outcome indicators: Food and fluid intake records, 24-hour recalls, food frequency questionnaire, intake and output data, observation, weight measurement records

Typically used with the following domains of nutrition interventions: Food and/or nutrient delivery, nutrition education, nutrition counseling, coordination of nutrition care by nutrition professional, population based nutrition action

Typically used to determine and monitor and evaluate change in the following nutrition diagnoses: Excessive or inadequate oral intake, food medication interaction, underweight, overweight/obesity, unintended weight loss, unintended weight gain, disordered eating pattern, unbalanced diet pattern, limited adherence to nutrition related recommendations, inability to manage self care, swallowing difficulty, breastfeeding difficulty, altered GI function

Note: Judgment must be used to select indicators and determine the appropriate measurement techniques and reference standards for a given client population and setting. Once identified, these indicators, measurement techniques, and reference standards should be identified in policies and procedures or other documents for use in client records, quality or performance improvement, or in formal research projects.

Client Example

Example of one (or more) of the nutrition care indicators (includes sample initial and reassessment documentation for one of the indicators)

Indicator(s) Selected

Fluid estimated intake from oral nutrition in 24 hours (mL/day)

Criteria for Evaluation

Comparison to reference standard, recommendation, or goal:

1. Reference standard: Reference intake standards
2. Recommendation: Client's fluid estimated intake from oral nutrition in 24 hours is 1,000 mL (33 oz). Recommended intake is 2,600 mL per 24 hours.
3. Goal: Client currently drinks 1,000 mL (33 oz) of oral fluids per day and has a personal goal of consuming 1,920 mL (64 oz) of fluid per day.

Fluid Intake

Sample Nutrition Assessment and Monitoring and Evaluation Documentation	
Initial nutrition assessment	Based on client's food diary, fluid estimated intake from oral nutrition in 24 hours is approximately 1,000 mL (33 oz). Goal is to consume approximately 1,920 mL (64 oz) of fluid per day. Will monitor fluid intake at next encounter.
Reassessment after nutrition intervention	Significant progress toward goal fluid intake. Based on fluid intake records, client increased consumption of fluids from 1,000 mL (33 oz) to 1,920 mL per day, exceeding goal and meeting recommended intake.

Food Intake

Definition

Amount, type, and pattern of food consumed and quality of diet.

> *Note:* Whenever possible, nutrient intake data should be considered in combination with clinical, biochemical, and anthropometric information, medical diagnosis, clinical status, and/or other factors to provide a valid assessment of nutritional status based on a totality of the evidence. (Institute of Medicine. *Dietary Reference Intakes: Applications in Dietary Assessment.* National Academies Press; 2000.)

Nutrition Assessment and Monitoring and Evaluation

Indicators

- Amount of food
- Estimated amount of food
  - Grains servings estimated in 24 hours (number/day)
  - Fruits servings estimated in 24 hours (number/day)
  - Vegetable servings estimated in 24 hours (number/day)
  - Mammalian milk products servings estimated in 24 hours (number/day)
  - Protein food servings estimated in 24 hours (number/day) (eg, meat, poultry, fish, eggs, beans, nut products)
  - Fat servings estimated in 24 hours (number/day)
  - Empty energy servings estimated in 24 hours (number/day)
  - Estimated percent of meals eaten in 24 hours (percent/day)—defined as the approximate proportion of all meals in one day that is consumed
- Measured amount of food
  - Grains servings measured in 24 hours (number/day)
  - Fruits servings measured in 24 hours (number/day)
  - Vegetable servings measured in 24 hours (number/day)
  - Mammalian milk products servings measured in 24 hours (number/day)
  - Protein food servings measured in 24 hours (number/day) (eg, meat, poultry, fish, eggs, beans, nut products)
  - Fat servings measured in 24 hours (number/day)
  - Empty energy servings measured in 24 hours (number/day)
  - Measured percent of meals eaten in 24 hours (percent/day)—defined as the known proportion of all meals in one day that is consumed
- Types of food
  - Fortified food intake (present/absent)—defined as oral intake of foods with extra nutrients added (eg, calcium-fortified orange juice)
  - Enriched food intake (present/absent)—defined as oral intake of foods that contain the nutrients that were added back after being lost during processing
  - Special dietary food intake (present/absent)—defined as oral intake of foods that have been modified for a nutrition purpose (eg, lactose free, gluten free, sugar free, low fat, nut free)

Food Intake

  - Medical food intake (present/absent)—defined as oral intake of foods for a special medical purpose to manage a nutrition related disease
  - Processed food intake (present/absent)—defined as oral intake of commercial convenience foods
  - Quick service food intake (present/absent)—defined as oral intake of fast foods
  - Self prepared food intake (present/absent)—defined as oral intake of foods prepared by the client or supportive individuals
  - Prepared food intake (present/absent)—defined as oral intake of food that is ready to eat, at or from a restaurant, market, food station, but excludes quick service food
- Meal/snack* pattern
- Estimated meal and snack pattern
  - Number of meals estimated in 24 hours (number/day)
  - Number of snacks estimated in 24 hours (number/day)
- Measured meal and snack pattern
  - Number of meals measured in 24 hours (number/day)
  - Number of snacks measured in 24 hours (number/day)
- Diet (food and beverages) Quality Index
  - Healthy Eating Index (HEI) 2015 score—defined as an assessment of how well reported food intake aligns with the 2015-2020 Dietary Guidelines for Americans
- Food variety (present/absent)—defined as consumption of a wide assortment of foods from different food groups on a regular basis

Note: Liquid meal replacements/supplements are found on the Fluid Intake reference sheet on page 32.

In almost all nutrition settings, food and nutrient intakes are estimates; therefore, estimated intake terms should be used. The exception is research settings where exact measurement of intake is done. Then, measured intake terms are appropriate.

Examples of the measurement methods or data sources for these outcome indicators: Food intake records, 24-hour recalls, food frequency questionnaire, menu analysis, dietary and physical activity assessment tool (eg, MyPlate), diet quality index (eg, Healthy Eating Index) or other reference intake standard tool

Typically used with the following domains of nutrition interventions: Food and/or nutrient delivery, nutrition education, nutrition counseling, coordination of nutrition care by nutrition professional, population based nutrition action

Typically used to determine and monitor and evaluate change in the following nutrition diagnoses: Excessive or inadequate oral intake, food medication interaction, underweight, overweight/obesity, disordered eating pattern, unintended weight gain, unintended weight loss, unbalanced diet pattern, limited adherence to nutrition related recommendations, inability to manage self care, food insecurity, intake of unsafe food, inadequate or excessive energy, macronutrient or micronutrient intake

Note: Judgment must be used to select indicators and determine the appropriate measurement techniques and reference standards for a given client population and setting. Once identified, these indicators, measurement techniques, and reference standards should be identified in policies and procedures or other documents for use in client records, quality or performance improvement, or in formal research projects.

---

* Snack is defined as food served between meals.

Food Intake

Client Example

Example(s) of one (or more) of the nutrition care indicators (includes sample initial and reassessment documentation for one of the indicators)

Indicator(s) Selected

Vegetable servings estimated in 24 hours and Fruit servings estimated in 24 hours

Criteria for Evaluation

Comparison to reference standard, recommendation, or goal:

1. Reference standard: Not applicable
2. Recommendation: Client's intake reflects an average of 1 to 2 servings vegetable servings in 24 hours and 1 fruit serving estimated in 24 hours, which is below the Dietary Approaches to Stop Hypertension (DASH) eating plan recommendation of 9 servings of fruits and vegetables per day.
3. Goal: Client's goal is to increase fruit and vegetable intake to 5 servings per day.

Sample Nutrition Assessment and Monitoring and Evaluation Documentation	
Initial encounter	Based on client's recalls, client's intake reflects an average of 1 to 2 vegetable servings estimated in 24 hours and 1 fruit serving estimated in 24 hours, which is below client goal of 5 servings of fruits and vegetables per day. Will monitor fruit and vegetable intake at next encounter.
Reassessment after nutrition intervention	Met goal of increasing fruit and vegetable intake to 5 servings per day.

Breastmilk* and Infant Formula Intake

Definition

Amount of human milk and/or the amount of infant formula consumed.

Nutrition Assessment and Monitoring and Evaluation

Indicators

Breastmilk intake

- Breastmilk feeding attempts in 24 hours (number/day)
- Adequacy of breastmilk intake (inadequate, adequate, excessive)
- Donor breastmilk intake (yes/no)—defined as human milk expressed by a lactating parent to feed an infant that is not the donor's infant
- Mother's† expressed breastmilk intake (yes/no)—defined as human milk expelled by a lactating parent to feed their own infant
- Estimated breastmilk intake
  - Breastmilk intake estimated volume in 24 hours (mL/day)—defined as the approximate intake in one day of human milk
  - Breastmilk intake estimated volume per kg in 24 hours (mL/kg/day)—defined as the approximate intake per kg of body weight in one day of human milk
- Measured breastmilk intake
  - Breastmilk intake measured volume in 24 hours (mL/day)—defined as the known quantity of intake in one day of human milk
  - Breastmilk intake measured volume per kg in 24 hours (mL/kg/day)—defined as the known quantity of intake per kg of body weight in one day of human milk

Infant formula intake (oz or mL/day)

- Infant formula feedings in 24 hours (number/day)
- Adequacy of infant formula intake (inadequate, adequate, excessive)
- Infant formula intake composition (eg, cow's milk, soy based)—defined as the formula characteristics and components
- Infant formula intake concentration (calories/oz, kcal/mL)—defined at the energy density of the infant formula
- Estimated infant formula intake
  - Infant formula intake estimated volume in 24 hours (mL/day)—defined as the approximate intake in one day of infant formula
  - Infant formula intake estimated volume per kg in 24 hours (mL/kg/day)—defined as the approximate intake per kg of body weight in one day of infant formula
- Measured infant formula intake
  - Infant formula intake measured volume in 24 hours (mL/day)—defined as the known quantity of intake in one day of infant formula
  - Infant formula intake measured volume per kg in 24 hours (mL/kg/day)—defined as the known quantity of intake per kg of body weight in one day of infant formula

---

* If a synonym for the term "breastmilk" is helpful or needed, an approved alternate is "human milk."

† If a synonym for the term "mother" is helpful or needed, an approved alternate is "lactating parent."

Breastmilk and Infant Formula Intake

Note: Breastfeeding* ability and capacity can be found on the Breastfeeding Assessment reference sheet on page 119.

Weight change can be found on the Body Composition/Growth/Weight History reference sheet on page 129.

Number of wet diapers per day can be found on the Urine Profile reference sheet on page 154.

Number/consistency of bowel movements can be found on the Nutrition Focused Physical Exam reference sheet on page 162.

If provided via tube, use the Enteral and Parenteral Nutrition Intake reference sheets on page 42 and 44.

In almost all nutrition settings, food and nutrient intakes are estimates; therefore, estimated intake terms should be used. The exception is research settings where exact measurement of intake is done. Then, measured intake terms are appropriate.

Examples of the measurement methods or data sources for these outcome indicators: Intake records, 24-hour recalls, usual intake recalls, observation of feeding, pre- and post-breastfeeding infant weights

Typically used with the following domains of nutrition interventions: Food and/or nutrient delivery, nutrition education, nutrition counseling, coordination of nutrition care by nutrition professional, population based nutrition action

Typically used to determine and monitor and evaluate change in the following nutrition diagnoses: Underweight, overweight, unintended weight gain, unintended weight loss, growth rate less than expected, limited adherence to nutrition related recommendations, inadequate or excessive energy intake, inadequate or excessive oral or fluid intake

Note: Judgment must be used to select indicators and determine the appropriate measurement techniques and reference standards for a given client population and setting. Once identified, these indicators, measurement techniques, and reference standards should be identified in policies and procedures or other documents for use in client records, quality or performance improvement, or in formal research projects.

Client Example

Example of one of the nutrition care indicators (includes sample initial and reassessment documentation for one of the indicators)

Indicator Selected

Infant formula intake volume estimated in 24 hours (mL/day)

Criteria for Evaluation

Comparison to reference standard, recommendation, or goal:

1. Reference standard: Client's infant formula volume estimated in 24 hours averages 410 mL (100 mL/kg body). This is below the reference standard of 150 mL/kg/day to support adequate growth.
2. Recommendation: Not applicable
3. Goal: Client currently consumes approximately 100 mL/kg/kg body weight infant formula per day. Client's goal is to increase intake to 150 mL/kg per day.

* If a synonym for the term "breastfeeding" is helpful or needed, an approved alternate is "chestfeeding."

Breastmilk and Infant Formula Intake

Sample Nutrition Assessment and Monitoring and Evaluation Documentation	
Initial nutrition assessment	Based on client's recalls, infant formula intake volume estimated in 24 hours is 410 mL (100 mL/kg/day), 33% below the reference standard of 150 mL/kg per day. Will monitor formula intake at next encounter.
Reassessment after nutrition intervention	Significant progress toward goal of consuming 150 mL/kg per day. Based on mother's records, infant formula intake volume estimated in 24 hours has increased to approximately 575 mL (140 mL/kg/day) over the past 7 days.

Enteral Nutrition Intake

Definition

Amount or type of enteral nutrition provided via a tube.

Note: Whenever possible, nutrient intake data should be considered in combination with clinical, biochemical, and anthropometric information, medical diagnosis, clinical status, and/or other factors to provide a valid assessment of nutritional status based on a totality of the evidence. (Institute of Medicine. *Dietary Reference Intakes: Applications in Dietary Assessment.* National Academies Press; 2000.)

Nutrition Assessment and Monitoring and Evaluation

Indicators

- Enteral nutrition formula/solution
  - Enteral nutrition formula composition (formula)
  - Enteral nutrition formula concentration (calories/kcal/kJ in each mL)
  - Enteral nutrition formula estimated volume in 24 hours (mL/day)
  - Enteral nutrition formula measured volume in 24 hours (mL/day)
  - Enteral tube feeding flush estimated volume in 24 hours (mL/day)
  - Enteral tube feeding flush measured volume in 24 hours (mL/day)

Note: Enteral nutrition tolerance can be found on the Nutrition Focused Physical Exam reference sheet on page 162 and/or the pertinent biochemical/sign or symptom reference sheet.

Examples of the measurement methods or data sources for these outcome indicators: Client report/recalls, client record, home evaluation, intake and output record

Typically used with the following domains of nutrition interventions: Food and/or nutrient delivery, nutrition education, coordination of nutrition care by nutrition professional

Typically used to determine and monitor and evaluate change in the following nutrition diagnoses: Inadequate or excessive intake of enteral nutrition, inadequate fluid intake, food medication interaction, unintended weight loss or gain

Note: Judgment must be used to select indicators and determine the appropriate measurement techniques and reference standards for a given client population and setting. Once identified, these indicators, measurement techniques, and reference standards should be identified in policies and procedures or other documents for use in client records, quality or performance improvement, or in formal research projects.

Client Example

Example of one of the nutrition care indicators (includes sample initial and reassessment documentation for one of the indicators)

Indicator Selected

Enteral nutrition formula volume in 24 hours (mL/day)

Enteral Nutrition Intake

Criteria for evaluation

Comparison to goal or reference standard:

1. Reference standard: Not applicable
2. Recommendation: Client's enteral nutrition formula volume in 24 hours meets the nutrition prescription of 80 mL/hour in 24 hours.
3. Goal: Not applicable

Sample Nutrition Assessment and Monitoring and Evaluation Documentation	
Initial nutrition assessment	Enteral nutrition formula volume in 24 hours meets 60% of recommended volume for 24 hours. Increase enteral nutrition rate to 80 mL/hour. Monitor enteral nutrition rate advancement.
Reassessment after nutrition intervention	Enteral nutrition formula volume in 24 hours meeting 85% estimated need. Progress toward nutrition prescription of 1 calorie or kcal per mL at 80 mL per hour in 24 hours.

Parenteral Nutrition Intake

Definition

Amount or type of parenteral nutrition and/or fluids provided intravenously.

Note: Whenever possible, nutrient intake data should be considered in combination with clinical, biochemical, and anthropometric information, medical diagnosis, clinical status, and/or other factors to provide a valid assessment of nutritional status based on a totality of the evidence. (Institute of Medicine. *Dietary Reference Intakes: Applications in Dietary Assessment.* National Academies Press; 2000.)

Nutrition Assessment and Monitoring and Evaluation

Indicators

- Parenteral nutrition formula/solution (specify)
  - Composition (formula or description)
  - Concentration (eg, percent, grams of solute per mL)
  - Rate (eg, mL/hour)
  - Schedule (eg, hours, timing, taper schedule)
- Intravenous fluids, eg, type; amount mL/day, mL/hr, mL with medications

Note: Parenteral nutrition tolerance can be accomplished with the Nutrition Focused Physical Exam reference sheet on page 162 and/or the pertinent biochemical/sign or symptom reference sheet.

Examples of the measurement methods or data sources for these outcome indicators: Client report/recalls, client record, home evaluation, intake and output record

Typically used with the following domains of nutrition interventions: Food and/or nutrient delivery, nutrition education, coordination of nutrition care by nutrition professional

Typically used to determine and monitor and evaluate change in the following nutrition diagnoses: Inadequate or excessive intake of parenteral nutrition, inadequate fluid intake, food medication interaction, unintended weight loss or gain

Note: Judgment must be used to select indicators and determine the appropriate measurement techniques and reference standards for a given client population and setting. Once identified, these indicators, measurement techniques, and reference standards should be identified in policies and procedures or other documents for use in client records, quality or performance improvement, or in formal research projects.

Criteria for Evaluation

Comparison to goal or reference standard:

1. Goal (tailored to patient/client's needs)
   OR
2. Reference standard

Parenteral Nutrition Intake

Client Example

Example(s) of one or two of the nutrition care indicators (includes sample initial and reassessment documentation for one of the indicators)

Indicator(s) Selected

Rate/schedule (mL/hour × number of hours)

Criteria for Evaluation

Comparison to goal or reference standard:

1. Goal: Patient/client's parenteral nutrition formula is at a rate of 50 mL per hour × 24 hours of standard solution compared to the nutrition prescription of 80 mL/hour × 24 hours to meet estimated nutrition requirements.
   OR
2. Reference standard: There is no reference standard for this outcome as the provision of enteral/parenteral nutrition is individualized.

Sample Nutrition Assessment Documentation	
Initial nutrition assessment with client	Parenteral nutrition formula rate of 25 mL per hour × 24 hours of standard solution compared to the nutrition prescription of 80 mL/hour to meet estimated nutrition requirements. Monitor nutrition initiation and rate advancement.
Reassessment after nutrition intervention	Parenteral nutrition formula at 70 mL per hour × 24 hours. Significant progress toward nutrition prescription of 80 mL per hour × 24 hours.

Alcohol Intake

Definition

Amount and pattern of alcohol (ethanol) consumption.

Nutrition Assessment and Monitoring and Evaluation

Indicators

- Alcohol intake in one week (g/week)—defined as the approximate intake over seven days of all sources of alcohol
- Alcohol intake in 24 hours (g/day)—defined as the approximate intake in one day of all sources of alcohol
- Beer intake in 24 hours (mL/day)—defined as the approximate intake in one day of beer
- Distilled alcohol intake in 24 hours (mL/day)—defined as the approximate intake in one day of distilled alcohol
- Wine intake in 24 hours (mL/day)—defined as the approximate intake in one day of wine
- Hard cider intake in 24 hours (mL/day)—defined as the approximate intake in one day of cider that contains alcohol
- Days per week alcoholic drinks consumed (number)—defined as usual or average number of days per week when alcohol containing drinks are consumed
- Alcohol intake pattern on drinking days (number)—defined as the typical number of standard alcohol-containing drinks on a drinking day

Note: One alcohol-containing drink is defined differently in countries around the world, with countries using grams, ounces, milliliters, and units. Where applicable in this reference sheet, one standard alcohol-containing drink equals 10 g of pure alcohol (ethanol). Professionals need to refer to guidelines in their respective countries to determine the alcohol content of one standard alcohol-containing drink.

Examples of the measurement methods or data sources for these outcome indicators: Client report/recalls, self-monitoring log

Typically used with the following domains of nutrition interventions: Nutrition education, nutrition counseling, coordination of nutrition care by a nutrition professional, population based nutrition action

Typically used to determine and monitor and evaluate change in the following nutrition diagnoses: Excessive intake of alcohol, excessive or inadequate intake of energy, altered nutrition related laboratory values, impaired nutrient utilization, overweight/obesity

Note: Judgment must be used to select indicators and determine the appropriate measurement techniques and reference standards for a given client population and setting. Once identified, these indicators, measurement techniques, and reference standards should be identified in policies and procedures or other documents for use in client records, quality or performance improvement, or in formal research projects.

Client Example

Example(s) of one (or more) of the nutrition care indicators (includes sample initial and reassessment documentation for one of the indicators)

Alcohol Intake

Indicator(s) Selected

Alcohol intake pattern on drinking days (number)

Criteria for Evaluation

Comparison to reference standard, recommendation, or goal:

1. Reference standard: Refer to country standards, if present, for alcohol reference standards.
2. Recommendation: Client's intake of three to four standard alcohol drinks on drinking days is significantly above the recommendation of one standard alcohol drink per day for adult females.
3. Goal: Client established a goal to reduce standard alcohol drink intake to one standard alcohol drink per day.

Sample Nutrition Assessment and Monitoring and Evaluation Documentation	
Initial encounter	Based on recalls, client's alcohol intake pattern on drinking days is three to four standard alcohol drinks, which is above the recommended amount for adult females. Client established goal to reduce intake to one standard alcohol drink on drinking days. Will monitor change in alcohol intake at next encounter
Reassessment after nutrition intervention	Progress toward goal. Alcohol intake pattern on drinking days, based on multiple 7-day records, is approximately two standard alcohol drinks on drinking days.

Bioactive Substance Intake

Definition

Amount and type of bioactive substances consumed.

Note: Bioactive substances are not part of the Dietary Reference Intakes, and therefore there are no established minimum requirements or Tolerable Upper Intake Levels. However, RDNs can assess whether estimated intakes are adequate or excessive using the client goal or nutrition prescription for comparison.

Working definition of bioactive substances—physiologically active components of foods that may have an effect on health. There is no scientific consensus about a definition for bioactive substances/components.

Nutrition Assessment and Monitoring and Evaluation

Indicators

- Estimated bioactive substance intake
- Plant stanol ester estimated intake in 24 hours (g/day)—defined as the approximate intake in one day of plant stanol esters
- Plant sterol ester estimated intake in 24 hours (g/day)—defined as the approximate intake in one day of plant sterol esters
- Soy protein estimated intake in 24 hours (g/day)—defined as the approximate intake in one day of soy protein
- Prebiotic estimated intake—defined as the approximate intake of a substrate that is selectively utilized by host microorganisms conferring a health benefit
- Psyllium estimated intake in 24 hours (g/day)—defined as the approximate intake in one day of psyllium
- Beta glucan estimated intake in 24 hours (g/day)—defined as the approximate intake in one day of beta glucan
- Measured bioactive substance intake
- Plant stanol ester measured intake in 24 hours (g/day)—defined as the known quantity of intake in one day of plant stanol esters
- Plant sterol ester measured intake in 24 hours (g/day)—defined as the known quantity of intake in one day of plant sterol esters
- Soy protein measured intake in 24 hours (g/day)—defined as the known quantity of intake in one day of soy protein
- Prebiotic measured intake—defined as the known intake of a substrate that is selectively utilized by host microorganisms conferring a health benefit
- Psyllium measured intake in 24 hours (g/day)—defined as the known quantity of intake in one day of psyllium
- Beta glucan measured intake in 24 hours (g/day)—defined as the known quantity of intake in one day of beta glucan
- Food additives intake (those thought to have an effect on a client's health)
- High intensity sweetener additive intake
- Excessive high intensity sweetener additive intake (present/absent)—defined as intake above the recommended acceptable daily intake (ADI) of high intensity sweeteners that contain nutritive and nonnutritive sugar substitutes
- Probiotic intake—defined as intake of live microorganisms in sufficient amounts* to confer a health benefit on the host

---

* While the definition of probiotic intake states the intake needs to be in "sufficient amounts," this is to remain consistent with the World Health Organization definition meaning of probiotic. How much probiotic intake would be considered "sufficient" to confer a health benefit on the host has not been determined.

Bioactive Substance Intake

Note: In almost all nutrition settings, food and nutrient intakes are estimates; therefore, estimated intake terms should be used. The exception is research settings where exact measurement of intake is done. Then, measured intake terms are appropriate.

Examples of the measurement methods or data sources for these outcome indicators: Client report/recalls, self-monitoring log

Typically used with the following domains of nutrition interventions: Nutrition education, nutrition counseling, population based nutrition action

Typically used to determine and monitor and evaluate change in the following nutrition diagnoses: Inadequate or excessive intake of bioactive substances, food medication interaction, altered GI function

Note: Judgment must be used to select indicators and determine the appropriate measurement techniques and reference standards for a given client population and setting. Once identified, these indicators, measurement techniques, and reference standards should be identified in policies and procedures or other documents for use in client records, quality or performance improvement, or in formal research projects.

Client Example

Example of one of the nutrition care indicators (includes sample initial and reassessment documentation for one of the indicators)

Indicator Selected

Plant sterol ester estimated intake in 24 hours (g/day)

Criteria for Evaluation

Comparison to reference standard, recommendation, or goal:

1. Reference standard: Not applicable
2. Recommendation: Client does not consume plant sterol esters compared to the recommended intake of 2 to 3 g per day.
3. Goal: Client established a goal to consume approximately 2 g of plant sterol esters per day 5 of 7 days per week.

Sample Nutrition Assessment and Monitoring and Evaluation Documentation	
Initial assessment	Based on recalls, client consuming 0 g of plant sterol ester per day. Goal intake of 2 g per day 5 out of 7 days per week established. Will monitor change in plant sterol ester intake at next encounter.
Reassessment after nutrition intervention	Good progress toward the goal of 2 g per day 5 out of 7 days per week of plant sterol ester. Based on diet records, plant sterol ester estimated intake in 24 hours is approximately 2 g per day 2 to 3 days per week.

Caffeine Intake

Definition

Amount of caffeine intake from all sources including food, beverages, supplements, medications, and via enteral and parenteral routes.

Nutrition Assessment and Monitoring and Evaluation

Indicators

- Total caffeine estimated intake in 24 hours (mg/day)—defined as the approximate intake in one day of caffeine
- Total caffeine measured intake in 24 hours (mg/day)—defined as the known quantity of intake in one day of caffeine

Note: In almost all nutrition settings, food and nutrient intakes are estimates; therefore, estimated intake terms should be used. The exception is research settings where exact measurement of intake is done. Then, measured intake terms are appropriate.

Examples of the measurement methods or data sources for these outcome indicators: Client report/recalls, self-monitoring log

Typically used with the following domains of nutrition interventions: Nutrition education, nutrition counseling

Typically used to determine and monitor and evaluate change in the following nutrition diagnoses: Food and nutrition related knowledge deficit, limited food and nutrition related skill

Note: Judgment must be used to select indicators and determine the appropriate measurement techniques and reference standards for a given client population and setting. Once identified, these indicators, measurement techniques, and reference standards should be identified in policies and procedures or other documents for use in client records, quality or performance improvement, or in formal research projects.

Client Example

Example of one of the nutrition care indicators (includes sample initial and reassessment documentation for one of the indicators)

Indicator Selected

Total caffeine estimated intake in 24 hours (mg/day)

Criteria for Evaluation

Comparison to reference standard, recommendation, or goal:

1. Reference standard: Client's intake is approximately 600 mg of caffeine per day, which is above the reference standard of 400 mg caffeine/day.
2. Recommendation: Not applicable
3. Goal: Client's total caffeine estimated intake in 24 hours is above the goal the client established of less than 400 mg caffeine/day.

Caffeine Intake

Sample Nutrition Assessment and Monitoring and Evaluation Documentation	
Initial nutrition assessment with client	Based on recalls, client total caffeine estimated intake in 24 hours is 600 mg of caffeine/day, which is above the reference standard of 400 mg/day. Will monitor change in caffeine intake at next encounter.
Reassessment after nutrition intervention	No progress toward the client's goal of 400 mg of caffeine/day. Based on diet records, client still consuming 600 mg of caffeine/day.

Fat Intake

Definition

Fat consumption from all sources including food, beverages, supplements, and via enteral and parenteral routes.

Note: Whenever possible, nutrient intake data should be considered in combination with clinical, biochemical, anthropometric information, medical diagnosis, clinical status, and/or other factors to provide a valid assessment of nutritional status based on a totality of the evidence. (Institute of Medicine. *Dietary Reference Intakes: Applications in Dietary Assessment.* National Academies Press; 2000.)

Nutrition Assessment and Monitoring and Evaluation

Indicators

Estimated fat intake

- Total fat estimated intake in 24 hours (g/day)—defined as the approximate intake in one day of all types of fat
- Saturated fat estimated intake in 24 hours (g/day)—defined as the approximate intake in one day of a fat that has no double bonds between carbon molecules
- *Trans* fatty acid estimated intake in 24 hours (g/day)—defined as the approximate intake in one day of an unsaturated fatty acid that is hydrogenated with the trans arrangement of the hydrogen atoms adjacent to its double bonds
- Polyunsaturated fat estimated intake in 24 hours (g/day)—defined as the approximate intake in one day of a fatty acid that contains more than one double bond
  - Linoleic acid (LA) estimated intake in 24 hours (g/day)—defined as the approximate intake in one day of a polyunsaturated, omega-6 and essential fatty acid with an 18-carbon chain length and two cis double bonds (18:2)
- Monounsaturated fat estimated intake in 24 hours (g/day)—defined as the approximate intake in one day of a fatty acid with one unsaturated (double) carbon bond
- Omega-3 fatty acid estimated intake in 24 hours (mg/day)—defined as the approximate intake in one day of a polyunsaturated fatty acid with a double bond at the third carbon atom from the methyl end of the carbon chain
  - Alpha linolenic acid estimated intake in 24 hours (mg/day)—defined as the approximate intake in one day of a polyunsaturated and essential omega-3 fatty acid with an 18-carbon chain and three cis double bonds (18:3)
  - Eicosapentaenoic acid (EPA) estimated intake in 24 hours (mg/day)—defined as the approximate intake in one day of a polyunsaturated, omega-3 fatty acid with a 20-carbon chain and five cis double bonds
  - Docosahexaenoic acid estimated intake in 24 hours (mg/day)—defined as the approximate intake in one day of a polyunsaturated, omega-3 fatty acid with a 22-carbon chain and six cis double bonds
- Essential fatty acid estimated intake in 24 hours (mg/day)—defined as the approximate intake in one day of a fatty acid (Linoleic acid [18:2] and Alpha linolenic acid [18:3]) that must be provided in the diet or enteral or parenteral nutrition because the human body cannot synthesize it
- Medium-chain triglyceride estimated intake in 24 hours (g/day)—defined as the approximate intake in one day of a triglyceride molecule with fatty acids having a carbon chain length of 6-12
- Fat estimated intake in one meal (g/meal)—defined as the approximate intake in one meal of all types of fat

Fat Intake

- Percent saturated fat estimated intake in 24 hours (percent/day)—defined as the approximate energy intake in one day from fat that has no double bonds between carbon molecules as a portion of total energy intake
- Fat estimated intake from oral nutrition in 24 hours (g/day)—defined as the estimated intake of fat in grams in one day derived from oral intake
- Fat estimated intake from enteral nutrition in 24 hours (g/day)—defined as the estimated intake of fat in grams in one day derived from enteral nutrition infusion
- Fat estimated intake from parenteral nutrition in 24 hours (g/day)—defined as the estimated intake of fat in grams in one day derived from parenteral nutrition infusion
- Fat estimated intake from intravenous fluids in 24 hours (g/day)—defined as the estimated intake of fat in grams in one day derived from intravenous fluid (IV) infusion
- Fat additive estimated intake in 24 hours (mL/day)—defined as the approximate intake in one day of fat additive
- Percent fat estimated intake in 24 hours (percent/day)—defined as the approximate energy intake in one day from fat intake

Measured fat intake

- Total fat measured intake in 24 hours (g/day)—defined as the known quantity of intake in one day of all types of fat
- Saturated fat measured intake in 24 hours (g/day)—defined as the known quantity of intake in one day of a fat that has no double bonds between carbon molecules
- *Trans* fatty acid measured intake in 24 hours (g/day)—defined as the known quantity of intake in one day of an unsaturated fatty acid that is hydrogenated with the trans arrangement of the hydrogen atoms adjacent to its double bonds
- Polyunsaturated fat measured intake in 24 hours (g/day)—defined as the known quantity of intake in one day of a fatty acid that contains more than one double bond
    - Linoleic acid (LA) measured intake in 24 hours (g/day)—defined as the known quantity of intake in one day of a polyunsaturated, omega-6 and essential fatty acid with an 18-carbon chain length and two cis double bonds (18:2)
- Monounsaturated fat measured intake in 24 hours (g/day)—defined as the known quantity of intake in one day of a fatty acid with one unsaturated (double) carbon bond
- Omega-3 fatty acid measured intake in 24 hours (mg/day)—defined as the known quantity of intake in one day of a polyunsaturated fatty acid with a double bond at the third carbon atom from the methyl end of the carbon chain
    - Alpha linolenic acid measured intake in 24 hours (mg/day)—defined as the known quantity of intake in one day of a polyunsaturated and essential omega-3 fatty acid with an 18-carbon chain and three cis double bonds (18:3)
    - Eicosapentaenoic acid (EPA) measured intake in 24 hours (mg/day)—defined as the known quantity of intake in one day of a polyunsaturated, omega-3 fatty acid with a 20-carbon chain and five cis double bonds
    - Docosahexaenoic acid (DHA) measured intake in 24 hours (mg/day)—defined as the known quantity of intake in one day of a polyunsaturated, omega-3 fatty acid with a 22-carbon chain and six cis double bonds
- Essential fatty acid measured intake in 24 hours (mg/day)—defined as the known quantity of intake in one day of a fatty acid (Linoleic acid [18:2] and Alphalinolenic acid [18:3]) that must be provided in the diet or enteral or parenteral nutrition because the human body cannot synthesize it

Fat Intake

- Medium chain triglyceride measured intake in 24 hours (g/day)—defined as the known quantity of intake in one day of a triglyceride molecule with fatty acids having a carbon chain length of 6-12
- Fat measured intake in one meal (g/meal)—defined as the known quantity of intake in one meal of all types of fat
- Percent saturated fat measured intake in 24 hours (percent/day)—defined as the known quantity of intake in one day of fat that has no double bonds between carbon molecules as a portion of total energy intake
- Fat measured intake from oral nutrition in 24 hours (g/day)—defined as the known quantity of intake of fat in grams in one day derived from oral intake
- Fat measured intake from enteral nutrition in 24 hours (g/day)—defined as the known quantity of intake of fat in grams in one day derived from enteral nutrition infusion
- Fat measured intake from parenteral nutrition in 24 hours (g/day)—defined as the known quantity of intake of fat in grams in one day derived from parenteral nutrition infusion
- Fat measured intake from intravenous fluids in 24 hours (g/day)—defined as the known quantity of intake of fat in grams in one day derived from intravenous fluid (IV) infusion
- Fat additive measured intake in 24 hours (mL/day)—defined as the known quantity of intake in one day of fat additive
- Percent fat measured intake in 24 hours (percent/day)—defined as the known quantity of energy intake in one day from fat intake

Note: Plant sterol and stanol esters can be found on the Bioactive Substance Intake reference sheet on page 48.

In almost all nutrition settings, food and nutrient intakes are estimates; therefore, estimated intake terms should be used. The exception is research settings where exact measurement of intake is done. Then, measured intake terms are appropriate.

Examples of the measurement methods or data sources for these outcome indicators: Food intake records, 24-hour recalls, food frequency questionnaires, qualitative intake assessment, menu analysis, fat and cholesterol targeted questionnaires and monitoring devices

Typically used with the following domains of nutrition interventions: Food and/or nutrient delivery, nutrition education, nutrition counseling

Typically used to determine and monitor and evaluate change in the following nutrition diagnoses: Inadequate and excessive fat intake, intake of types of fats inconsistent with needs, overweight/obesity, altered nutrition related lab values, food and nutrition related knowledge deficit

Note: Judgment must be used to select indicators and determine the appropriate measurement techniques and reference standards for a given client population and setting. Once identified, these indicators, measurement techniques, and reference standards should be identified in policies and procedures or other documents for use in client records, quality or performance improvement, or in formal research projects.

Client Example

Example(s) of one of the nutrition care indicators (includes sample initial and reassessment documentation for one of the indicators)

Indicator Selected

Total fat estimated intake in 24 hours (g/day)

Fat Intake

Criteria for Evaluation

Comparison to reference standard, recommendation, or goal:

1. Reference standard: Not applicable
2. Recommendation: Not applicable
3. Goal: Client's total fat estimated intake in 24 hours is 120 g. Client's goal is to decrease total fat estimated intake in 24 hours to less than 80 g.

Sample Nutrition Assessment and Monitoring and Evaluation Documentation	
Initial encounter	Based on food diary, client's total fat estimated intake in 24 hours is 120 g. Client's goal is to decrease total fat estimated intake in 24 hours to less than 80 g. Will monitor fat intake at next appointment.
Reassessment after nutrition intervention	Significant progress toward the goal intake of less than 80 g of total fat estimated intake in 24 hours. Based on food diary, client's total fat estimated intake in 24 hours decreased from 120 g to 85 g of fat in 1 day. Will continue to monitor progress at next encounter in 6 weeks.

Cholesterol Intake

Definition

Dietary cholesterol consumption from all sources including food, beverages, supplements, and via enteral and parenteral routes.

Note: Whenever possible, nutrient intake data should be considered in combination with clinical, biochemical, anthropometric information, medical diagnosis, clinical status, and/or other factors to provide a valid assessment of nutritional status based on a totality of the evidence. (Institute of Medicine. *Dietary Reference Intakes: Applications in Dietary Assessment.* National Academies Press; 2000.)

Nutrition Assessment and Monitoring and Evaluation

Indicators

- Cholesterol estimated intake in 24 hours (mg/day)—defined as the approximate intake in one day of cholesterol
- Cholesterol measured intake in 24 hours (mg/day)—defined as the known quantity of intake in one day of cholesterol

Note: Plant sterol and stanol esters can be found on the Bioactive Substance Intake reference sheet on page 48.

Note: In almost all nutrition settings, food and nutrient intakes are estimates; therefore, estimated intake terms should be used. The exception is research settings where exact measurement of intake is done. Then, measured intake terms are appropriate.

Examples of the measurement methods or data sources for these outcome indicators: Food intake records, 24-hour recalls, food frequency questionnaires, qualitative intake assessment, menu analysis, fat- and cholesterol-targeted questionnaires and monitoring devices

Typically used with the following domains of nutrition interventions: Food and/or nutrient delivery, nutrition education, nutrition counseling

Typically used to determine and monitor and evaluate change in the following nutrition diagnoses: Excessive fat intake, excessive cholesterol intake, overweight/obesity, altered nutrition related lab values, altered food and nutrition related knowledge deficit, limited food and nutrient related skill

Note: Judgment must be used to select indicators and determine the appropriate measurement techniques and reference standards for a given client population and setting. Once identified, these indicators, measurement techniques, and reference standards should be identified in policies and procedures or other documents for use in client records, quality or performance improvement, or in formal research projects.

Client Example

Example(s) of one of the nutrition care indicators (includes sample initial and reassessment documentation for one of the indicators)

Indicator Selected

Cholesterol estimated intake in 24 hours (mg/day)

Cholesterol Intake

Criteria for Evaluation

Comparison to goal or reference standard:

1. Reference standard: Not applicable
2. Recommendation: Not applicable
3. Goal: Client cholesterol estimated intake is 24 hours is 350 mg/day. Client's goal is to decrease intake to within Healthy US-Style Eating Pattern (100 to 300 mg/day).

Sample Nutrition Assessment and Monitoring and Evaluation Documentation	
Initial nutrition assessment	Based on food diary, client's cholesterol estimated intake in 24 hours is 350 mg/day. Client's goal is to reduce cholesterol estimated intake in 24 hours to 100 to 300 mg/day. Will monitor cholesterol intake at next appointment.
Reassessment after nutrition intervention	Progress toward the goal of 100 to 300 mg/day of cholesterol. Based on food diary, client's cholesterol estimated intake in 24 hours decreased from 350 mg/day to 250 mg/day. Will continue to monitor progress at next encounter in 6 weeks.

Protein Intake

Definition

Protein intake from all sources including food, beverages, supplements, and via enteral and parenteral routes.

Note: Whenever possible, nutrient intake data should be considered in combination with clinical, biochemical, anthropometric information, medical diagnosis, clinical status, and/or other factors to provide a valid assessment of nutritional status based on a totality of the evidence. (Institute of Medicine. *Dietary Reference Intakes: Applications in Dietary Assessment.* National Academies Press; 2000.)

Nutrition Assessment and Monitoring and Evaluation

Indicators

Estimated protein intake

- Total protein estimated intake in 24 hours (g/day)—defined as the approximate intake in one day of all protein
- High biological value protein estimated intake in 24 hours (g/day)—defined as the approximate intake in one day from proteins which contain a ratio of essential amino acids that are needed for humans
- Casein estimated intake in 24 hours (g/day)—defined as the approximate intake in one day from the phosphoprotein component in milk and milk products that can also be an ingredient in food
- Whey protein estimated intake in 24 hours (g/day)—defined as the approximate intake in one day of the complete protein component in milk and milk products that can also be an ingredient in food
- Gluten estimated intake in 24 hours (g/day)—defined as the approximate intake in one day of the protein found primarily in cereal grains and contains gliadin and a glutenin
- Protein estimated intake per kg body weight in 24 hours (g/kg/day)—defined as the approximate intake per kg of body weight in one day of all protein
- Natural protein estimated intake in 24 hours (specify, g/day)—defined as the approximate intake of the portion of total protein that comes from food sources
- Protein estimated intake in one meal (g/meal)—defined as the approximate intake in one meal of all types of protein
- Percent protein estimated intake in 24 hours (percent/day)—defined as the approximate intake in one day from protein intake
- Protein estimated intake from oral nutrition in 24 hours (specify, g/day)—defined as the approximate intake of protein in grams per day derived from oral intake
- Protein estimated intake from enteral nutrition in 24 hours (specify, g/day)—defined as the approximate intake of protein in grams per day derived from intact or semi-elemental protein enteral nutrition infusion
- Protein additive estimated intake in 24 hours (g/day and mL/day)—defined as the approximate intake in one day of protein additive

Measured protein intake

- Total protein measured intake in 24 hours (g/day)—defined as the known quantity of intake in one day of all protein
- High biological value protein measured intake in 24 hours (g/day)—defined as the known quantity of intake in one day from proteins which contain a ratio of essential amino acids that are needed for humans

Protein Intake

- Casein measured intake in 24 hours (g/day)—defined as the known quantity of intake in one day from the phosphoprotein component in milk and milk products that can also be an ingredient in food
- Whey protein measured intake in 24 hours (g/day)—defined as the known quantity of intake in one day of the complete protein component in milk and milk products that can also be an ingredient in food
- Gluten measured intake in 24 hours (g/day)—defined as the known quantity of intake in one day of the protein found primarily in cereal grains and contains gliadin and a glutenin
- Protein measured intake per kg body weight in 24 hours (g/kg/day)—defined as the known quantity of intake per kg of body weight in one day of all protein
- Natural protein measured intake in 24 hours (specify, g/day)—defined as the known quantity of intake of the portion of total protein that comes from food sources
- Protein measured intake in one meal (g/meal)—defined as the known quantity of intake in one meal of all types of protein
- Percent protein measured intake in 24 hours (percent/day)—defined as the known quantity of intake in one day from protein intake
- Protein measured intake from oral nutrition in 24 hours (specify, g/day)—defined as the known quantity of intake of protein in grams per day derived from oral intake
- Protein measured intake from enteral nutrition in 24 hours (specify, g/day)—defined as the known quantity of intake of protein in grams per day derived from intact or semi-elemental protein enteral nutrition infusion
- Protein additive measured intake in 24 hours (g/day and mL/day)—defined as the known quantity of intake in one day of protein additive

Note: Soy protein can be found on the Bioactive Substance Intake reference sheet on page 48. Amino acid intake from elemental enteral nutrition, parenteral nutrition, or intravenous (IV) fluids can be documented using terms on the Amino Acid Intake reference sheet on page 61.

In almost all nutrition settings, food and nutrient intakes are estimates; therefore, estimated intake terms should be used. The exception is research settings where exact measurement of intake is done. Then, measured intake terms are appropriate.

Examples of the measurement methods or data sources for these outcome indicators: Food intake records, 24-hour recalls, food frequency questionnaires, qualitative protein intake collection tools, nutrition fact labels, other product information, nutrient composition tables

Typically used with the following domains of nutrition interventions: Food and/or nutrient delivery, nutrition education, nutrition counseling, coordination of nutrition care by nutrition professional

Typically used to determine and monitor and evaluate change in the following nutrition diagnoses: Inadequate and excessive protein intake, intake of types of proteins or amino acids inconsistent with needs, malnutrition, inadequate protein energy intake, altered GI function, limited adherence to nutrition related recommendations

Note: Judgment must be used to select indicators and determine the appropriate measurement techniques and reference standards for a given client population and setting. Once identified, these indicators, measurement techniques, and reference standards should be identified in policies and procedures or other documents for use in client records, quality or performance improvement, or in formal research projects.

Protein Intake

Client Example

Example(s) of one of the nutrition care indicators (includes sample initial and reassessment documentation for one of the indicators)

Indicator Selected

Total protein estimated intake in 24 hours (g/day)

Criteria for Evaluation

Comparison to reference standard, recommendation, or goal:

1. Reference standard: Client's total protein estimated intake in 24 hours of 25 g/day is less than the DRI of 53 g/day (0.8 g/kg body weight).
2. Recommendation: 55 to 65 g/day (1 to 1.2 g/kg body weight)
3. Goal: Client's goal is to increase enteral nutrition feeding to provide at least 45 g/day protein.

Sample Nutrition Assessment and Monitoring and Evaluation Documentation	
Initial encounter	Enteral feeding currently providing 25 g/day of protein, below the recommended level of 55 to 65 g/day (1 to 1.2 g/kg body weight). Client established a goal to increase enteral nutrition feeding to provide total protein estimated intake in 24 hours of at least 45 g/day. Will continue to monitor protein intake daily.
Reassessment after nutrition intervention	Some progress toward goal intake of 45 g protein/day. Current total protein estimated intake in 24 hours is 30 g protein/day. Will continue to monitor protein intake daily.

Amino Acid Intake

Definition

Amino acid intake from all sources including food, beverages, supplements, and via enteral and parenteral routes.

Note: Whenever possible, nutrient intake data should be considered in combination with clinical, biochemical, anthropometric information, medical diagnosis, clinical status, and/or other factors to provide a valid assessment of nutritional status based on a totality of the evidence. (Institute of Medicine. *Dietary Reference Intakes: Applications in Dietary Assessment.* National Academies Press; 2000.)

Nutrition Assessment and Monitoring and Evaluation

Indicators

Estimated amino acid intake

- Total amino acid estimated intake in 24 hours (mg/day)—defined as the approximate intake in one day of total amino acids
- Essential amino acid estimated intake in 24 hours (mg/day)—defined as the approximate intake in one day of amino acids that cannot be synthesized by humans and must be provided by the diet or by enteral or parenteral nutrition
- Histidine estimated intake in 24 hours (mg/day)—defined as the approximate intake in one day of an essential amino acid with the formula $C_6H_9N_3O_2$
- Methionine estimated intake in 24 hours (mg/day)—defined as the approximate intake in one day of an essential amino acid with the formula $C_5H_{11}NO_2S$
- Isoleucine estimated intake in 24 hours (mg/day)—defined as the approximate intake in one day of an essential amino acid and branched-chain amino acid with the formula $C_6H_{13}NO_2$, (2S,3S)-2-amino-3-methylpentanoic acid
- Leucine estimated intake in 24 hours (mg/day)—defined as the approximate intake in one day of an essential amino acid and branched-chain amino acid with the formula $C_6H_{13}NO_2$, L-2-amino-4-methylpentanoic
- Lysine estimated intake in 24 hours (mg/day)—defined as the approximate intake in one day of an essential amino acid with the formula $C_5H_{11}NO_2$
- Threonine estimated intake in 24 hours (mg/day)—defined as the approximate intake in one day of an essential amino acid with the formula $C_4H_9NO_3$
- Tryptophan estimated intake in 24 hours (mg/day)—defined as the approximate intake in one day of an essential amino acid with the formula $C_{11}H_{12}N_2O_2$
- Phenylalanine estimated intake in 24 hours (mg/day)—defined as the approximate intake in one day of an essential amino acid with the formula $C_9H_{11}NO_2$
- Valine estimated intake in 24 hours (mg/day)—defined as the approximate intake in one day of an essential amino acid and branched-chain amino acid with the formula $C_5H_{11}NO_2$
- Nonessential amino acid estimated intake in 24 hours (mg/day)—defined as the approximate intake in one day of amino acids that can be synthesized by humans
- Arginine estimated intake in 24 hours (mg/day)—defined as the approximate intake in one day of a nonessential amino acid with the formula $C_6H_{14}N_4O_2$
- Glutamine estimated intake in 24 hours (mg/day)—defined as the approximate intake in one day of a nonessential amino acid with the formula $C_5H_{10}N_2O_3$

Amino Acid Intake

- Homocysteine estimated intake in 24 hours (mg/day)—defined as the approximate intake in one day of a nonessential amino acid with the formula $C_4H_9NO_2S$
- Tyramine estimated intake in 24 hours (mg/day)—defined as the approximate intake in one day of a nonessential amino acid with the formula $C_8H_{11}NO$
- Tyrosine estimated intake in 24 hours (mg/day)—defined as the approximate intake in one day of a nonessential amino acid with the formula $C_9H_{11}NO_3$
- Estimated amino acid intake from enteral nutrition in 24 hours (specify g/day)—defined as the approximate intake of amino acids in grams in one day derived from elemental enteral nutrition infusion
- Estimated amino acid intake from parenteral nutrition in 24 hours (specify g/day)—defined as the approximate intake of amino acids in grams in one day derived from parenteral nutrition infusion
- Estimated amino acid intake from intravenous fluids in 24 hours (specify g/day)—defined as the approximate intake of amino acids in grams in one day derived from intravenous (IV) infusion

Measured amino acid intake

- Total amino acid measured intake in 24 hours (mg/day)—defined as the known quantity of intake in one day of total amino acids
- Essential amino acid measured intake in 24 hours (mg/day)—defined as the known quantity of intake in one day of amino acids that cannot be synthesized by humans and must be provided by the diet or by enteral or parenteral nutrition
- Histidine measured intake in 24 hours (mg/day)—defined as the known quantity of intake in one day of an essential amino acid with the formula $C_6H_9N_3O_2$
- Methionine measured intake in 24 hours (mg/day)—defined as the known quantity of intake in one day of an essential amino acid with the formula $C_5H_{11}NO_2S$
- Isoleucine measured intake in 24 hours (mg/day)—defined as the known quantity of intake in one day of an essential amino acid and branched-chain amino acid with the formula $C_6H_{13}NO_2$, (2S,3S)-2-Amino-3-methylpentanoic acid
- Leucine measured intake in 24 hours (mg/day)—defined as the known quantity of intake in one day of an essential amino acid and branched-chain amino acid with the formula $C_6H_{13}NO_2$, L-2-Amino-4-methylpentanoic
- Lysine measured intake in 24 hours (mg/day)—defined as the known quantity of intake in one day of an essential amino acid with the formula $C_5H_{11}NO_2$
- Threonine measured intake in 24 hours (mg/day)—defined as the known quantity of intake in one day of an essential amino acid with the formula $C_4H_9NO_3$
- Tryptophan measured intake in 24 hours (mg/day)—defined as the known quantity of intake in one day of an essential amino acid with the formula $C_{11}H_{12}N_2O_2$
- Phenylalanine measured intake in 24 hours (mg/day)—defined as the known quantity of intake in one day of an essential amino acid with the formula $C_9H_{11}NO_2$
- Valine measured intake in 24 hours (mg/day)—defined as the approximate intake in one day of an essential amino acid and branched-chain amino acid with the formula $C_5H_{11}NO_2$
- Nonessential amino acid measured intake in 24 hours (mg/day)—defined as the known quantity of intake in one day of amino acids that can be synthesized by humans
- Arginine measured intake in 24 hours (mg/day)—defined as the known quantity of intake in one day of a nonessential amino acid with the formula $C_6H_{14}N_4O_2$
- Glutamine measured intake in 24 hours (mg/day)—defined as the known quantity of intake in one day of a nonessential amino acid with the formula $C_5H_{10}N_2O_3$

Amino Acid Intake

- Homocysteine measured intake in 24 hours (mg/day)—defined as the known quantity of intake in one day of a nonessential amino acid with the formula $C_4H_9NO_2S$
- Tyramine measured intake in 24 hours (mg/day)—defined as the known quantity of intake in one day of a nonessential amino acid with the formula $C_8H_{11}NO$
- Tyrosine measured intake in 24 hours (mg/day)—defined as the known quantity of intake in one day of a nonessential amino acid with the formula $C_9H_{11}NO_3$
- Measured amino acid intake from enteral nutrition in 24 hours (specify g/day)—defined as the known intake of amino acids in grams in one day derived from elemental enteral nutrition infusion
- Measured amino acid intake from parenteral nutrition in 24 hours (specify g/day)—defined as the known intake of amino acids in grams in one day derived from parenteral nutrition infusion
- Measured amino acid intake from intravenous fluids in 24 hours (specify g/day)—defined as the known intake of amino acids in grams inone day derived from intravenous (IV) infusion

Note: In almost all nutrition settings, food and nutrient intakes are estimates; therefore, estimated intake terms should be used. The exception is research settings where exact measurement of intake is done. Then, measured intake terms are appropriate.

Examples of the measurement methods or data sources for these outcome indicators: Food intake records, 24-hour recalls, food frequency questionnaires, qualitative amino acid intake collection tools, nutrition fact labels, other product information, nutrient composition tables

Typically used with the following domains of nutrition interventions: Food and/or nutrient delivery, nutrition education, nutrition counseling, coordination of nutrition care by nutrition professional

Typically used to determine and monitor and evaluate change in the following nutrition diagnoses: Intake of types of amino acids inconsistent with needs, malnutrition, inadequate protein energy intake, altered gastrointestinal (GI) function, limited adherence to nutrition related recommendations

Note: Judgment must be used to select indicators and determine the appropriate measurement techniques and reference standards for a given client population and setting. Once identified, these indicators, measurement techniques, and reference standards should be identified in policies and procedures or other documents for use in client records, quality or performance improvement, or in formal research projects.

Client Example

Example(s) of one of the nutrition care indicators (includes sample initial and reassessment documentation for one of the indicators)

Indicator(s) Selected

Histidine estimated intake in 24 hours (mg/kg/day)

Criteria for Evaluation

Comparison to reference standard, recommendation, or goal:

1. Reference standard: Client's current intake of histidine per day is 520 mg/day (8 mg/kg/day) below the EAR level of 11 mg/kg/day of histidine.
2. Recommendation: Not applicable
3. Goal: Client established a goal of histidine estimated intake in 24 hours of at least 715 mg/day (11 mg/kg/day).

Amino Acid Intake

Sample Nutrition Assessment and Monitoring and Evaluation Documentation	
Initial nutrition assessment	Histidine estimated intake in 24 hours averages 520 mg/day (8 mg/kg/day) which is below the EAR of 715 mg/day (11 mg/kg/day) for a person 19 years of age or older. Will continue to monitor histidine intake daily.
Reassessment after nutrition intervention	Histidine estimated intake in 24 hours averages 675 mg/day. Significant progress toward goal intake of 715 mg/day (11 mg/kg/day) for a person 19 years of age or older.

Carbohydrate Intake

Definition

Carbohydrate consumption from all sources including food, beverages, supplements, and via enteral and parenteral routes, including relative measures of the quantity and/or type of carbohydrate consumed.

> *Note:* Whenever possible, nutrient intake data should be considered in combination with clinical, biochemical, anthropometric information, medical diagnosis, clinical status, and/or other factors to provide a valid assessment of nutritional status based on a totality of the evidence. (Institute of Medicine. *Dietary Reference Intakes: Applications in Dietary Assessment.* Washington, DC: National Academies Press; 2000.)

Nutrition Assessment and Monitoring and Evaluation

Indicators

Estimated carbohydrate intake

- Total carbohydrate estimated intake in 24 hours (g/day)—defined as the approximate intake in one day of total carbohydrate
- Complex carbohydrate estimated intake in 24 hours (g/day)—defined as the approximate intake in one day of a polysaccharide that is comprised of three or more sugars; also called starch
- Simple carbohydrate estimated intake in 24 hours (g/day)—defined as the approximate intake in one day of mono- and disaccharides
- Galactose estimated intake in 24 hours (g/day)—defined as the approximate intake in one day of a monosaccharide which is a common component of lactose
- Lactose estimated intake in 24 hours (g/day)—defined as the approximate intake in one day of a disaccharide sugar of galactose and glucose; present in milk
- Fructose estimated intake in 24 hours (g/day)—defined as the approximate intake in one day of a monosaccharide sugar found in fruit and honey
- Carbohydrate estimated intake per kg body weight in 24 hours (g/kg/day)—defined as the approximate intake per kg of body weight in one day of all carbohydrate
- Carbohydrate estimated intake in one meal (g/meal)—defined as the approximate intake in one meal of all types of carbohydrate
- Percent carbohydrate estimated intake in 24 hours (percent/day)—defined as the approximate energy intake in one day from carbohydrate intake
- Carbohydrate estimated intake from oral nutrition in 24 hours (g/day)—defined as the estimated intake of carbohydrate in grams in one day derived from oral intake
- Carbohydrate estimated intake from enteral nutrition in 24 hours (g/day)—defined as the estimated intake of carbohydrate in grams in one day derived from enteral nutrition infusion
- Carbohydrate estimated intake from parenteral nutrition in 24 hours (g/day)—defined as the estimated intake of carbohydrate in grams in one day derived from parenteral nutrition infusion
- Carbohydrate estimated intake from intravenous fluids in 24 hours (g/day)—defined as the estimated intake of carbohydrate in grams in one day derived from intravenous (IV) infusion
- Carbohydrate additive estimated intake in 24 hours (g/day)—defined as the approximate intake in one day of carbohydrate additive
- Estimated daily glycemic index value (number)—defined as the estimated measure in one day reflecting the consumption of all carbohydrate

Carbohydrate Intake

- Estimated daily glycemic load (number)—defined as the estimated measure in one day reflecting the quantity and type of all carbohydrate consumed
- Insulin to carbohydrate ratio (ratio)—defined as the estimated number of grams of carbohydrate covered by one unit of rapid-acting (or short-acting) insulin

Measured carbohydrate intake

- Total carbohydrate measured intake in 24 hours (g/day)—defined as the known quantity of intake in one day of total carbohydrate
- Complex carbohydrate measured intake in 24 hours (g/day)—defined as the known quantity of intake in one day of a polysaccharide that is comprised of three or more sugars; also called starch
- Simple carbohydrate measured intake in 24 hours (g/day)—defined as the known quantity of intake in one day of monosaccharides and disaccharides
- Galactose measured intake in 24 hours (g/day)—defined as the known quantity of intake in one day of a monosaccharide which is a common component of lactose
- Lactose measured intake in 24 hours (g/day)—defined as the known quantity of intake in one day of a disaccharide sugar of galactose and glucose; present in milk
- Fructose measured intake in 24 hours (g/day)—defined as the known quantity of intake in one day of a monosaccharide sugar found in fruit and honey
- Carbohydrate measured intake per kg body weight in 24 hours (g/kg/day)—defined as the known quantity of intake per kg of body weight in one day of all carbohydrate
- Carbohydrate measured intake in one meal (g/meal)—defined as the known quantity of intake in one meal of all types of carbohydrate
- Percent carbohydrate measured intake in 24 hours (percent/day)—defined as the known quantity of energy intake in one day from carbohydrate intake
- Carbohydrate measured intake from oral nutrition in 24 hours (g/day)—defined as the known quantity of intake of carbohydrate in grams in one day derived from oral intake
- Carbohydrate measured intake from enteral nutrition (g/day)—defined as the known quantity of intake of carbohydrate in grams in one day derived from enteral nutrition infusion
- Carbohydrate measured intake from parenteral nutrition (g/day)—defined as the known quantity of intake of carbohydrate in grams in one day derived from parenteral nutrition infusion
- Carbohydrate measured intake from intravenous fluids (g/day)—defined as the known quantity of intake of carbohydrate in grams in one day derived from intravenous (IV) infusion
- Carbohydrate additive measured intake in 24 hours (g/day)—defined as the known quantity of intake in one day of carbohydrate additive

Note: Fiber intake can be found on the Fiber Intake reference sheet on page 68.
Psyllium and beta glucan can be found on the Bioactive Substance Intake reference sheet on page 48.

Examples of the measurement methods or data sources for these outcome indicators: Food intake records, 24-hour or typical day's recalls, food frequency questionnaires, qualitative intake assessment, menu analysis, carbohydrate counting tools, intake/output sheets (for tube feeding or parenteral nutrition)

Typically used with the following domains of nutrition interventions: Food and/or nutrient delivery, nutrition education, nutrition counseling, coordination of nutrition care by nutrition professional

Carbohydrate Intake

Typically used to determine and monitor and evaluate change in the following nutrition diagnoses: Inadequate and excessive carbohydrate intake, intake of types of carbohydrate inconsistent with needs, inconsistent carbohydrate intake, altered nutrition related laboratory values, food medication interaction

Note: Judgment must be used to select indicators and determine the appropriate measurement techniques and reference standards for a given client population and setting. Once identified, these indicators, measurement techniques, and reference standards should be identified in policies and procedures or other documents for use in client records, quality or performance improvement, or in formal research projects.

Client Example

Example of one of the nutrition care indicators (includes sample initial and reassessment documentation for one of the indicators)

Indicator Selected

Total carbohydrate estimated intake in 24 hours (g/day)

Criteria for Evaluation

Comparison to reference standard, recommendation, or goal:

1. Reference standard: Not applicable
2. Recommendation: Client's total carbohydrate estimated intake in 24 hours averages 295 g/day.
3. Goal: Client's goal intake is 225 g/day.

Sample Nutrition Assessment and Monitoring and Evaluation Documentation	
Initial encounter	Based on 3-day diet records, client's total carbohydrate estimated intake in 24 hours averages 295 g/day, above the client's goal of 225 g/day.
Reassessment after nutrition intervention	Good progress made toward goal. Client's total carbohydrate estimated intake in 24 hours averages 245 g/day. Will monitor carbohydrate intake at next encounter.

Fiber Intake

Definition

Amount and/or type of plant source matter consumed that is not completely digested but may be at least partially fermented in the distal bowel and is derived from all sources, including food, beverages, supplements, and via enteral routes.

Note: Whenever possible, nutrient intake data should be considered in combination with clinical, biochemical, and anthropometric information, medical diagnosis, clinical status, and/or other factors to provide a valid assessment of nutritional status based on a totality of the evidence. (Institute of Medicine. *Dietary Reference Intakes: Applications in Dietary Assessment*. National Academies Press; 2000.)

Nutrition Assessment and Monitoring and Evaluation

Indicators

Estimated fiber intake

- Total fiber estimated intake in 24 hours (g/day)—defined as the approximate intake in one day of total fiber
- Soluble fiber estimated intake in 24 hours (g/day)—defined as the approximate intake in one day of soluble fiber
- Insoluble fiber estimated intake in 24 hours (g/day)—defined as the approximate intake in one day of insoluble fiber
- Fiber estimated intake from oral intake in 24 hours (g/day)—defined as the approximate intake of fiber in grams in one day derived from oral intake
- Fiber estimated intake from enteral nutrition in 24 hours (g/day)—defined as the approximate intake of fiber in grams in one day derived from enteral nutrition infusion
- Fiber additive estimated intake in 24 hours (g or mL/day)—defined as the approximate intake in one day of fiber additive

Measured fiber intake

- Total fiber measured intake in 24 hours (g/day)—defined as the known quantity of intake in one day of total fiber
- Soluble fiber measured intake in 24 hours (g/day)—defined as the known quantity of intake in one day of soluble fiber
- Insoluble fiber measured intake in 24 hours (g/day)—defined as the known quantity of intake in one day of insoluble fiber
- Fiber measured intake from oral nutrition in 24 hours (g/day)—defined as the known quantity of intake of fiber in grams in one day derived from oral intake
- Fiber measured intake from enteral nutrition (g/day)—defined as the known quantity of intake of fiber in grams in one day derived from enteral nutrition infusion
- Fiber additive measured intake in 24 hours (g or mL/day)—defined as the known quantity of intake in one day of fiber additive

Note: Psyllium and beta glucan can be found on the Bioactive Substance Intake reference sheet on page 48.

In almost all nutrition settings, food and nutrient intakes are estimates; therefore, estimated intake terms should be used. The exception is research settings where exact measurement of intake is done. Then, measured intake terms are appropriate.

Fiber Intake

Examples of the measurement methods or data sources for these outcome indicators: Food intake records, 24-hour recalls, food frequency questionnaires, qualitative intake assessment, menu analysis, fiber counting tools, nutrition fact labels, other product information, nutrient composition tables

Typically used with the following domains of nutrition interventions: Food and/or nutrient delivery, nutrition education, nutrition counseling, coordination of nutrition care by nutrition professional

Typically used to determine and monitor and evaluate change in the following nutrition diagnoses: Inadequate and excessive fiber intake, altered GI function, disordered eating pattern, inadequate bioactive substance intake

Note: Judgment must be used to select indicators and determine the appropriate measurement techniques and reference standards for a given client population and setting. Once identified, these indicators, measurement techniques, and reference standards should be identified in policies and procedures or other documents for use in client records, quality or performance improvement, or in formal research projects.

Client Example

Example of one of the nutrition care indicators (includes sample initial and reassessment documentation for one of the indicators)

Indicator Selected

Total fiber estimated intake in 24 hours (g/day)

Criteria for Evaluation

Comparison to reference standard, recommendation, or goal:

1. Reference standard: Client's total fiber estimated intake in 24 hours averages 15 g/day, which is below the DRI of 25 g/day for a 40-year-old woman.
2. Recommendation: Not applicable
3. Goal: Client's goal is to increase fiber intake to approximately 25 g/day.

Sample Nutrition Assessment and Monitoring and Evaluation Documentation	
Initial encounter	Based on food diary, client's total fiber estimated intake in 24 hours averages 15 g/day. Will monitor fiber intake at next encounter in 3 weeks.
Reassessment after nutrition intervention	Goal achieved. Client's total fiber estimated intake in 24 hours averages 27 g/day, which meets the goal intake of 25 g/day. Will continue to monitor to ensure that success is sustained.

Vitamin Intake

Definition

Vitamin intake from all sources including food, beverages, supplements, and via enteral and parenteral routes.

Note: Whenever possible, nutrient intake data should be considered in combination with clinical, biochemical, and anthropometric information, medical diagnosis, clinical status, and/or other factors to provide a valid assessment of nutritional status based on a totality of the evidence. (Institute of Medicine. *Dietary Reference Intakes: Applications in Dietary Assessment*. National Academies Press; 2000.)

Nutrition Assessment and Monitoring and Evaluation

Indicators

Estimated vitamin intake

- Vitamin A estimated intake in 24 hours (µg/day)—defined as the approximate intake in one day of vitamin A
- Vitamin C estimated intake in 24 hours (mg/day)—defined as the approximate intake in one day of vitamin C
- Vitamin D estimated intake in 24 hours (µg/day)—defined as the approximate intake in one day of vitamin D
- Vitamin E estimated intake in 24 hours (mg/day)—defined as the approximate intake in one day of vitamin E
- Vitamin K estimated intake in 24 hours (µg/day)—defined as the approximate intake in one day of vitamin K
- Thiamin estimated intake in 24 hours (mg/day)—defined as the approximate intake in one day of thiamin
- Riboflavin estimated intake in 24 hours (mg/day)—defined as the approximate intake in one day of riboflavin
- Niacin estimated intake in 24 hours (mg/day)—defined as the approximate intake in one day of niacin
- Folate estimated intake in 24 hours (µg/day)—defined as the approximate intake in one day of folate
- Vitamin B6 estimated intake in 24 hours (mg/day)—defined as the approximate intake in one day of vitamin B6
- Vitamin B12 estimated intake in 24 hours (µg/day)—defined as the approximate intake in one day of vitamin B12
- Pantothenic acid estimated intake in 24 hours (mg/day)—defined as the approximate intake in one day of pantothenic acid
- Biotin estimated intake in 24 hours (µg/day)—defined as the approximate intake in one day of biotin
- Multivitamin estimated intake in 24 hours (yes/no)—defined as the approximate intake in one day of a multivitamin

Measured vitamin intake

- Vitamin A measured intake in 24 hours (µg/day)—defined as the known quantity of intake in one day of vitamin A
- Vitamin C measured intake in 24 hours (mg/day)—defined as the known quantity of intake in one day of vitamin C

Vitamin Intake

- Vitamin D measured intake in 24 hours (µg/day)—defined as the known quantity of intake in one day of vitamin D
- Vitamin E measured intake in 24 hours (mg/day)—defined as the known quantity of intake in one day of vitamin E
- Vitamin K measured intake in 24 hours (µg/day)—defined as the known quantity of intake in one day of vitamin K
- Thiamin measured intake in 24 hours (mg/day)—defined as the known quantity of intake in one day of thiamin
- Riboflavin measured intake in 24 hours (mg/day)—defined as the known quantity of intake in one day of riboflavin
- Niacin measured intake in 24 hours (mg/day)—defined as the known quantity of intake in one day of niacin
- Folate measured intake in 24 hours (µg/day)—defined as the known quantity of intake in one day of folate
- Vitamin B6 measured intake in 24 hours (mg/day)—defined as the known quantity of intake in one day of vitamin B6
- Vitamin B12 measured intake in 24 hours (µg/day)—defined as the known quantity of intake in one day of vitamin B12
- Pantothenic acid measured intake in 24 hours (mg/day)—defined as the known quantity of intake in one day of pantothenic acid
- Biotin measured intake in 24 hours (µg/day)—defined as the known quantity of intake in one day of biotin
- Multivitamin measured intake in 24 hours (yes/no)—defined as the known quantity of intake in one day of a multivitamin

Note: Laboratory measures associated with body vitamin status can be found on the Vitamin Profile reference sheet on page 156.

In almost all nutrition settings, food and nutrient intakes are estimates; therefore, estimated intake terms should be used. The exception is research settings where exact measurement of intake is done. Then, measured intake terms are appropriate.

Examples of the measurement methods or data sources for these outcome indicators: Client report or recalls, food frequency, qualitative intake assessment, home evaluation, supplement use questionnaire

Typically used with the following domains of nutrition interventions: Food and/or nutrient delivery, nutrition education, nutrition counseling, coordination of nutrition care by nutrition professional

Typically used to determine and monitor and evaluate change in the following nutrition diagnoses: Excessive or inadequate intake of vitamins, parenteral, or enteral nutrition; unbalanced diet

Note: Judgment must be used to select indicators and determine the appropriate measurement techniques and reference standards for a given client population and setting. Once identified, these indicators, measurement techniques, and reference standards should be identified in policies and procedures or other documents for use in client records, quality or performance improvement, or in formal research projects.

Vitamin Intake

Client Example

Example of one or two of the nutrition care indicators (includes sample initial and reassessment documentation for one of the indicators)

Indicator(s) Selected

Vitamin D estimated intake in 24 hours (μg/day)

Criteria for Evaluation

Comparison to reference standard, recommendation, or goal:

1. Reference standard: Client's vitamin D estimated intake in 24 hours is 4 μg/day (160 IU), which is below the EAR of 10 μg (400 IU) and the RDA of 15 μg (600 IU) for a 15-year-old male.
2. Recommendation: Not applicable
3. Goal: Client established a goal to resume vitamin D supplement 4 out of 7 days per week.

Sample Nutrition Assessment and Monitoring and Evaluation Documentation	
Initial nutrition assessment	Based on recalls, client with cystic fibrosis has vitamin D estimated intake in 24 hours of 4 μg/day, which is below the EAR of 10 μg (400 IU) and the RDA of 15 ug (600 IU) per day for vitamin D for a 15-year old male. Client has also discontinued fat-soluble vitamin supplement but has established a goal to take supplement 4 out of 7 days per week. Will monitor vitamin D intake at next encounter and intake of fat-soluble vitamin supplement and request 25 hydroxy, vitamin D level (Vitamin Profile reference sheet).
Reassessment after nutrition intervention	25 Hydroxy, vitamin D level below expected range (from Vitamin Profile reference sheet). Progress toward the EAR of 10 μg (400 IU) and RDA of 15 ug (600 IU). Based on diet record, client's vitamin D estimated intake in 24 hours from food sources is 5 to 7 μg/day (200-280 IU), and client is taking fat-soluble vitamin supplement 5 days per week on average. Despite progress, because client has cystic fibrosis; client will need to continue fat-soluble vitamin supplementation in addition to food sources. Repeat lab in 3 months.

Mineral/Element Intake

Definition

Mineral/element intake from all sources including food, beverages, supplements, and via enteral and parenteral routes.

Note: Whenever possible, nutrient intake data should be considered in combination with clinical, biochemical, and anthropometric information, medical diagnosis, clinical status, and/or other factors to provide a valid assessment of nutritional status based on a totality of the evidence. (Institute of Medicine. *Dietary Reference Intakes: Applications in Dietary Assessment.* National Academies Press; 2000.)

Nutrition Assessment and Monitoring and Evaluation

Indicators

Estimated mineral intake

- Calcium estimated intake in 24 hours (mg/day)—defined as the approximate intake in one day of calcium
- Chloride estimated intake in 24 hours (mg/day)—defined as the approximate intake in one day of calcium
- Iron estimated intake in 24 hours (mg/day)—defined as the approximate intake in one day of iron
- Magnesium estimated intake in 24 hours (mg/day)—defined as the approximate intake in one day of magnesium
- Potassium estimated intake in 24 hours (g/day)—defined as the approximate intake in one day of potassium
- Phosphorus estimated intake in 24 hours (mg/day)—defined as the approximate intake in one day of phosphorus
- Sodium estimated intake in 24 hours (g/day)—defined as the approximate intake in one day of sodium
- Zinc estimated intake in 24 hours (mg/day)—defined as the approximate intake in one day of zinc
- Sulfate estimated intake in 24 hours (g/day)—defined as the approximate intake in one day of sulfate
- Fluoride estimated intake in 24 hours (mg/day)—defined as the approximate intake in one day of fluoride
- Copper estimated intake in 24 hours (μg/day)—defined as the approximate intake in one day of copper
- Iodine estimated intake in 24 hours (μg/day)—defined as the approximate intake in one day of iodine
- Selenium estimated intake in 24 hours (μg/day)—defined as the approximate intake in one day of selenium
- Manganese estimated intake in 24 hours (mg/day)—defined as the approximate intake in one day of manganese
- Chromium estimated intake in 24 hours (μg/day)—defined as the approximate intake in one day of chromium
- Molybdenum estimated intake in 24 hours (μg/day)—defined as the approximate intake in one day of molybdenum
- Boron estimated intake in 24 hours (mg/day)—defined as the approximate intake in one day of boron
- Cobalt estimated intake in 24 hours (μg/day)—defined as the approximate intake in one day of cobalt
- Multimineral estimated intake in 24 hours (yes/no)—defined as the approximate intake in one day of a multimineral
- Multitrace element estimated intake in 24 hours (yes/no)—defined as the approximate intake in one day of a multitrace element

Mineral/Element Intake

Measured mineral intake

- Calcium measured intake in 24 hours (mg/day)—defined as the known quantity of intake in one day of calcium
- Chloride measured intake in 24 hours (mg/day)—defined as the known quantity of intake in one day of calcium
- Iron measured intake in 24 hours (mg/day)—defined as the known quantity of intake in one day of iron
- Magnesium measured intake in 24 hours (mg/day)—defined as the known quantity of intake in one day of magnesium
- Potassium measured intake in 24 hours (g/day)—defined as the known quantity of intake in one day of potassium
- Phosphorus measured intake in 24 hours (mg/day)—defined as the known quantity of intake in one day of phosphorus
- Sodium measured intake in 24 hours (g/day)—defined as the known quantity of intake in one day of sodium
- Zinc measured intake in 24 hours (mg/day)—defined as the known quantity of intake in one day of zinc
- Sulfate measured intake in 24 hours (g/day)—defined as the known quantity of intake in one day of sulfate
- Fluoride measured intake in 24 hours (mg/day)—defined as the known quantity of intake in one day of fluoride
- Copper measured intake in 24 hours (µg/day)—defined as the known quantity of intake in one day of copper
- Iodine measured intake in 24 hours (µg/day)—defined as the known quantity of intake in one day of iodine
- Selenium measured intake in 24 hours (µg/day)—defined as the known quantity of intake in one day of selenium
- Manganese measured intake in 24 hours (mg/day)—defined as the known quantity of intake in one day of manganese
- Chromium measured intake in 24 hours (µg/day)—defined as the known quantity of intake in one day of chromium
- Molybdenum measured intake in 24 hours (µg/day)—defined as the known quantity of intake in one day of molybdenum
- Boron measured intake in 24 hours (mg/day)—defined as the known quantity of intake in one day of boron
- Cobalt measured intake in 24 hours (µg/day)—defined as the known quantity of intake in one day of cobalt
- Multimineral measured intake in 24 hours (yes/no)—defined as the known quantity of intake in one day of a multimineral
- Multitrace element measured intake in 24 hours (yes/no)—defined as the known quantity of intake in one day of a multitrace element

Note: In almost all nutrition settings, food and nutrient intakes are estimates; therefore, estimated intake terms should be used. The exception is research settings where exact measurement of intake is done. Then, measured intake terms are appropriate.

Mineral/Element Intake

Examples of the measurement methods or data sources for these outcome indicators: Client report or recalls, food frequency, qualitative intake assessment, home evaluation, home care or pharmacy report, supplement use questionnaire

Typically used with the following domains of nutrition interventions: Food and/or nutrient delivery, nutrition education, nutrition counseling, coordination of nutrition care by nutrition professional

Typically used to determine and monitor and evaluate change in the following nutrition diagnoses: Excessive or inadequate intake of minerals, food medication interaction, altered nutrition related laboratory values, impaired nutrient utilization, unbalanced diet pattern, limited adherence to nutrition related recommendations

Note: Judgment must be used to select indicators and determine the appropriate measurement techniques and reference standards for a given client population and setting. Once identified, these indicators, measurement techniques, and reference standards should be identified in policies and procedures or other documents for use in client records, quality or performance improvement, or in formal research projects.

Client Example

Example of one of the nutrition care indicators (includes sample initial and reassessment documentation for one of the indicators)

Indicator Selected

Calcium estimated intake in 24 hours (mg/day)

Criteria for Evaluation

Comparison to reference standard, recommendation, or goal:

1. Reference standard: The client's calcium estimated intake in 24 hours averages 500 mg/day, which is 50% of the RDA for women 31 to 50 years of age.
2. Recommendation: Not applicable
3. Goal: Client's goal is to increase calcium intake via food to 1,000 mg/day.

Sample Nutrition Assessment and Monitoring and Evaluation Documentation	
Initial nutrition assessment with client	Based on recalls, client's calcium estimated intake in 24 hours is 500 g/day, which is below the RDA for women 31 to 50 years of age. Client's goal is to increase intake of calcium to 1,000 mg/day via calcium-rich foods. Will monitor calcium intake at next encounter.
Reassessment after nutrition intervention	Significant progress toward RDA. Based on diet record, client's calcium estimated intake in 24 hours is 750 mg/day, 75% of the RDA.

Consistency Modifier Intake

Definition

Intake of substances used to change the consistency of food, fluids, and breastmilk and infant formula feedings.

Nutrition Assessment and Monitoring and Evaluation

Indicators

Estimated consistency modifier intake

- Thickener additive estimated intake in 24 hours (g/day and mL/day)—defined as the approximate intake in one day of thickener additive used to change the consistency of food, fluids, and breastmilk and infant formula feedings

Measured consistency modifier intake

- Thickener additive measured intake in 24 hours (g/day and mL/day)—defined as the known quantity of intake in one day of thickener additive used to change the consistency of food, fluids, and breastmilk and infant formula feedings

Note: In almost all nutrition settings, food and nutrient intakes are estimates; therefore, estimated intake terms should be used. The exception is research settings where exact measurement of intake is done. Then, measured intake terms are appropriate.

Examples of the measurement methods or data sources for these outcome indicators: Food intake records, 24-hour recalls, intake records, qualitative intake assessment

Typically used to determine and to monitor and evaluate change in the following nutrition interventions: Food and/or nutrient delivery, nutrition education, nutrition counseling, coordination of nutrition care by nutrition professional

Typically used to determine and to monitor and evaluate change in the following nutrition diagnoses: Swallowing difficulty; inadequate oral intake; inadequate energy, macronutrient or micronutrient intake

Note: Judgment must be used to select indicators and determine the appropriate measurement techniques and reference standards for a given client population and setting. Once identified, these indicators, measurement techniques, and reference standards should be identified in policies and procedures or other documents for use in client records, quality or performance improvement, or in formal research projects.

Client Example(s)

Example of one of the nutrition care indicators (includes sample initial and reassessment of documentation for one of the indicators)

Indicator(s) Selected

Thickener additive estimated intake in 24 hours (g/day and mL/day)

Consistency Modifier Intake

Criteria for Evaluation

Comparison to reference standard, recommendation, or goal:

1. Reference standard: Not applicable
2. Recommendation: Add 128 g/day of thickener to fluids each day or 16 g (4 teaspoons) to each 240 mL (8 oz) serving of water, juice, coffee, and tea.
3. Goal: Client goal is to consistently and accurately add thickener to oral fluids.

Sample Nutrition Assessment and Monitoring and Evaluation Documentation	
Initial encounter	Based on recalls, thickener additive estimated intake in 24 hours is 128 g/day, 16 g of thickener added to each 240 mL (8 oz) serving of water, juice, coffee, and tea. This meets the recommendation by the speech-language pathologist.
Reassessment after nutrition intervention	Client continues to meet goal and recommendation. Thickener additive estimated intake in 24 hours is 128 g/day, to accurately thicken oral fluids.

Diet Order

Definition

A general or modified diet prescribed and documented in a client medical record by a credentialed provider as part of a medical treatment plan.

Nutrition Assessment

Indicators

General healthful diet order

- Modified diet order (eg, type, amount of energy and/or nutrients/day, distribution, texture)
- Enteral nutrition order (eg, formula, rate/schedule, access)
- Parenteral nutrition order (eg, solution, access, rate)

Examples of the measurement methods or data sources for these outcome indicators: Medical record, referring health care provider or agency, client history

Typically used with the following domains of nutrition interventions: Food and/or nutrient delivery, nutrition education, nutrition counseling, coordination of nutrition care by nutrition professional

Typically used to determine and monitor and evaluate change in the following nutrition diagnoses: Inadequate or excessive energy, macronutrient or micronutrient intake, inadequate or excessive oral intake, swallowing difficulty

Note: Judgment must be used to select indicators and determine the appropriate measurement techniques and reference standards for a given client population and setting. Once identified, these indicators, measurement techniques, and reference standards should be identified in policies and procedures or other documents for use in client records, quality or performance improvement, or in formal research projects.

Client Example

Example of one (or more) of the nutrition care indicators (includes sample initial assessment documentation for one of the indicators)

Indicator(s) Selected

Modified diet order

Criteria for Evaluation

Comparison to reference standard, recommendation, or goal:

1. Reference standard: No validated standard exists.
2. Recommendation: Customized to client.
3. Goal: Not applicable

	Sample Nutrition Assessment Documentation
Initial encounter	Client prescribed a 2,400 calorie or kcal (11,000 kJ) diet.

Diet Experience

Definition

Previous nutrition/diet orders, diet education/counseling, and diet characteristics that influence patient/client's dietary intake.

Nutrition Assessment

Indicators

- Previously prescribed diets
  - Previous modified diet (specify, eg, type, amount of energy and/or nutrients/day, distribution, texture)
  - Enteral nutrition order (specify)
  - Parenteral nutrition order (specify)
- Previous diet/nutrition education/counseling (specify, eg, type, year)
- Self-selected diets followed (specify, eg, commercial diets, diet books, culturally directed)
- Dieting attempts
  - Number of past diet attempts (number)
  - Results (specify, eg, successful/unsuccessful, pounds or kilograms lost)
  - Successful strategies (specify, eg, no snacking, self-monitoring)
- Food allergies
  - Previous modified diet (specify, eg, type and/or foods/food group) followed as a result of diagnosed or reported food allergy
- Food intolerance
  - Previous modified diet (specify, eg, type and/or foods/food group) followed as a result of diagnosed or reported food intolerance

Examples of the measurement methods or data sources for these outcome indicators: Patient/client report, medical record, patient/client history, food and nutrition delivery coordination of care

Typically used with the following domains of nutrition interventions: Nutrition education, nutrition counseling

Typically used to determine and monitor and evaluate change in the following nutrition diagnoses: Disordered eating pattern, not ready for diet/lifestyle change, excessive oral intake, food- and nutrition-related knowledge deficit, unsupported beliefs/attitudes about food- or nutrition-related topics, undesirable food choices, swallowing difficulty, intake of unsafe food

Note: Judgment must be used to select indicators and determine the appropriate measurement techniques and reference standards for a given client population and setting. Once identified, these indicators, measurement techniques, and reference standards should be identified in policies and procedures or other documents for use in client records, quality or performance improvement, or in formal research projects.

Criteria for Evaluation

Comparison to goal or reference standard:

1. Goal (tailored to patient/client's needs)
   OR
2. Reference standard

Diet Experience

Client Example

Example(s) of one or two of the nutrition care indicators (includes sample initial assessment documentation for one of the indicators)

Indicator(s) Selected

Previous diet/nutrition education/counseling

Criteria for Evaluation

Comparison to goal or reference standard:

1. Goal: Not generally used
   OR
2. Reference standard: No validated standard exists.

	Sample Nutrition Assessment Documentation
Initial nutrition assessment with client	Patient/client completed a 6-week diabetic education class 2 years ago.

Eating Environment

Definition

The aggregate of surrounding things, conditions, or influences that affect food intake.

Nutrition Assessment and Monitoring and Evaluation

Indicators

- Location (specify, e.g., home, school, day care, restaurant, nursing home, senior center)
- Atmosphere
  - Acceptable noise level (yes/no)
  - Appropriate lighting (yes/no)
  - Appropriate room temperature (yes/no)
  - Appropriate table height (yes/no)
  - Appropriate table service (eg, plates, napkins)/meal service (type of service, eg, table service, buffet)/set-up (make food accessible for consumption) (yes/no)
  - Eats at designated eating location (does not wander) (yes/no)
  - Eats without distractions (eg, watching TV/reading) (yes/no)
  - No unpleasant odors (yes/no)
- Caregiver/companion
  - Allowed to select foods (often, sometimes, never)
  - Caregiver influences/controls what client eats (eg, encourages, forces) (yes/no)
  - Caregiver models expected eating behavior (yes/no)
  - Caretaker presence (present/not present)
  - Favorite food is offered or withheld to influence behavior (reward/punishment) (yes/no)
  - Has companionship while eating (another or others present) (yes/no)
  - Meal/snacks offered at consistent times ("grazing" discouraged) (yes/no)
- Appropriate breastfeeding accommodations/facility (yes/no)
- Eats alone (specify reason, frequency)

Examples of the measurement methods or data sources for these outcome indicators: Patient/client report, medical record, referring health care provider or agency, observation

Typically used with the following domains of nutrition interventions: Food and/or nutrient delivery, nutrition education, nutrition counseling, coordination of nutrition care by nutrition professional

Typically used to determine and monitor and evaluate change in the following nutrition diagnoses: Inadequate oral intake, self-feeding difficulty, poor nutrition quality of life, limited access to food

Note: Judgment must be used to select indicators and determine the appropriate measurement techniques and reference standards for a given client population and setting. Once identified, these indicators, measurement techniques, and reference standards should be identified in policies and procedures or other documents for use in client records, quality or performance improvement, or in formal research projects.

Eating Environment

Evaluation

Criteria for Evaluation

Comparison to goal or reference standard:

1. Goal (tailored to patient/client's needs)
   OR
2. Reference standard

Client Example

Example(s) of one or two of the nutrition care indicators (includes sample initial and reassessment documentation for one of the indicators)

Indicator(s) Selected

Eats at designated eating location

Criteria for Evaluation

Comparison to goal or reference standard:

1. Goal: Two-year-old child with inadequate intake of calories/kcal/kJ and/or nutrients. Goal is to improve intake through modifications in feeding environment and meal pattern.
   OR
2. Reference standard: No validated standard exists.

Sample Nutrition Assessment and Monitoring and Evaluation Documentation	
Initial nutrition assessment with client	Caregiver completed 3-day food record indicating multiple (10) feeding opportunities throughout the day. Child consumes mostly juice, dry cereal, and chips. Prefers foods that can be consumed from bottle or finger foods. Child does not sit at the table to eat, but wanders the house and is allowed to request and receive snacks ad lib. Energy and nutrient intake is less than 75% of standard. Referral to behavioral specialist offered.
Reassessment after nutrition intervention	Caregiver completed follow-up 3-day food record indicating reduced number of feeding opportunities throughout the day (six to seven). States child resisted at first but now eats at table at regular meal/snack times. Caregiver is continuing to work with behavioral specialist for both mealtime and other behavior issues. Energy and nutrient intake have improved to 85% to 90% of standard.

Enteral and Parenteral Nutrition Administration

Definition

Delivery of nutrition via enteral and/or parenteral access.

Nutrition Assessment and Monitoring and Evaluation

Indicators

- Enteral nutrition administration assessment—evaluation of the delivery technique for infusion of nutrients distal to the oral cavity via a tube inserted into the gastrointestinal (GI) tract
- Method of enteral nutrition feeding administration—defined as the delivery technique for infusion of nutrients distal to the oral cavity via a tube inserted into the GI tract
- Orogastric enteral nutrition feeding administration (present/absent)—defined as the delivery technique for infusion of nutrients via a tube that is introduced into the oral cavity and terminates in the stomach
- Oroenteric enteral nutrition feeding administration (present/absent)—defined as the delivery technique for infusion of nutrients via a tube that is introduced into the oral cavity and terminates in the small intestine
- Nasogastric enteral nutrition feeding administration (present/absent)—defined as the delivery technique for infusion of nutrients via a tube that is introduced into the nasal cavity and terminates in the stomach
- Nasoduodenal enteral nutrition feeding administration (present/absent)—defined as the delivery technique for infusion of nutrients via a tube that is introduced into the nasal cavity and terminates in the duodenum
- Nasojejunal enteral nutrition feeding administration (present/absent)—defined as the delivery technique for infusion of nutrients via a tube that is introduced into the nasal cavity and terminates in the jejunum
- Gastrostomy enteral nutrition feeding administration (present/absent)—defined as the delivery technique for infusion of nutrients via a feeding tube percutaneously or surgically placed in the stomach
- Jejunostomy enteral nutrition feeding administration (present/absent)—defined as the delivery technique for infusion of nutrients via a feeding tube percutaneously or surgically placed in the jejunum
- Continuous enteral nutrition feeding (present/absent)—defined as minimally interrupted, hourly infusion of enteral nutrition formula
- Bolus enteral nutrition feeding (present/absent)—defined as a larger volume of enteral nutrition formula via syringe over a short (eg, 10-30 minute) time period
- Intermittent enteral nutrition feeding (present/absent)—defined as intermittent (over 2-3 hours) and/or cyclic infusion (over 8-16 hours) of enteral nutrition formula via a feeding bag
- Enteral nutrition feeding access device patency status (patent/not patent)—defined as the condition of the enteral nutrition feeding access device
- Body position for enteral nutrition administration—defined as the direction of the chest of the body during delivery of enteral nutrition feeding
- Supine body position for enteral nutrition administration (present/absent)—defined as lying with the chest of the body facing upward during delivery of enteral nutrition feeding
- Prone body position for enteral nutrition administration (present/absent)—defined as lying with the chest of the body facing downward during delivery of enteral nutrition feeding

Enteral and Parenteral Nutrition Administration

- Degree elevation of head of bed for enteral nutrition administration (number)—defined as the angle, in degrees, that the head of the bed is raised during delivery of enteral nutrition feeding
- Parenteral nutrition administration assessment—evaluation of the delivery technique for nutrients infused via a route other than the GI tract (ie, intravenous and/or intraperitoneal infusion)
- Method of parenteral nutrition administration—defined as the delivery technique for intravenous and/or intraperitoneal infusion of nutrients
- Peripheral venous parenteral nutrition administration (present/absent)—defined as intravenous infusion of nutrients directly into a peripheral vein
- Central venous parenteral nutrition administration (present/absent)—defined as intravenous infusion of nutrients into the vena cava or right atrium
- Intradialytic parenteral nutrition administration (present/absent)—defined as infusion of nutrients via venous access during hemodialysis treatment
- Intraperitoneal parenteral nutrition administration (present/absent)—defined as infusion of nutrients during peritoneal dialysis treatment
- Continuous parenteral nutrition administration (present/absent)—defined as uninterrupted hourly infusion of parenteral nutrition solution
- Cyclic parenteral nutrition administration (present/absent)—defined as infusion, typically over 6-20 ours, of parenteral nutrition solution
- Parenteral nutrition access device patency status (patent/not patent)—defined as the condition of the parenteral nutrition access device

Examples of the measurement methods or data sources for these outcome indicators: Client report/recalls, health record, client nutrition focused physical exam, provider referral

Typically used with the following domains of nutrition interventions: Food and/or nutrient delivery, nutrition education, nutrition counseling, coordination of nutrition care by nutrition professional, population based nutrition action

Typically used to determine and monitor and evaluate change in the following nutrition diagnoses: Enteral nutrition administration inconsistent with needs, parenteral nutrition administration inconsistent with needs, inadequate or excessive enteral or parenteral nutrition infusion, inadequate fluid intake, predicted food medication interaction

Note: Judgment must be used to select indicators and determine the appropriate measurement techniques and reference standards for a given client population and setting. Once identified, these indicators, measurement techniques, and reference standards should be identified in policies and procedures or other documents for use in client records, quality or performance improvement, or in formal research projects.

Client Example

Example(s) of one or two of the nutrition care indicators (includes sample initial and reassessment documentation for one of the indicators)

Indicator(s) Selected

Gastrostomy enteral nutrition feeding administration (present/absent)

Enteral and Parenteral Nutrition Administration

Criteria for Evaluation

Comparison to reference standard, recommendation, or goal:

1. Reference standard: Refer to enteral nutrition guidelines.
2. Recommendation: Consider access for gastrostomy enteral nutrition feeding administration because client is a candidate for long-term enteral support to meet nutrition needs.
3. Goal: Not applicable

Sample Nutrition Assessment and Monitoring and Evaluation Documentation	
Initial nutrition assessment	Client enteral nutrition is via nasogastric feeding tube; however, with long-term enteral nutrition support anticipated, recommend evaluation for gastrostomy enteral nutrition feeding administration. Monitor enteral nutrition feeding delivery technique.
Reassessment after nutrition intervention	Percutaneous endoscopic gastrostomy (PEG) access procedure planned for tomorrow. Will provide follow-up care regarding enteral nutrition administration via PEG.

Fasting Determination

Definition

The pattern of and tolerance to absence of nutrient administration from all sources.

Nutrition Assessment and Monitoring and Evaluation

Indicators

- Reported fasting pattern in one calendar day—defined as the timing within one calendar day when the client does not take in or infuse nutrients (e.g., overnight fast, fast between meals)
- Reported fasting pattern in one calendar week—defined as the timing within one calendar week when the client does not take in or infuse nutrients (e.g., Friday evening)
- Reported fasting pattern in one calendar month—defined as the timing within one calendar month when the client does not take in or infuse nutrients (e.g., every Sabbath)
- Reported fasting pattern in one calendar year—defined as the timing within one calendar year when the client does not take in or infuse nutrients (e.g., Lent, Passover, Ramadan, occasional fasting)
- Reported fasting tolerance—defined as the length of time a client can endure a lack of nutrient intake or nutrient infusion without physiological consequence (specify in hours)

Examples of the measurement methods or data sources for these outcome indicators: Client report, medical record, client history, food and nutrition delivery coordination of care

Typically used with the following domains of nutrition interventions: Nutrition education, nutrition counseling

Typically used to determine and monitor and evaluate change in the following nutrition diagnoses: Inadequate oral intake, inadequate carbohydrate intake, food and nutrition related knowledge deficit, belief finding that hinders food and/or nutrition behavior change, attitude finding that hinders food and/or nutrition behavior change

Note: Judgment must be used to select indicators and determine the appropriate measurement techniques and reference standards for a given client population and setting. Once identified, these indicators, measurement techniques, and reference standards should be identified in policies and procedures or other documents for use in client records, quality or performance improvement, or in formal research projects.

Client Example

Example(s) of one or two of the nutrition care indicators (includes sample initial assessment documentation for one of the indicators)

Indicator(s) Selected

Reported fasting tolerance: reported fasting pattern in one calendar day

Criteria for Evaluation

Comparison to reference standard, recommendation, or goal:

1. Reference standard: No validated standard exists.
2. Recommendation: Limit or avoid fasting longer than 5 hours for this client with an inborn error of metabolism where limiting fasting is recommended.
3. Goal: Limit or avoid fasting longer than 4 hours, 7 of 7 nights per week because longer periods result in physiological consequence for this client with an inborn error of metabolism.

Fasting Determination

Sample Nutrition Assessment Documentation	
Initial nutrition assessment with client	The client's (with an inborn error of metabolism) reported fasting tolerance is approximately 5 hours, at which time the client must take in nutrients to avoid hypoglycemia. The client identified that they will limit fasting daily to no longer than 4 hours, 7 of 7 nights per week. [New goal identified]
Reassessment after nutrition intervention	Goal achieved. Client's reported fasting pattern in one calendar day is no longer than 4 hours on 7 of 7 nights per week.

Medications

Definition

Prescription and over-the-counter (OTC) medications that may impact nutritional status.

Nutrition Assessment and Monitoring and Evaluation

Indicators

Prescription medication use

- Current prescriptions with nutrient/food medication interactions, specify
- Insulin or insulin secretagogues, specify
    - Insulin sensitivity factor (mg/dL)—defined as the estimated reduction in blood glucose in mg/dL per unit of rapid-acting (or short-acting) insulin, also referred to as the correction insulin
- Medication, alter blood pressure, specify
- Medication, alter breastmilk production, specify
- Medication, lipid lowering, specify
- Medications, alter glucose levels, specify
- Other, specify

Over-the-counter (OTC) medications use

- Current OTC products with nutrient/food medication implications, specify
- Medication, alter blood pressure, specify
- Medication, alter breastmilk production, specify
- Medication, lipid lowering, specify
- Medications, alter glucose levels, specify
- Other, specify

Misuse of medications (e.g., accidental overdose, illegal drugs, laxatives, diuretics, drug use during pregnancy), specify

> *Note:* Vitamin and mineral supplements can be found on the Vitamin Intake and Mineral/Element Intake reference sheets on pages 70 and 73. Alcohol is found on the Alcohol Intake reference sheet on page 46.

Examples of the measurement methods or data sources for these outcome indicators: Client report, medical record, referring health care provider or agency

Typically used with the following domains of nutrition interventions: Food and/or nutrient delivery, nutrition education, nutrition counseling, coordination of nutrition care by nutrition professional

Typically used to determine and monitor and evaluate change in the following nutrition diagnoses: Food medication interaction; increased energy expenditure; malnutrition (undernutrition); inadequate or excessive energy; oral, fluid, carbohydrate, protein, fat, vitamin, and mineral intake; unintended weight gain or loss; overweight/obesity; underweight; disordered eating pattern

> *Note:* Judgment must be used to select indicators and determine the appropriate measurement techniques and reference standards for a given client population and setting. Once identified, these indicators, measurement techniques, and reference standards should be identified in policies and procedures or other documents for use in client records, quality or performance improvement, or in formal research projects.

Medications

Client Example

Example(s) of one or two of the nutrition care indicators (includes sample initial and reassessment documentation for one of the indicators)

Indicator(s) Selected

Prescription medication with nutrient/food medication interactions: Prednisone

Criteria for Evaluation

Comparison reference standard, recommendation, or goal:

1. Reference standard: Not applicable
2. Recommendation: Client with prescription for 50 mg/d prednisone and concerned about concurrent weight gain caused by increased appetite and fluid retention.
3. Goal: Client goal is to track hunger and intake and implement mitigation strategies identified in collaboration with nutrition professional during prednisone therapy.

Sample Nutrition Assessment and Monitoring and Evaluation Documentation	
Initial nutrition assessment with client	Client's prescription medication is 50 mg/d prednisone for rheumatoid arthritis. Current weight 182 lb (83 kg). Long-term therapy may result in a need for protein, calcium, potassium, phosphorus, folate and vitamin A, C, and D supplementation. Client currently taking a vitamin/mineral supplement and concerned about weight gain caused by increased appetite and fluid retention. Client goal to implement hunger and intake tracking and mitigation strategies as identified collaboratively with nutrition professional.
Reassessment after nutrition intervention	Client's prescription medication prednisone dose reduced to 25 mg/d. Currently taking a one-a-day multivitamin/multimineral, tracking hunger and intake on most days, and snacking on raw vegetables between meals. Weight stable.

Complementary/Alternative Medicine

Definition

Complementary and alternative medicine products, including herbal preparations that may impact nutritional status

Nutrition Assessment and Monitoring and Evaluation

Indicators

- Nutrition related complementary/alternative medicine use (e.g., gingko, St. John's Wart, elderberry, garlic, ephedra, probiotics)

Note: Vitamin and mineral supplements can be found on the Vitamin and Mineral/Element Intake reference sheets on pages 70 and 73, respectively. Alcohol is found on the Alcohol Intake reference sheet on page 46.

Examples of the measurement methods or data sources for these outcome indicators: Patient/client report, medical record, referring health care provider or agency

Typically used with the following domains of nutrition interventions: Food and/or nutrient delivery, nutrition education, nutrition counseling, coordination of nutrition care by nutrition professional

Typically used to determine and monitor and evaluate change in the following nutrition diagnoses: Food medication interaction, increased energy expenditure, malnutrition (undernutrition), unintended weight gain or loss, overweight/obesity, intake of unsafe foods, disordered eating pattern

Note: Judgment must be used to select indicators and determine the appropriate measurement techniques and reference standards for a given client population and setting. Once identified, these indicators, measurement techniques, and reference standards should be identified in policies and procedures or other documents for use in client records, quality or performance improvement, or in formal research projects.

Criteria for Evaluation

Comparison to goal or reference standard:

1. Goal (tailored to patient/client's needs)
   OR
2. Reference standard

Client Example

Example(s) of one or two of the nutrition care indicators (includes sample initial and reassessment documentation for one of the indicators)

Indicator(s) Selected

Complementary/alternative medicine use—ephedra

Complementary/Alternative Medicine

Criteria for Evaluation

Comparison to goal or reference standard:

1. Goal: Patient/client taking ephedra with the hope that it will promote weight loss. Goal is to have patient/client eliminate ephedra for safety reasons and engage in nutrition counseling for weight management.
OR
2. Reference standard: Not applicable

Sample Nutrition Assessment and Monitoring and Evaluation Documentation	
Initial nutrition assessment with client	Patient/client complementary/alternative medicine use of ephedra is for weight loss. Patient/client reports being unaware of safety concerns.
Reassessment after nutrition intervention	Patient/client complementary/alternative medicine use of ephedra has stopped and had success with weight loss as a result of nutrition counseling.

Food and Nutrition Knowledge

Definition

Level of understanding about food, nutrition, and health or nutrition related information and guidelines relevant to client needs.

Nutrition Assessment and Monitoring and Evaluation

Indicators

- Nutrition knowledge of community (no knowledge, minimal knowledge, basic knowledge, intermediate knowledge, advanced knowledge)—defined as the assessed level of knowledge of a community, subpopulation, or population
- Nutrition knowledge of supportive individuals (eg, family, caregivers) (no knowledge, minimal knowledge, basic knowledge, intermediate knowledge, advanced knowledge)—defined as the assessed level of knowledge of those who give or support care
- Nutrition knowledge of individual client (no knowledge, minimal knowledge, basic knowledge, intermediate knowledge, advanced knowledge)—defined as the assessed level of knowledge of an individual client

Examples of the measurement methods or data sources for these indicators: Pre- and/or posttests administered orally, on paper, or by computer, scenario discussions, client restates key information, review of food records, practical demonstration/test, survey, nutrition quotient, nutrition questionnaire, nutrition assessment inventory

Typically used with the following domains of nutrition interventions: Nutrition education, nutrition counseling, population based nutrition action

Typically used to determine and to monitor and evaluate change in the following nutrition diagnoses: Food and nutrition related knowledge deficit, limited adherence to nutrition related recommendations, undesirable food choices, breastfeeding difficulty, overweight/obesity, intake domain nutrition diagnoses.

Note: Judgment must be used to select indicators and determine the appropriate measurement techniques and reference standards for a given client population and setting. Once identified, these indicators, measurement techniques, and reference standards should be identified in policies and procedures or other documents for use in client records, quality or performance improvement, or in formal research projects.

Client Example

Example of one of the nutrition care indicators (includes sample initial and reassessment documentation for one of the indicators)

Indicator(s) Selected

Nutrition knowledge of individual client

Criteria for Evaluation

Comparison to goal or reference standard:

1. Recommendation: Not applicable
2. Goal: Client established a goal to learn how to accurately read a food label and identify the total number of grams of carbohydrate per serving of food.
3. Recommendation: Not applicable

Food and Nutrition Knowledge

Sample Nutrition Assessment and Monitoring and Evaluation Documentation	
Initial nutrition assessment with client	Individual client with newly diagnosed diabetes with no knowledge of carbohydrate counting. Client established a goal to learn how to accurately read a food label and identify the total number of grams of carbohydrate per serving of food
Reassessment after nutrition intervention	Client has intermediate knowledge of how to read food labels and state grams of carbohydrate in individual food items. Client has basic knowledge of how to consistently apply this knowledge to food intake and distribution of carbohydrate throughout the day. Will continue to monitor at next encounter.

Food and Nutrition Skill

Definition

Level of food, nutrition, and health or nutrition related skills relevant to client needs.

Nutrition Assessment and Monitoring and Evaluation

Indicators

- Nutrition skill of community (no skill, minimal skill, basic skill, intermediate skill, advanced skill)—defined as the assessed level of skill of a community, subpopulation, or population
- Nutrition skill of supportive individuals (eg, family, caregivers) (no skill, minimal skill, basic skill, intermediate skill, advanced skill)—defined as the assessed level of skill of family and those who give or support care
- Nutrition skill of individual client (no skill, minimal skill, basic skill, intermediate skill, advanced skill)—defined as the assessed level of skill of an individual client

Examples of the measurement methods or data sources for these outcome indicators: Pre- and/or post-tests administered orally, on paper, or by computer, scenario discussions, client restates key information, review of food records, practical demonstration, survey, nutrition questionnaire, nutrition assessment inventory

Typically used to determine and monitor and evaluate change in the following domains of nutrition interventions: Nutrition education, nutrition counseling, population based nutrition action

Typically used to determine and to monitor and evaluate change in the following nutrition diagnoses: Food and nutrition related knowledge deficit, limited adherence to nutrition related recommendations, self feeding difficulty, breastfeeding difficulty, intake domain nutrition diagnoses.

Note: Judgment must be used to select indicators and determine the appropriate measurement techniques and reference standards for a given client population and setting. Once identified, these indicators, measurement techniques, and reference standards should be identified in policies and procedures or other documents for use in client records, quality or performance improvement, or in formal research projects.

Client Example

Example of one of the nutrition care indicators (includes sample initial and reassessment documentation for one of the indicators)

Indicator(s) Selected

Nutrition skill of individual client

Criteria for Evaluation

Comparison to goal or reference standard:

1. Reference standard: Not applicable
2. Recommendation: Not applicable
3. Goal: Individual client established a goal to learn to guide baby's lips and mouth for a successful latch.

Food and Nutrition Skill

Sample Nutrition Assessment and Monitoring and Evaluation Documentation	
Initial nutrition assessment	Individual client with newborn infant and no nutrition skill related to breast-feeding. Individual client established a goal to guide baby's lips and mouth for a successful latch.
Reassessment after nutrition intervention	Individual client with basic skill guiding baby's lips and mouth for successful latch. Able to demonstrate successful latch three out of five times. Will continue to monitor at next encounter.

Belief and Attitude Determination

Definition

Ascertaining of the client's acceptance of the truth about (belief) or way of thinking or feeling about (attitude) food- or nutrition-related phenomenon or behavior, which influences food or nutrition-related behavior.

Nutrition Assessment and Monitoring and Evaluation

Indicators

- Nutrition priority of individual client (present/absent)—defined as the individual client's beliefs and attitudes about food and nutrition that are believed to be of prime concern
- Nutrition priority of client's supportive individuals (present/absent)—defined as the client's supportive individuals (eg, family, caregiver) beliefs and attitudes about food and nutrition that are believed to be of prime concern
- Nutrition priority of client's supportive structures (present/absent)—defined as the client's supportive structures' (eg, social service agencies and faith-based organizations) beliefs and attitudes about food and nutrition that are believed to be of prime concern
- Nutrition priority of client's stakeholders (present/absent)—defined as the client's stakeholders' (eg, constituencies with impact on client nutrition) beliefs and attitudes about food and nutrition that are believed to be of prime concern
- Conflict with individual client's value system (present/absent)—defined as the individual client's beliefs and attitudes that are incongruent with the client's values
- Conflict with client's supportive individuals' value system (present/absent)—defined as the client's beliefs and attitudes that are incongruent with the values of the client's supportive individuals (eg, family and caregivers)
- Conflict with client's supportive structures' value system (present/absent)—defined as the client's beliefs and attitudes that are incongruent with the values of the client's supportive structures (eg, social service agencies and faith based organizations)
- Conflict with stakeholders' value system (present/absent)—defined as the client's beliefs and attitudes that are incongruent with the values of stakeholders (eg, constituencies with impact on client nutrition)
- Behavioral beliefs—defined as factors (motivation, control, norms, readiness) that influence the client's food- and nutrition-related behaviors
  - Perceived susceptibility to nutrition related health problems score (self-rated on a scale of 1 to 7; 1 = very low to 7 = very high perceived susceptibility)—defined as a client's belief that they have a health condition or are at high risk for developing a health condition
  - Perceived severity of risk to health score (self-rated on a scale of 1 to 7; 1 = very low to 7 = very high perceived severity of risk)—defined as a client's belief about the severity of their risk of a health condition
  - Likelihood of performing nutrition related behavior score (self-rated on a scale of 1 to 7; 1 = unlikely to perform behavior to 7 = very likely to perform behavior)—defined as the probability of the client performing the behavior(s)
  - Perceived control over nutrition related behavior score (self-rated on a scale of 1 to 7; 1 = very low to 7 = very high perceived control)—defined as the client's belief in their power to change nutrition related behavior(s)
  - Nutrition self efficacy score (self-rated on a scale of 1 to 7; 1 = very low confidence to 7 = very high confidence in ability)—defined as the client's confidence in their ability to change nutrition related behavior(s)

Belief and Attitude Determination

  - Perceived barrier to nutrition related behavior score (self-rated on a scale of 1 to 7; 1 = very low to 7 = very high perceived barriers)—defined as the client's belief about barriers to adopting nutrition related behaviors
- Readiness to change nutrition related behavior stage
  - Precontemplation stage for readiness to change (present/absent)
  - Contemplation stage for readiness to change (present/absent)
  - Preparation stage for readiness to change (present/absent)
  - Action stage for readiness to change (present/absent)
  - Maintenance stage for readiness to change (present/absent)
  - Relapse stage for readiness to change (present/absent)
- Readiness to change nutrition related behavior score (self-rated on scale of 1 to 10; 1 = not ready to 10 = fully ready to change)—defined as a client assessment of their preparedness to change nutrition related behaviors
- Negative emotions about food and nutrition (present/absent)—defined as negative feelings about food and/or nutrition
- Positive emotions about food and nutrition (present/absent)—defined as positive feelings about food and/or nutrition
- Unrealistic nutrition related goals (present/absent)—defined as client food and/or nutrition expectations that may not be achievable
- Unscientific nutrition belief (present/absent)—defined as client acceptance of the truth about food and/or nutrition that is incongruent with scientific evidence
- Body image disturbance (present/absent)—defined as client's distressing or impairing preoccupation with defects in their body that are not apparent to others
- Preoccupation with food (present/absent)—defined as thoughts about food that dominate the client's thinking
- Preoccupation with body weight (present/absent)—defined as thoughts about body weight that dominate the client's thinking
- Preoccupation with body shape (present/absent)—defined as thoughts about body shape that dominate the client's thinking
- Negative nutrition self talk (present/absent)—defined as negative thoughts about oneself related to food and nutrition
- Positive nutrition self talk (present/absent)—defined as positive thoughts about oneself related to food and nutrition
- Preference for food (yes/no)—defined as a liking of specific food stuffs consumed
- Preferences for beverages (yes/no)—defined as a liking of specific liquids consumed
- Craving for nonfood item (yes/no)—defined as a yearning for a substance not generally considered edible

Examples of the measurement methods or data sources for these outcome indicators: Client self-report, client assessment questionnaire or interview, medical record, referring health care provider or agency, survey data

Typically used to monitor and evaluate change in the following domains of nutrition interventions: Food and/or nutrient delivery, nutrition education, nutrition counseling, population based nutrition action

Belief and Attitude Determination

Typically used to determine and monitor and evaluate change in the following nutrition diagnoses: Belief finding that hinders food and/or nutrition behavior change; attitude finding that hinders food and/or nutrition behavior change; not ready for nutrition related behavior change; inability to manage self-care; self-monitoring deficit, excessive or inadequate oral, energy, macronutrient, micronutrient, or bioactive substance intake; imbalance of nutrients; intake of types of fats inconsistent with needs; intake of types of proteins inconsistent with needs; intake of types of carbohydrate inconsistent with needs; inadequate/excessive fiber intake; unbalanced diet pattern; underweight; overweight/obesity; disordered eating pattern; physical inactivity; excess physical activity; food insecurity; limited access to potable water

Note: Judgment must be used to select indicators and determine the appropriate measurement techniques and reference standards for a given client population and setting. Once identified, these indicators, measurement techniques, and reference standards should be identified in policies and procedures or other documents for use in client records, quality or performance improvement, or in formal research projects.

Client Example

Example(s) of one of the nutrition care indicators (includes sample initial and reassessment documentation for one of the indicators)

Indicator(s) Selected

Readiness to change nutrition related behavior stage

Criteria for Evaluation

Comparison to goal or reference standard:

1. Reference standard: Not applicable
2. Recommendation: Not applicable
3. Goal: Client is currently in the precontemplation stage of change. Client goal is to move to the preparation stage of change within 3 months.

Sample Nutrition Assessment and Monitoring and Evaluation Documentation	
Initial nutrition assessment	Assessment results indicate client is currently in the precontemplation stage of change related to need for nutrition changes. Will initiate motivational interviewing and reassess in 2 weeks.
Reassessment after nutrition intervention	Significant progress toward goal. Reassessment indicates that client has moved from the precontemplation stage to the contemplation stage related to need for nutrition changes. Will reassess in 2 weeks.

Adherence Behavior

Definition

Level of congruence with nutrition-related recommendations or behavioral changes agreed upon by client to achieve nutrition-related goals.

Nutrition Assessment and Monitoring and Evaluation

Indicators

- Self reported nutrition adherence score (self-rated on a scale of 1 to 10; 1 = not adherent to 10 = completely adherent)—defined as a client assessment of their congruence to agreed upon nutrition related goals
- Nutrition encounter ratio (ratio)—defined as the ratio of actual nutrition encounters to the total planned nutrition encounters
- Ability to recall nutrition goals (very able to recall goals, somewhat able to recall goals, unable to recall goals)—defined as the degree to which a client can describe previously agreed upon nutrition objectives
- Nutrition self monitoring at agreed upon rate (self rated on a scale of 1 to 10; 1 = not adherent to 10 = completely adherent)—defined as a client assessment of their congruence to agreed upon, nutrition related self monitoring
- Nutrition self management as agreed upon (self rated on a scale of 1 to 10; 1 = not adherent to 10 = completely adherent)—defined as a client assessment of their congruence with agreed upon, nutrition related self management

Note: Use in conjunction with appropriate Food and Nutrition Intake, Anthropometric Data, and Biochemical Data reference sheets.

May be useful in relapse prevention treatment (analyze and control factors that caused the lapse).

Examples of the measurement methods or data sources for these outcome indicators: Nutrition encounter attendance, self-monitoring records (eg, food record to evaluate fat, sodium, calories/kcal/kJ, diet quality, binge eating), client self-report, adherence tools or questionnaires, provider assessment, self-efficacy assessment, readiness to change assessment

Typically used with the following domains of nutrition interventions: Food and/or nutrient delivery, nutrition education, nutrition counseling, population based nutrition action

Typically used to determine and monitor and evaluate change in the following nutrition diagnoses: Limited adherence to nutrition-related recommendations, self monitoring deficit, not ready for nutrition-related behavior change

Note: Judgment must be used to select indicators and determine the appropriate measurement techniques and reference standards for a given client population and setting. Once identified, these indicators, measurement techniques, and reference standards should be identified in policies and procedures or other documents for use in client records, quality or performance improvement, or in formal research projects.

Adherence Behavior

Client Example

Example(s) of one (or more) of the nutrition care indicators (includes sample initial and reassessment documentation for one of the indicators)

Indicator(s) Selected

Self reported nutrition adherence score (self rated on a scale of 1 to 10)

Criteria for Evaluation

Comparison to reference standard, recommendations, or goal:

1. Reference standard: Not applicable
2. Recommendations: Not applicable
3. Goal: Client rates self 4/10 (1 = not adherent to 10 = completely adherent) on ability to adhere to meal plan.

Sample Nutrition Assessment and Monitoring and Evaluation Documentation	
Initial encounter	Client rates self 4/10 on ability to adhere to meal plan developed in collaboration with dietitian. Discussions with client regarding barrier(s) to achieving goals and strategies to improve adherence. Goal set to adhere to meal plan 5 days per week. Client will evaluate progress toward goal at the next encounter and rate adherence.
Reassessment after nutrition intervention	Some progress toward goal. Client rated self 6/10 on ability to adhere to meal plan 5 days per week. Client is doing well on weekdays but verbalizes need to improve on weekends. Discussed strategies to improve adherence to meal plan on the weekends. Client will monitor progress and adherence at next encounter.

Avoidance Behavior

Definition

Keeping away from something or someone to postpone an outcome or perceived consequence.

Nutrition Assessment and Monitoring and Evaluation

Indicators

- Avoidance
  - Specific foods (specify, eg, grapefruit, seeds)
  - Food groups (specify, eg, milk/milk products)
  - Fluids (specify)
  - Textures (specify)
  - Social situations (specify)
  - Other (specify)
  - Restrictive eating (yes/no)
- Cause of avoidance behavior (e.g., personal choice, prescribed dietary restriction, GI distress, suspected allergy, eating disorder, cancer treatment side effects, medications, mental illness, Parkinson's disease)

Examples of the measurement methods or data sources for these outcome indicators: Self-monitoring records, client interview

Typically used with the following domains of nutrition interventions: Nutrition counseling

Typically used to determine and monitor and evaluate change in the following nutrition diagnoses: Disordered eating pattern, overweight/obesity, underweight, altered GI function

Note: Judgment must be used to select indicators and determine the appropriate measurement techniques and reference standards for a given client population and setting. Once identified, these indicators, measurement techniques, and reference standards should be identified in policies and procedures or other documents for use in client records, quality or performance improvement, or in formal research projects.

Evaluation

Criteria for Evaluation

Comparison to goal or reference standard:

1. Goal (tailored to patient/client's needs)
   OR
2. Reference standard

Client Example

Example(s) of one or two of the nutrition care indicators (includes sample initial and reassessment documentation for one of the indicators)

Avoidance Behavior

Indicator(s) Selected

Avoidance of social situations

Criteria for Evaluation

Comparison to goal or reference standard:

1. Goal: Patient/client avoiding social situations in an effort to avoid overeating. Goal is to learn strategies to control eating in social situations.
   OR
2. Reference standard: No validated standard exists.

Sample Nutrition Assessment and Monitoring and Evaluation Documentation	
Initial nutrition assessment	Client avoids social situations because they are afraid they will overeat. Reviewed client's food diary and client brainstormed strategies which may help them control eating in social situations. Client will preplan food intake on days they have social engagements, will have a piece of fruit before going to help curb their appetite, and will maintain a food diary.
Reassessment after nutrition intervention	Client made some progress toward goal. Attended two of four social engagements where food was served and successfully controlled food intake both times. Client will continue to use strategies. Will reevaluate avoidance behavior at next encounter.

Binge Eating and Purging Behavior

Definition

Recurrent episodes of excessive eating over a short time accompanied by a feeling of lack of control during the binge episode. This may be followed by compensatory behavior to make up for the excessive eating, referred to as purging. Purging behavior, actions to create physical or psychological relief of the fear, may also occur independent of binge eating.

Nutrition Assessment and Monitoring and Evaluation

Indicators

- Binge eating behavior (present/absent)—defined as eating a larger portion of food than what most people would consume during a short period of time (within any two-hour period) accompanied by a feeling of lack of control over eating during the binge episode
- Self induced purging behavior (present/absent)—defined as a behavior to create physical or psychological relief of the fear of weight gain
- Number of binge eating episodes per week (number/week)—defined as the typical number of binge-eating episodes in one week
- Number of self-induced purging episodes per week (number/week)—defined as the typical number of self-induced episodes intended to create physical or psychological relief in one week

Note: Misuse of laxatives, diuretics, or other drugs is found on the Medication reference sheet on page 88. Amount and type of physical activity is found on the Physical Activity reference sheet on page 123. Fasting terms can be found on the Fasting Determination reference sheet on page 86.

Examples of the measurement methods or data sources for these outcome indicators: Client interview, health record, referring health care provider or agency, self-monitoring records

Typically used with the following domains of nutrition interventions: Food and/or nutrient delivery, nutrition education, nutrition counseling, coordination of nutrition care

Typically used to determine and monitor and evaluate change in the following nutrition diagnoses: Excessive oral intake, disordered eating pattern, overweight/obesity, altered nutrition related laboratory values, poor food and/or nutrition quality of life, underweight

Note: Judgment must be used to select indicators and determine the appropriate measurement techniques and reference standards for a given client population and setting. Once identified, these indicators, measurement techniques, and reference standards should be identified in policies and procedures or other documents for use in client records, quality or performance improvement, or in formal research projects.

Client Example

Example(s) of one or two of the nutrition care indicators (includes sample initial and reassessment documentation for one of the indicators)

Indicator(s) Selected

Number of binge eating episodes per week

Binge Eating and Purging Behavior

Criteria for Evaluation

Comparison to reference standard, recommendation, or goal:

1. Reference standard: Less than one binge eating episode per week for 3 months.
2. Recommendation: No binge eating episodes.
3. Goal: Client reports three binge eating episodes per week with a goal to reduce binge eating to one episode per week in 2 months.

Sample Nutrition Assessment and Monitoring and Evaluation Documentation	
Initial encounter	Client reports three binge eating episodes this week.
Reassessment after nutrition intervention	Some progress toward goal. Client reported two binge eating episodes this week for the past month. Will continue to monitor at next encounter.

Eating Behavior

Definition

Manner of acting and/or conduct while consuming food that influences food (ie, solid and liquid) intake.

Nutrition Assessment and Monitoring and Evaluation

Indicators

- Duration of typical eating occasion (minutes)—defined as the usual length of time from beginning to end of an eating episode
- Percentage of typical eating occasion spent consuming food (percentage)—defined as the usual estimated amount of time in minutes the client spends eating as a percentage of the duration of a typical eating occasion in minutes
- Refusing food (present/absent)—defined as rejecting food consumption
- Fatigue during eating (present/absent)—defined as tiredness while consuming food (ie, solid and liquid) that results in inadequate intake of food and/or nutrients
- Readiness to consume new food (present/absent)—defined as an indication of willingness to eat a wider variety of food
- Aversion to particular food (present/absent)—defined as a significant dislike of a solid food
- Sensory aversion to particular food (present/absent)—defined as rejection of food (ie, solid or liquid) due to heightened sensation (eg, taste, visual appearance, temperature, texture) from the food
- Aversion to particular beverage (present/absent)—defined as a significant dislike for liquid food
- Distracted during eating (present/absent)—defined as decreased attention to food consumption during an eating occasion

Examples of the measurement methods or data sources for these outcome indicators: Observation, health record, referring health care provider or agency, caregiver observation, client interview

Typically used with the following domains of nutrition interventions: Food and/or nutrient delivery, coordination of nutrition care by nutrition professional, population based nutrition action

Typically used to determine and monitor and evaluate change in the following nutrition diagnoses: Self feeding difficulty, inadequate and excessive oral intake, limited food acceptance, unbalanced diet pattern, inadequate mineral intake, inadequate fiber intake, disordered eating pattern, inadequate vitamin intake, inadequate protein intake, inadequate fluid intake

> *Note:* Judgment must be used to select indicators and determine the appropriate measurement techniques and reference standards for a given client population and setting. Once identified, these indicators, measurement techniques, and reference standards should be identified in policies and procedures or other documents for use in client records, quality or performance improvement, or in formal research projects.

Client Example

Example(s) of one nutrition care indicator (includes sample initial and reassessment documentation for one of the indicators)

Indicator(s) Selected

Percent of typical eating occasion spent consuming food (percentage). Distracted during eating

Eating Behavior

Criteria for Evaluation

Comparison to reference standard, recommendation, or goal:

1. Reference standard: No validated standard exists.
2. Recommendation: No validated standard exists.
3. Goal: Lunch meal observation of 4-year-old client is distracted during eating. Goal identified with client's supportive individual (eg, family, caregiver) is to reduce environmental disruptions and eat with client to promote improvement in meeting energy needs to at least 50%.

Sample Nutrition Assessment and Monitoring and Evaluation Documentation	
Initial nutrition assessment	Lunch meal observation revealed that client is distracted during eating and consumed only 10% of estimated energy needs.
Reassessment after nutrition intervention	Significant progress toward goal. Additional observation and records demonstrate reduction in environmental distractions and caregiver eats meals with client. Observation reveals that percent of typical eating occasion spent consuming food is now approximately 40%. Will monitor at next encounter.

Social Network Behavior

Definition

Ability to build and utilize a network of family, friends, colleagues, health professionals, and community resources for encouragement, emotional support, and to enhance one's environment to support behavior change.

Nutrition Assessment and Monitoring and Evaluation

Indicators

- Ability to build and utilize social networks (e.g., may include perceived social support, social integration, and assertiveness)

Examples of the measurement methods or data sources for these outcome indicators: Self-monitoring records, client self-report, goal-tracking tools

Typically used with the following domains of nutrition interventions: Nutrition counseling

Typically used to determine and monitor and evaluate change in the following nutrition diagnoses: Intake domain nutrition diagnoses, underweight, overweight/obesity, disordered eating pattern, unbalanced diet pattern, inability to manage self-care, breastfeeding difficulty, not ready for nutrition related behavior change, limited adherence to nutrition-related recommendations

Note: Judgment must be used to select indicators and determine the appropriate measurement techniques and reference standards for a given client population and setting. Once identified, these indicators, measurement techniques, and reference standards should be identified in policies and procedures or other documents for use in client records, quality or performance improvement, or in formal research projects.

Client Example

Example(s) of one or two of the nutrition care indicator (includes sample initial and reassessment documentation for one of the indicators)

Indicator(s) Selected

Ability to build and utilize social support (e.g., may include perceived social support, social integration, and assertiveness)

Criteria for Evaluation

Comparison to reference standard, recommendation, or goal:

1. Reference standard: No validated standard exists.
2. Recommendation: No validated standard exists
3. Goal: Client expresses goal to improve Ability to build and utilize social support.

Social Network Behavior

Sample Nutrition Assessment and Monitoring and Evaluation Documentation	
Initial nutrition assessment	Client states that they rarely verbalizes their nutrition-related desires/needs to their family and rates their ability to elicit support from their social network as limited. They are willing to work on their Ability to build and utilize social support by communicating nutrition needs before the next encounter. Will evaluate at the next encounter.
Reassessment after nutrition intervention	Some progress toward goal. Client is making attempts to improve their ability to build and utilize social support. They have begun to verbalize their needs. They are researching restaurants that will meets their needs that others will enjoy. Will monitor at next encounter in 2 weeks.

Food and Nutrition Program Participation

Definition

Client participation in supportive food and nutrition programs for which the client may be eligible.

Nutrition Assessment and Monitoring and Evaluation

Indicators

- Eligibility for government nutrition programs (yes/no)—defined as qualification status for national, provincial, regional, or state-based nutrition programs that offer food support and/or nutrition intervention
- Enrollment in government nutrition programs (yes/no)—defined as active recipient of or involvement in services from national, provincial, regional, or state-based nutrition programs that offer food support and/or nutrition intervention
- Eligibility for community nutrition programs (yes/no)—defined as qualification status for nutrition programs that offer food support and/or nutrition intervention
- Enrollment in community nutrition programs (yes/no)—defined as active recipient of or involvement in services from nutrition programs that offer food support and/or nutrition intervention
- Awareness of programs offering food support and nutrition intervention (yes/no)—defined as client ability to name or recognize programs related to the client's needs

Examples of the measurement methods or data sources for these outcome indicators: Client report of eligibility and enrollment, program referral completion information, client setting evaluation, survey data on program participation rates among eligible households

Typically used with the following domains of nutrition interventions: Food and/or nutrient delivery, nutrition education, nutrition counseling, coordination of nutrition care by nutrition professional, population based nutrition action

Typically used to determine and monitor and evaluate change in the following nutrition diagnoses: Food insecurity, limited access to potable water, limited access to nutrition related supplies, inadequate or excessive energy intake, inadequate protein intake, inadequate vitamin intake, inadequate mineral intake, food and nutrition related knowledge deficit

Note: Judgment must be used to select indicators and determine the appropriate measurement techniques and reference standards for a given client population and setting. Once identified, these indicators, measurement techniques, and reference standards should be identified in policies and procedures or other documents for use in client records, quality or performance improvement, or in formal research projects.

Client Example

Example(s) of one of the nutrition care indicators (includes sample initial and reassessment documentation for one of the indicators)

Indicator(s) Selected

Enrollment in government nutrition programs

Food and Nutrition Program Participation

Criteria for Evaluation

Comparison to reference standard, recommendation, or goal:

1. Reference standard: Not applicable
2. Recommendation: Recommend enrollment in government nutrition program because client is eligible and willing to enroll.
3. Goal: Client was unaware of eligibility requirement and is willing to complete required documentation to allow enrollment in government nutrition program (school lunch).

Sample Nutrition Assessment and Monitoring and Evaluation Documentation	
Initial nutrition assessment with client	The client's parent was not aware of required documentation for enrollment in government nutrition program (school lunch) and parent aims to complete them. Will follow up with parent and monitor change in school lunch program participation at next encounter.
Reassessment after nutrition intervention	Progress toward goal as client's family/guardian has completed and submitted school lunch program forms. Review for enrollment in program at future encounter.

Safe Food Availability

Definition

Reliable acquisition of safe and acceptable food to meet nutrition needs for an active, healthy life.

Nutrition Assessment and Monitoring and Evaluation

Indicators

- Availability of shopping facilities (yes/no)—defined as access to affordable sources of acceptable and safe food to meet nutrition needs
- Ability to procure safe food (yes/no)—defined as the capacity to source (eg, grocery stores, growing, hunting, fishing, food relief agencies) acceptable and safe foods to select a wide variety of food to meet nutrition needs
- Access to food preparation equipment (yes/no)—defined as ability to obtain and use equipment necessary to prepare food to meals or snacks
- Availability of food refrigeration (yes/no)—defined as access to cold food storage
- Ability to store food safely (yes/no)—defined as the capacity to keep food safe for consumption
- Ability to identify safe food (yes/no)—defined as the capacity to select foods for consumption that are free from spoilage or contaminants
- Individual client food security level (high, marginal, low, and very low)—defined as the degree to which an individual client in the household has reliable availability of food to meet nutrition needs from socially acceptable sources without running out
- Household food security level (high, marginal, low, and very low)—defined as the degree to which the household has reliable availability of food to meet nutrition needs from socially acceptable sources without running out
- Situational food insecurity (present/absent)—defined as short-term instability in food security
- Chronic food insecurity (present/absent)—defined as medium- to long-term instability in food security

Examples of the measurement methods or data sources for these outcome indicators: Client report overall food availability/food consumed during the week, referral information, setting evaluation, survey data

Typically used with the following domains of nutrition interventions: Food and/or nutrition delivery, nutrition education, nutrition counseling, coordination of nutrition care by nutrition professional, population based nutrition action

Typically used to determine and monitor and evaluate change in the following nutrition diagnoses: Food insecurity, intake of unsafe food, inadequate or excessive energy intake, inadequate or excessive oral intake, inadequate vitamin and mineral intake

Note: Judgment must be used to select indicators and determine the appropriate measurement techniques and reference standards for a given client population and setting. Once identified, these indicators, measurement techniques, and reference standards should be identified in policies and procedures or other documents for use in client records, quality or performance improvement, or in formal research projects.

Safe Food Availability

Client Example

Example(s) of one of the nutrition care indicators (includes sample initial and reassessment documentation for one of the indicators)

Indicator(s) Selected

Access to food preparation equipment (yes/no)

Criteria for Evaluation

Comparison to goal or reference standard:

1. Reference standard: Not applicable
2. Recommendation: Reliable Access to food preparation equipment
3. Goal: Client establishes goal to complete appointment with relevant professional regarding Access to food preparation equipment.

Sample Nutrition Assessment and Monitoring and Evaluation Documentation	
Initial nutrition assessment with client	The client's Access to food preparation equipment is not reliable. Will monitor change in access at next encounter after coordination of nutrition care with relevant professional.
Reassessment after nutrition intervention	Achieved goal as client has reliable Access to food preparation equipment.

Safe Water Availability

Definition

Reliable acquisition of water that can be safely consumed.

Nutrition Assessment and Monitoring and Evaluation

Indicators

- Availability of potable water (yes/no)—defined as ready access to water that meets guidelines for safe drinking water
- Ability to decontaminate water (yes/no)—defined as the capacity to interpret public health warnings and use of strategies to treat water for consumption
- Awareness of public health water alert (yes/no)—defined as attentiveness of warnings issued by public health authorities regarding drinking water

Examples of the measurement methods or data sources for these outcome indicators: Client report of potable water availability and/or decontamination strategies, referral information, setting evaluation, survey data, government issued reports and warnings

Typically used with the following domains of nutrition interventions: Nutrition education, nutrition counseling, coordination of nutrition care by nutrition professional, population based nutrition action

Typically used to determine and monitor and evaluate change in the following nutrition diagnoses: Limited access to potable water, Inadequate fluid intake, Intake of unsafe water

Note: Judgment must be used to select indicators and determine the appropriate measurement techniques and reference standards for a given client population and setting. Once identified, these indicators, measurement techniques, and reference standards should be identified in policies and procedures or other documents for use in client records, quality or performance improvement, or in formal research projects.

Client Example

Example(s) of one of the nutrition care indicators (includes sample initial and reassessment documentation for one of the indicators)

Indicator(s) Selected

Awareness of public health water alert (yes/no)

Criteria for Evaluation

Comparison to reference standard, recommendation, or goal:

1. Reference standard: Not applicable
2. Recommendation: Awareness of public health water alert
3. Goal: Client reports limited awareness of water decontamination public health warnings.

Safe Water Availability

Sample Nutrition Assessment and Monitoring and Evaluation Documentation	
Initial nutrition assessment	The client has limited awareness of the current public health alert for water decontamination (eg, community has a boil water alert for water used for drinking and cooking). Education provided. Client establishes goal to decontaminate water for duration of alert. Will monitor change in decontamination practices.
Reassessment after nutrition intervention	Substantial progress toward goal as client is decontaminating water consistent with public health alert.

Food and Nutrition Related Supplies Availability

Definition

Reliable ability to obtain necessary supplies to support food consumption and nutrition needs.

Nutrition Assessment and Monitoring and Evaluation

Indicators

- Access to food and nutrition related supplies (yes/no)—defined as ability to obtain nutrition related supplies for providing, assessing, and monitoring and evaluating nutrition interventions to administer, self-monitor, and meet food and nutrition needs (eg, glucose monitor, monitoring strips, lancets, pedometer, parenteral/enteral nutrition supplies, thickeners, blood pressure–related devices)
- Access to assistive eating devices (equipment or utensils; specify, eg, modified utensils, plates, bowls, gavage feeding supplies)
- Access to assistive food preparation devices (specify, eg, modified utensils for food preparation, electric can openers, rocking knives, one-handed devices)

Examples of the measurement methods or data sources for these outcome indicators: Client report, referral information, setting evaluation

Typically used with the following domains of nutrition interventions: Food and/or nutrient delivery, nutrition education, nutrition counseling, coordination of nutrition care by nutrition professional, population based nutrition action

Typically used to determine and monitor and evaluate change in the following nutrition diagnoses: Limited availability to nutrition related supplies, inability to manage self care, inadequate oral intake, self feeding difficulty, limited adherence to nutrition related recommendations, not ready for diet/lifestyle change, self monitoring deficit

> *Note:* Judgment must be used to select indicators and determine the appropriate measurement techniques and reference standards for a given client population and setting. Once identified, these indicators, measurement techniques, and reference standards should be identified in policies and procedures or other documents for use in client records, quality or performance improvement, or in formal research projects.

Client Example

Example(s) of one of the nutrition care indicators (includes sample initial and reassessment documentation for one of the indicators)

Indicator(s) Selected

Access to food and nutrition related supplies (yes/no)

Food and Nutrition Related Supplies Availability

Criteria for Evaluation

Comparison to reference standard, recommendation, or goal:

1. Reference: Standard American Diabetes Association Standards of Care (2019).
2. Recommendation: Client does not have access to nutrition related supplies for regular glucose monitoring.
3. Goal: Client establishes goal to attend appointment with relevant professional who will assist with obtaining glucose monitoring supplies.

Sample Nutrition Assessment and Monitoring and Evaluation Documentation	
Initial nutrition assessment with client	The client does not have access to nutrition related supplies (glucose monitoring strips). Referral to relevant professional. Will monitor change in access to nutrition related supplies (glucose monitoring strips) availability at next encounter.
Reassessment after nutrition intervention	Goal met as client met with relevant professional and has access to nutrition related supplies (glucose monitoring strips).

Food and Nutrition Sanitation

Definition

Reliable and accessible sanitation and hygiene to keep food, water, and nutrition related supplies safe and reduce spread of disease.

Nutrition Assessment and Monitoring and Evaluation

Indicators

- Availability of suitable sanitation facilities (yes/no)—defined as the availability of suitable sanitation facilities and the capacity to use these facilities to ensure that waste (ie, human and animal) is kept separate and does not contaminate food, water, and nutrition related supplies
- Ability to wash hands with soap and water (yes/no)—defined as the availability of handwashing facilities and the capacity to use these facilities to reduce contamination and the spread of disease to food, water, and nutrition related supplies

Examples of the measurement methods or data sources for these outcome indicators: Client report referral information, setting evaluation, survey data, microorganism culture results

Typically used with the following domains of nutrition interventions: Food and/or nutrition delivery, nutrition education, nutrition counseling, coordination of nutrition care by nutrition professional, population based nutrition action

Typically used to determine and monitor and evaluate change in the following nutrition diagnoses: Food insecurity, intake of unsafe food, limited access to potable water, food and nutrition related knowledge deficit

> *Note:* Judgment must be used to select indicators and determine the appropriate measurement techniques and reference standards for a given client population and setting. Once identified, these indicators, measurement techniques, and reference standards should be identified in policies and procedures or other documents for use in client records, quality or performance improvement, or in formal research projects.

Client Example

Example(s) of one of the nutrition care indicators (includes sample initial and reassessment documentation for one of the indicators)

Indicator(s) Selected

Ability to wash hands with soap and water (yes/no) and Availability of suitable sanitation facilities (yes/no)

Criteria for Evaluation

Comparison to goal or reference standard:

1. Reference standard: International and national standards for hand washing.
2. Recommendation: Ability to wash hands with soap and water and Availability of suitable sanitation facilities.
3. Goal: Client establishes goal to identify suitable sanitation facility during work to use for washing hands prior to eating.

Food and Nutrition Sanitation

Sample Nutrition Assessment and Monitoring and Evaluation Documentation	
Initial nutrition assessment with client	The client has limited ability to wash hands with soap and water prior to eating due to limited availability of suitable sanitation facilities. Soap is lacking in working environment. Client will identify suitable sanitation facility during work and use prior to eating.
Reassessment after nutrition intervention	Client has identified suitable sanitation facilities during working hours and reports consistent ability to wash hands with soap and water prior to eating.

Breastfeeding* Assessment

Definition

Evaluation of breastfeeding ability and capacity to support the nutritional and other needs of the infant and mother.

Nutrition Assessment and Monitoring and Evaluation

Indicators

- Initiation of breastfeeding
  - Start breastfeeding (date)—defined as the day breastfeeding was initiated
  - Stop breastfeeding (date)—defined as the day breastfeeding ceased
- Breastfeeding approach
  - Exclusive breastfeeding (yes/no)—defined as nourishment, all nutrients and fluid, provided via human milk† for the first 6 months of life; permits oral vitamin and mineral supplements and medicines
  - Predominant breastfeeding (yes/no)—defined as nourishment primarily from human milk, including expressed mother's‡ or donor human milk; permits infant formula and other liquids, oral vitamin and mineral supplements and medicines
  - Partial breastfeeding (yes/no)—defined as nourishment partially from human milk, including expressed mother's or donor human milk, with nourishment from infant formula and other sources
- Breastfeeding difficulties
  - Infant able to latch on to nipple for feeding (yes/no)
  - Infant unable to latch on to nipple for feeding (yes/no)
  - Difficulty latching on to nipple for feeding (yes/no)
  - Abscess of breast associated with lactation (yes/no)
  - Cracked nipple associated with lactation (yes/no)
  - Infection of nipple associated with lactation (yes/no)
  - Non purulent mastitis associated with lactation (yes/no)
  - Retracted nipple associated with lactation (yes/no)
  - Inversion of nipple associated with lactation (yes/no)
  - Breast tissue with lactating capability engorged (yes/no)
  - Previous surgery on breast tissue with lactating capability (yes/no)
  - Breast abnormality associated with lactation (yes/no)
  - Inadequate flow of human milk (yes/no)
- Finding related to infant's ability to suck
  - Infant able to suck (yes/no)
  - Infant unable to suck (yes/no)
  - Difficulty sucking (yes/no)

Note: Infant/child growth can be found on the Body Composition/Growth/Weight History reference sheet on page 129.

---

*If a synonym for the term "breastfeeding" is helpful or needed, an approved alternate is "chestfeeding."

† If a synonym for the term "human milk" is helpful or needed, an approved alternate is "breast milk."

‡ If a synonym for the term "mother" is helpful or needed, an approved alternate is "lactating parent."

Breastfeeding Assessment

Note: Breastfeeding self-efficacy and intention can be found on the Belief and Attitude Determination reference sheet on page 96.

Examples of the measurement methods or data sources for these outcome indicators: Client report, practitioner observation of breastfeeding, self-monitoring records, infant weight trends

Typically used with the following domains of nutrition interventions: Nutrition education, nutrition counseling, coordination of nutrition care by nutrition professional, population based nutrition action

Typically used to determine and monitor and evaluate change in the following nutrition diagnoses: Breastfeeding difficulty, predicted breastfeeding difficulty, food and nutrition related knowledge deficit, limited food and nutrition related skill, unsupported beliefs/attitudes about food or nutrition related topics, unintended weight loss, inadequate fluid intake

Note: Judgment must be used to select indicators and determine the appropriate measurement techniques and reference standards for a given client population and setting. Once identified, these indicators, measurement techniques, and reference standards should be identified in policies and procedures or other documents for use in client records, quality or performance improvement, or in formal research projects.

Client Example

Example(s) of one (or more) of the nutrition care indicators (includes sample initial and reassessment documentation for one of the indicators)

Indicator(s) Selected

Exclusive breastfeeding (yes/no)

Criteria for Evaluation

Comparison to reference standard, recommendation, or goal:

1. Reference standard: Not applicable
2. Recommendation: Not applicable
3. Goal: Client fears breastfeeding will be difficult upon return to work. Client goal is exclusive breastfeeding until returning to work when client will add supplemental infant formula to breastfeeding.

Sample Nutrition Assessment and Monitoring and Evaluation Documentation	
Initial encounter	Postpartum client states goal of exclusive breastfeeding and then a combination of formula and breastfeeding upon return to work. Will provide nutrition education, promotion of exclusive breastfeeding and discussing with employer accommodation for pumping human milk at work, and refer to lactation support group.
Reassessment after nutrition intervention	Client reports exclusive breastfeeding for 3 months. Promotion of exclusive breastfeeding and nutrition education. Continue to monitor.

Nutrition Related Activities of Daily Living and Instrumental Activities of Daily Living

Definition

Level of ability to perform nutrition-related activities of grocery shopping, meal preparation, and self-feeding (also called self-dining).

Nutrition Assessment and Monitoring and Evaluation

Indicators

- Ability to perform shopping activities (able, able with difficulty, unable)
- Ability to plan meals (able, able with difficulty, unable)
- Ability to prepare food for eating (able, able with difficulty, unable)
- Ability to prepare meal (able, able with difficulty, unable)
- Ability to self feed (yes/no)
- Ability to position self in relation to food (able, able with difficulty, unable)—defined as the capacity to place the body in proximity to food intended for consumption
- Feeding assisted (yes/no)
- Ability to use cutlery to feed self (able, able with difficulty, unable)
- Ability to use adaptive eating devices for self feeding (able, able with difficulty, unable)—defined as the capacity to use modified assistive eating utensils to consume food
- Ability to self administer enteral nutrition feeding (able, able with difficulty, unable)—defined as the capacity to infuse enteral nutrition as defined in a nutrition care plan
- Ability to self administer parenteral nutrition (able, able with difficulty, unable)—defined as the capacity to infuse parenteral nutrition as defined in a nutrition care plan
- Ability to remember to eat (yes/no, able, able with difficulty, unable)—defined as the memory recall capacity to eat food and/or supplements as defined in a nutrition care plan
- Ability to remember to infuse enteral nutrition (able, able with difficulty, unable)—defined as the memory recall capacity to administer enteral nutrition as defined in a nutrition care plan
- Ability to remember to infuse parenteral nutrition (able, able with difficulty, unable)—defined as the memory recall capacity to administer parenteral nutrition as defined in a nutrition care plan
- Nutrition related activities of daily living (ADL) score (score)
- Nutrition related instrumental activities of daily living (IADL) score (score)
- Ability to open and close containers (able, able with difficulty, unable)—defined as the capacity to unseal and seal a container

Note: Sufficient intake of food can be found on the Food Intake reference sheet on page 36.

Sufficient intake of fluid can be found on the Fluid Intake reference sheet on page 32.

Food security can be found on the Safe Food Availability reference sheet on page 111.

Ability to maintain sanitation can be found on the Food and Nutrition Sanitation reference sheet on page 117.

Ability to maintain weight can be found on the Body Composition/Growth/Weight History reference sheet on page 129.

Nutrition Related Activities of Daily Living and Instrumental Activities of Daily Living

Examples of the measurement methods or data sources for these outcome indicators: Self-report, caregiver report, home visit, surveys, monitoring devices, ADL and/or IADL measurement tool, meal site attendance records

Typically used with the following domains of nutrition interventions: Food and/or nutrient delivery, coordination of nutrition care by nutrition professional

Typically used to determine and monitor and evaluate change in the following nutrition diagnoses: Inability to manage self care, impaired ability to prepare foods/meals, self feeding difficulty

Note: Judgment must be used to select indicators and determine the appropriate measurement techniques and reference standards for a given client population and setting. Once identified, these indicators, measurement techniques, and reference standards should be identified in policies and procedures or other documents for use in client records, quality or performance improvement, or in formal research projects.

Client Example

Example(s) of one or two of the nutrition care indicators (includes sample initial and reassessment documentation for one of the indicators)

Indicator(s) Selected

Ability to prepare meals (able, able with difficulty, unable)

Criteria for Evaluation

Comparison to reference standard, recommendation, or goal:

1. Reference standard: ADL and IADL tools that are validated.
2. Recommendation: Able to prepare meals.
3. Goal: Client's short-term goal is to complete meal preparation 2 days per week.

Sample Nutrition Assessment and Monitoring and Evaluation Documentation	
Initial encounter	Client with difficulty performing ADLs and IADLs due to illness. Client goal is to complete meal preparation 2 days per week and use community resource, senior center meals, five times per week.
Reassessment after nutrition intervention	Client meeting goal to prepare meals 2 days per week and attending community resource senior center for remaining meals. Will work on preparing meals 3 days per week with senior center meals 4 days per week. Will reassess at next encounter.

Physical Activity

Definition

Level of physical activity and/or amount of exercise performed.

Nutrition Assessment and Monitoring and Evaluation

Indicators

- Physical activity history (e.g, activities, preferences, attitudes)
- Consistency (yes/no)
- Frequency (number times/week)
- Duration (number minutes/session, number of total minutes/day)
- Intensity (e.g., talk test, Borg Rating of Perceived Exertion, % of predetermined max heart rate)
- Type of physical activity (e.g., cardiovascular, muscular strength/endurance, flexibility; lifestyle, programmed)
- Strength (e.g., handgrip strength or other muscle strength measure)
- Handgrip strength (normal, measurably reduced) defined as a proxy measure of upper extremity muscle function
- TV/screen time (minutes/day)
- Other sedentary activity time (e.g., commuting; sitting at desk, in meetings, at sporting or arts events) (minutes/day)
- Involuntary physical movement (present/absent)
- Non exercise activity thermogensis (NEAT) (present/absent, level)

Examples of the measurement methods or data sources for these outcome indicators: History interview/ questionnaire, physical activity log, step counter, accelerometer, attendance at strength training, balance training (for older adults), and/or aerobic classes, caretaker records, medical record, dynamometer

Typically used with the following domains of nutrition interventions: Nutrition education, nutrition counseling

Typically used to determine and monitor and evaluate change in the following nutrition diagnoses: Physical inactivity, excessive exercise, underweight, overweight/obesity, unintended weight loss or weight gain

Note: Judgment must be used to select indicators and determine the appropriate measurement techniques and reference standards for a given client population and setting. Once identified, these indicators, measurement techniques, and reference standards should be identified in policies and procedures or other documents for use in client records, quality or performance improvement, or in formal research projects.

Evaluation

Criteria for Evaluation

Comparison to goal or reference standard:

1. Goal (tailored to patient/client's needs)
   OR
2. Reference standard

Physical Activity

Client Example

Example(s) of one or two of the nutrition care indicators (includes sample initial and reassessment documentation for one of the indicators)

Indicator(s) Selected

Consistency and duration

Criteria for Evaluation

Comparison to goal or reference standard:

1. Goal: Patient/client typically walks approximately 10 minutes, twice per week. Patient/client goal is to walk approximately 15 minutes, 5 days per week.
   OR
2. Reference standard: Patient/client's typical 10-minute walk, twice a week is well below the recommended at least 30 minutes of moderate-intensity physical activity (in bouts 10 minutes or longer), 5 days per week or at least 20 minutes of vigorous intensity physical activity (in bouts 10 minutes or longer), 3 days per week (American College of Sports Medicine [ACSM]/American Heart Association [AHA] Recommendations: Physical Activity and Public Health for adults and seniors)

Sample Nutrition Assessment and Monitoring and Evaluation Documentation	
Initial encounter with patient/client	Based on exercise log, patient/client doing moderate intensity physical activities 30 minutes/day, 2 days/week. Goal is to do at least 30 minutes/day (in bouts 10 minutes or longer), moderate-intensity activities, 5 or more days/wk. Will monitor physical activity level at next appointment.
Reassessment after nutrition intervention	Significant progress toward goal of exercising at 30 minutes/day, moderate intensity activities, 5 or more days/wk. Patient/client reports doing moderate-intensity activities 30 minutes per day, 4 days/week.

Factors Affecting Access to Physical Activity

Definition

Factors influencing access to physical activity opportunities and physical activity participation.

Nutrition Assessment and Monitoring and Evaluation

Indicators

- Perceived neighborhood safety(self-rated on scale of 1 to 10; 1 = unsafe to 10 = safe)—defined as the client's perception of crime and traffic, presence of gangs, witness to physical attacks, presence of community members walking or playing outside, and feeling it is safe to walk outside
- Perceived walkability of neighborhood (self-rated on a scale of 1 to 10; 1 = not walkable to 10 = very walkable)—defined as the client's perception of their ability to walk in a neighborhood related to street connectivity, road type, dwelling density, and land use attributes (ie, residential, commercial, institutional or industrial land use)
- Perceived proximity to parks (self-rated on a scale of 1 to 10; 1 = large distance to nearest park/green space to 10 = small distance to nearest park)—defined as the client's perception of the distance from the client's home/workplace to the nearest park
- Access to physical activity facility (self-rated on a scale of 1 to 10; 1 = no availability of facility to 10 = excellent availability of facility)—defined as the client's perception of the availability of a physical activity facility in the client's environment

Note: Physical disability, mobility, and socioeconomic factors affecting physical activity can be documented in the Personal Data and Social History reference sheets on pages 168 and 176, respectively.

Examples of the measurement methods or data sources for these outcome indicators: Client perception, neighborhood crime statistics, neighborhood traffic statistics, geographic information systems data to map a neighborhood, availability of retail establishments within walking distance

Typically used with the following domains of nutrition interventions: Nutrition education, nutrition counseling and coordination of care, population based nutrition action

Typically used to determine and monitor and evaluate change in the following nutrition diagnoses: overweight/obesity, physical inactivity, not ready for nutrition related behavior change

Note: Judgment must be used to select indicators and determine the appropriate measurement techniques and reference standards for a given client population and setting. Once identified, these indicators, measurement techniques, and reference standards should be identified in policies and procedures or other documents for use in client records, quality or performance improvement, or in formal research projects.

Client Example

Example(s) of one of the nutrition care indicators (includes sample initial and reassessment documentation for one of the indicators)

Indicator(s) Selected

Perceived neighborhood safety

Factors Affecting Access to Physical Activity

Criteria for Evaluation

Comparison to goal or reference standard, recommendation, or goal:

1. Reference standard: Not applicable
2. Recommendation: Not applicable
3. Goal: Client perceived neighborhood safety is 2 when increased physical activity in neighborhood is client's goal.

Sample Nutrition Assessment and Monitoring and Evaluation Documentation	
Initial encounter	Client's perceived neighborhood safety is rating of a 2 out of 10 for an individual to engage in outdoor exercise alone because of environmental factors (eg, crime, traffic, gang presence, witness to physical attack). This has limited ability to adhere to goal of increasing physical activity.
Reassessment after nutrition intervention	Client has joined a neighborhood outdoor exercise group and the perceived neighborhood safety is rated a 7 out of 10 and client has increasing adherence with regular physical activity.

Food and/or Nutrition Quality of Life

Definition

Extent to which the Nutrition Care Process impacts a client's physical, mental, and/or social well-being.

Nutrition Assessment and Monitoring and Evaluation

Indicators

- Food and/or nutrition quality of life responses—defined as the expressed quality of life feeling related to food and/or nutrition
- Primary food and/or nutrition related concern—defined as the main food and/or nutrition matter valued by the client
- Client reported experience measure*—defined as the client's perspective of their care as it relates to food and/or nutrition
- Client reported outcome measure†—defined as outcome data that helps the client assess their health as it relates to food and/or nutrition

Examples of the measurement methods or data sources for these outcome indicators: Nutrition Quality of Life measurement tool, other quality of life tools, client survey

Typically used with the following domains of nutrition interventions: Food and/or nutrient delivery, nutrition education, nutrition counseling, coordination of nutrition care by nutrition professional, population based nutrition action

Typically used to determine and monitor and evaluate change in the following nutrition diagnoses: Poor food and/or nutrition quality of life, inadequate or excessive energy or macronutrient intake, underweight, unintended weight loss, overweight/obesity, unintended weight gain, disordered eating pattern, inability to manage self-care, swallowing difficulty, chewing difficulty, self-feeding difficulty, altered GI function, food insecurity.

Note: Judgment must be used to select indicators and determine the appropriate measurement techniques and reference standards for a given client population and setting. Once identified, these indicators, measurement techniques, and reference standards should be identified in policies and procedures or other documents for use in client records, quality or performance improvement, or in formal research projects.

Client Example

Example(s) of one or two of the nutrition care indicators (includes sample initial and reassessment documentation for one of the indicators)

Indicator(s) Selected

Food and/or nutrition related concern

* If a synonym for the term "client-reported experience measure" is helpful or needed, an approved alternate is "patient-reported experience measure (PREM)."

† If a synonym for the term "Client-reported outcome measure" is helpful or needed, an approved alternate is "patient-reported outcome (PRO)" and/or "patient-reported outcome measure (PROM)"

Food and/or Nutrition Quality of Life

Criteria for Evaluation

Comparison to reference standard, recommendation, or goal:

1. Reference standard: Not applicable
2. Recommendation: Not applicable
3. Goal: New goal identified to increase estimated vegetable serving intake in 24 hours by trying one new vegetable serving per day on 3 of 7 days per week. The goal is to resolve food and/or nutrition related concern of limited food options on kidney disease diet.

Sample Nutrition Assessment and Monitoring and Evaluation Documentation	
Initial encounter	Client's food and/or nutrition related concern is limited food options on diet for kidney disease. Increase estimated vegetable serving intake in 24 hours: Client identified goal that they will try one new vegetable serving per day on 3 of 7 days per week by next encounter in 3 weeks. Will monitor food and/or nutrition related concern in 3 weeks.
Reassessment after nutrition intervention	Goal achieved. Client reports that their food and/or nutrition related concern is lessened. Will continue to monitor and reassess in 3 months.

Body Composition/Growth/Weight History

Definition

Measures of the body, including fat, muscle, and bone components and growth

Nutrition Assessment and Monitoring and Evaluation

Indicators

- Body height—defined as measures of a body's length, typically from head to foot
  - Measured body height (in/cm)—defined as measured standing height
  - Measured body length (in/cm)—defined as measured recumbent length
  - Birth length (in/cm)—defined as measured recumbent length at birth
  - Preamputation measured body height (in/cm)—defined as body height prior to removal of a limb or part of a limb
  - Preamputation estimated body height (in/cm)—defined as estimated body height prior to removal of a limb or part of a limb
  - Estimated body height (in/cm)—defined as estimated body height
  - Stated body height (in/cm)—defined as stated body height
  - Measured peak adult body height (in/cm)—defined as tallest measured height recorded in adulthood
  - Stated peak adult body height (in/cm)—defined as stated body height at age 25
  - Knee height measure (in/cm)—defined as the measured distance from the posterior surface of the thigh, just proximal to the patella, to the sole of the foot when the knee is bent at a 90 degree angle
  - Tibia length measure (cm)—defined as the measured distance from the superomedial edge of the tibia to the inferior edge of the medial malleolus
  - Arm span measure (in/cm)—defined as the measured distance of outstretched arms between the tip of the middle finger to the tip of the other middle finger with arms parallel to the ground
  - Arm demispan measure (cm)—defined as the measured distance from the midline at the sternal notch to the web between the middle and ring fingers along outstretched arm (Mini Nutrition Assessment)
  - Arm halfspan measure (cm)—defined as the measured distance from the midline at the sternal notch to the tip of the middle finger (Mini Nutrition Assessment)
  - Height measurement device—defined as the tool used to measure height or length
- Body weight—defined as measures of a body's mass, heaviness, or lightness of a body
  - Measured body weight (lb, oz, kg, g)—defined as measured body weight
  - Stated body weight (lb, oz, kg, g)—defined as reported body weight
  - Stated peak body weight (lb, kg)—defined as reported maximum body weight
  - Measured peak body weight (lb, kg)—defined as the measured maximum body weight
  - Usual stated body weight (UBW) (lb, oz, kg, g)—defined as the reported body weight that is typical for the individual
  - Usual stated body weight St (UBW) percentage (%)—defined as the calculation using actual body weight divided by usual weight and then multiplied by 100
  - Birth weight (lb, oz, kg, g)—defined as the measured body weight at birth
  - Stated prepregnancy body weight (lb, oz, kg, g)—defined as the reported weight prior to pregnancy
  - Dosing body weight (lb, oz, kg, g)—defined as the calculated body weight that may be used to determine the appropriate dose for medications, enteral nutrition, parenteral nutrition, and intravenous fluids (IVs)

Body Composition/Growth/Weight History

- Estimated dry body weight (lb, oz, kg, g)—defined as the estimated body weight without excess fluid volume (euvolemic)
- Preamputation measured body weight (lb, oz, kg, g)—defined as the measured body weight prior to removal of a limb or part of a limb
- Preamputation estimated body weight (lb, oz, kg, g)—defined as the estimated body weight prior to removal of a limb or part of a limb
- Postamputation measured body weight (lb, oz, kg, g)—defined as the measured body weight after removal of a limb or part of a limb
- Postamputation estimated body weight (lb, oz, kg, g)—defined as the estimated body weight after removal of a limb or part of a limb
- Predialysis body weight (lb, oz, kg, g)—defined as measured body weight prior to dialysis
- Postdialysis body weight (lb, oz, kg, g)—defined as measured body weight after dialysis

- Body frame—defined as an estimate of a body frame based upon height and wrist measure
  - Body frame size (small/medium/large)—defined as calculation using measured wrist circumference and measured height to estimate frame size
  - Wrist joint circumference (in/cm)—defined as the measured circumference of the wrist
- Body weight change—defined as measures of the difference in body weight typically over time
  - Weight gain (lb, kg, oz, g)—defined as the measured increase in body weight over a specified period of time
  - Weight loss (lb, kg, oz, g)—defined as the measured decrease in body weight over a specified period of time
  - Body weight change percentage (%)—defined as the weight change value divided by the original weight and multiplied by 100
  - Measured interdialytic body weight gain (lb, oz, kg, g)—defined as the measured increase in body weight between dialysis treatments
  - Measured interdialytic body weight loss (lb, oz, kg, g)—defined as the measured decrease in body weight between dialysis treatments
  - Measured gestational body weight gain (lb, oz, kg, g)—defined as measured weight increase during pregnancy
  - Measured gestational body weight loss (lb, oz, kg, g)—defined as measured weight decrease during pregnancy
  - Body weight change intent (intentional/unintentional)—defined as the purpose of weight gain or weight loss
- Body mass—defined as measures of a body's or a specific part of a body's weight
  - Body mass index (BMI) (kg/m2)—defined as weight in kilograms divided by the square height in meters
  - BMI prime ratio (ratio)—defined as the ratio of actual BMI to the upper limit BMI of 25
  - Appendicular skeletal muscle mass (SM or ASMM) (kg)—defined as the sum of the lean soft tissue mass of both arms and legs without bone minerals
  - Appendicular skeletal muscle mass index (ASMI) (kg/m^2)—defined as appendicular muscle mass divided by height squared
  - Fat free mass (kg)
  - Fat free mass index (kg/m^2)—defined as lean soft tissue and bone minerals when measured with dual energy x-ray absorptiometry (DXA), fat free mass when measured with bioelectrical impedance analysis (BIA) divided by height squared

Body Composition/Growth/Weight History

- Skeletal muscle mass (kg [DXA or BIA] or cm^2 [CT])—defined as skeletal muscle which can be derived via dual energy x-ray absorptiometry (DXA) bioelectrical impedance analysis (BIA), or computed tomography (CT)
- Skeletal muscle mass index (SMI) (kg/m^2 [DXA or BIA] or cm^2/m^2 [CT])—defined as skeletal muscle area (SMA) divided by height squared; psoas, paraspinal muscles, and abdominal wall muscles can also sometimes be included
- Lean soft tissue mass (LST) (kg)—defined as the sum of body water, total body protein, carbohydrates, nonfat lipids, and soft tissue mineral (fat and bone mineral compartments are excluded)
- Method for assessing muscle mass (eg, bioelectrical impedance analysis [BIA], dual energy X-ray absorptiometry [DXA], computed tomography [CT])

- Growth pattern indices—defined as measures used to monitor growth
  - BMI for age percentile (percentile)—defined as weight in kilograms divided by the square of height in meters at the child's age
  - BMI for age *z* score (*z* score)—defined as the standard deviation score for BMI at the child's age
  - Head occipital-frontal circumference (in/cm)—defined as the largest occipital-frontal circumference
  - Birth head occipital-frontal circumference (in/cm)—defined as the largest occipital-frontal circumference at birth
  - Head occipital-frontal circumference for age percentile (percentile)—defined as attained head circumference at the child's age
  - Head occipital-frontal circumference-for-age *z* score (*z* score)—defined as the standard deviation score for attained head circumference at the child's age
  - Body length for age percentile (percentile)—defined as attained growth in recumbent length at the child's age
  - Body length for age *z* score (*z* score)—defined as the standard deviation score for attained length at the child's age
  - Body stature for age percentile (percentile)—defined as attained growth in standing height at the child's age
  - Stature for age *z* score (*z* score)—defined as the standard deviation score for attained height at the child's age
  - Body weight for length percentile (percentile)—defined as body weight in proportion to attained growth in recumbent length
  - Body weight for length *z* score (*z* score)—defined as the standard deviation score for body weight in proportion to attained growth in recumbent length
  - Body weight for age percentile (percentile)—defined as body weight relative to the child's age
  - Body weight for age *z* score (*z* score)—defined as the standard deviation score for attained body weight at the child's age
  - Body weight for stature percentile (percentile)—defined as body weight in proportion to attained growth in standing height
  - Body weight for stature *z* score (*z* score)—defined as the standard deviation score for body weight in proportion to attained growth in height
  - Mid parental body height comparator (in/cm)—defined as the parental heights used to predict a child's expected adult height percentile
- Body compartment estimates—defined as measures of fat, muscle, and bone components of a body
  - Body fat percentage (%)—defined as the portion of the body attributed to body fat and excludes muscle, fluids, bone, or organs

Body Composition/Growth/Weight History

- Body fat percentage technique—defined as the tool used to estimate body fat
- Body surface area (m^2)—defined as the measured surface area of a human body
- Calculated body surface area (m^2)—defined at the calculated surface area of a human body
- Bone maturation age (years)—defined as the degree of maturation of a child's skeleton
- Bone mineral density t score (t score)—defined as the measure of bone density compared with a relevant standard
- Bone mineral density *z* score (*z* score)—defined as the standard deviation score for the minerals in bone compared with a relevant standard
- Bone mineral density technique—defined as the test to measure bone mineral density
- Mid arm muscle circumference (in/cm/mm)—defined as the measure of the muscle area of the upper arm
- Mid arm muscle circumference percentile (percentile)—defined as the rank of the muscle area of the upper arm
- Triceps skin fold thickness (in/cm/mm)—defined as measure of the fold of skin taken over the tricep muscle
- Triceps skin fold percentile (percentile)—defined as the percentile rank of the skin fold thickness over the tricep muscle
- Triceps skin fold *z* score (*z* score)—defined as the standard deviation score for the skin fold thickness over the tricep muscle
- Waist circumference (in/cm)—defined as the circumference around the waist measured at the umbilicus
- Waist circumference narrowest point (in/cm)—defined as the circumference around the waist measured at the narrowest point
- Waist circumference iliac crest (in/cm)—defined as the circumference around the waist measured at the midpoint between the lower margin of the least palpable rib and the top of the iliac crest
- Hip circumference (in/cm)—defined as the circumference of the hips measure at the widest portion of the buttocks
- Waist to hip ratio (ratio)—defined as the calculated ratio of the measured waist circumference at the iliac crest divided by the measured hip circumference
- Mid upper arm circumference (in/cm/mm)—defined as the circumference of the upper right arm measured between the tip of the shoulder and the tip of the elbow
- Mid upper arm circumference, left arm (in/cm/mm)—defined as the circumference of the upper left arm measured between the tip of the shoulder and the tip of the elbow
- Mid upper arm circumference *z* score (*z* score)—defined as the standard deviation score for mid upper arm circumference
- Waist circumference to body height ratio (ratio)—defined as the calculated ratio of the measured waist circumference at the iliac crest divided by measured body height
- Left calf circumference (cm)
- Right calf circumference (cm)
- Lumbar muscle cross section area (cm^2)—defined as a measure of skeletal muscle area (SMA) at the specified level of the lumbar vertebra
- Muscle thickness (cm)—defined as depth of measured muscle thickness, which is generally measured at the thickest part of the muscle chosen via ultrasound
- Thigh circumference (cm)—defined as thigh girth measurement taken 1 cm below the level of the gluteal fold, perpendicular to the long axis of the thigh

Body Composition/Growth/Weight History

Examples of the measurement methods or data sources for these outcome indicators: Referring health care provider or agency, direct measurement, client report, health record

Typically used with the following domains of nutrition interventions: Food and nutrient delivery, nutrition education, nutrition counseling, coordination of nutrition care by nutrition professional population based nutrition action

Typically used to determine and monitor and evaluate change in the following nutrition diagnoses: Excessive or inadequate intake of energy, fat, protein, carbohydrate, alcohol, and/or mineral intake; underweight, overweight, physical inactivity, excessive exercise, sarcopenia

Client Example

Example(s) of one or two of the nutrition care indicators (includes sample initial and reassessment documentation for one of the indicators)

Indicator(s) Selected

Body mass index (BMI) for age percentile

Criteria for Evaluation

Comparison to reference standard, recommendation, or goal:

1. Reference standard: Child's (> age 3 years) Body mass index (BMI) for age percentile per growth curves has crossed two percentile channels from 50% to 10% in last 6 months.
2. Recommendation: Recommended weight gain of 20 to 30 g per day.
3. Goal: Not applicable

Sample Nutrition Assessment and Monitoring and Evaluation Documentation	
Initial nutrition assessment	Child's Body mass index (BMI) for age percentile per growth curves has crossed two percentile channels from 50% to 10% in last 6 months. Will monitor BMI percentile/age at next encounter.
Reassessment after nutrition intervention	Child's Body mass index (BMI) for age percentile per growth curves is unchanged from baseline measure.

Acid Base Balance

Definition

Balance between acids and bases in the body fluids. The pH (hydrogen ion concentration) of the arterial blood provides an index for the total body acid-base balance.

Nutrition Assessment

Indicators

- pH (number)
- Arterial bicarbonate, HCO_3 (mmol/L)
- Partial pressure of carbon dioxide in arterial blood, $PaCO_2$ (mmHg)
- Partial pressure of oxygen in arterial blood, PaO_2 (mmHg)
- Venous pH (number)
- Venous bicarbonate, CO_2 (mmol/L)

Note: Sodium and chloride can be found on the Electrolyte and Renal Profile reference sheet on page 135.

Examples of the measurement methods or data sources for these outcome indicators: Biochemical measurement, laboratory report

Typically used with the following domains of nutrition interventions: Food and/or nutrient delivery, coordination of nutrition care by nutrition professional

Typically used to determine and monitor and evaluate change in the following nutrition diagnoses: Altered nutrition-related laboratory values

Client Example

Example(s) of one or two of the nutrition care indicators (includes sample initial and reassessment documentation for one of the indicators)

Indicator(s) Selected

pH, serum (number)

Criteria for Evaluation

Comparison to goal or reference standard:

1. Goal: Not generally used
   OR
2. Reference standard: The patient/client pH is 7.48 which is above (above, below, or within expected range) the reference standard (7.35 to 7.45).

	Sample Nutrition Assessment Documentation
Initial nutrition assessment with client	Patient/client's pH is 7.48, which is above expected range. Will monitor change in pH at next arterial blood gas.
Reassessment after nutrition intervention	Significant progress toward reference standard. Patient/client's pH is 7.40, within expected range.

Electrolyte and Renal Profile

Definition

Laboratory measures associated with electrolyte balance and kidney function

Nutrition Assessment and Monitoring and Evaluation

Indicators

- BUN (mg/dL or mmol/L)
- Creatinine (mg/dL or µmol/L)
- BUN: creatinine/ratio (ratio number)
- GFR (mL/min/1.73 m^2)
- Sodium (mEq/L or mmol/L)
- Chloride (mEq/L or mmol/L)
- Potassium (mEq/L or mmol/L)
- Magnesium (mEq/L or mmol/L)
- Calcium, serum (mg/dL or mmol/L)
- Calcium, ionized (mg/dL or mmol/L)
- Phosphorus (mg/dL or mmol/L)
- Serum osmolality (mOsm/kg or mmol/kg)
- Parathyroid hormone (pg/mL or ng/L)

Note: Bicarbonate can be found on the Acid Base Balance reference sheet on page 134.

Serum albumin can be found on the Protein Profile reference sheet on page 152 for adjustment of serum calcium.

Examples of the measurement methods or data sources for these outcome indicators: Biochemical measurement, laboratory report

Typically used with the following domains of nutrition interventions: Food and/or nutrient delivery, coordination of nutrition care by nutrition professional

Typically used to determine and monitor and evaluate change in the following nutrition diagnoses: Excessive or inadequate intake of protein or minerals

Client Example

Example(s) of one or two of the nutrition care indicators (includes sample initial and reassessment documentation for one of the indicators)

Indicator(s) Selected

Potassium (mEq/L)

Criteria for Evaluation

Comparison to goal or reference standard:

1. Goal: A goal of serum K+ 3.5 to 5.5 mEq/L in patient/client on medications that block the renin-angiotensin system
   OR
2. Reference standard: The patient/client's potassium is 2.9 mEq/L, which is below (above, below, within expected range) the expected range (3.5 to 5.0 mEq/L).

Electrolyte and Renal Profile

Sample Nutrition Assessment and Monitoring and Evaluation Documentation	
Initial nutrition assessment with client	Patient/client's serum potassium is 2.9 mEq/L, which is below the expected range. Will monitor change in potassium at next encounter.
Reassessment after nutrition intervention	Regression from reference standard. Patient/client's potassium is 2.7 mEq/L, below the expected range.

Essential Fatty Acid Profile

Definition

Laboratory measures of essential fatty acids

Nutrition Assessment and Monitoring and Evaluation

Indicators

- Triene:tetraene ratio (ratio number)

Examples of the measurement methods or data sources for these outcome indicators: Biochemical measurement, laboratory report/record

Typically used with the following domains of nutrition interventions: Food and/or nutrient delivery, coordination of nutrition care by nutrition professional

Typically used to determine and monitor and evaluate change in the following nutrition diagnoses: Inadequate intake of fat, parenteral nutrition; parenteral nutrition composition inconsistent with needs; parenteral nutrition administration inconsistent with needs; altered nutrition-related laboratory values; impaired nutrient utilization

> *Note:* Judgment must be used to select indicators and determine the appropriate measurement techniques and reference standards for a given client population and setting. Once identified, these indicators, measurement techniques, and reference standards should be identified in policies and procedures or other documents for use in client records, quality or performance improvement, or in formal research projects.

Evaluation

Criteria for Evaluation

Comparison to goal or reference standard:

1. Goal (tailored to patient/client's needs)
   OR
2. Reference standard

Client Example

Example(s) of one or two of the nutrition care indicators (includes sample initial and reassessment documentation for one of the indicators)

Indicator(s) Selected

Triene:tetraene ratio (ratio number)

Criteria for Evaluation

Comparison to goal or reference standard:

1. Goal: Not generally used
   OR
2. Reference standard: The patient/client triene:tetraene ratio is 0.45, which is (above, below, or within expected range) above expected range (> 0.2 to 0.4 essential fatty acid deficiency).

Essential Fatty Acid Profile

Sample Nutrition Assessment and Monitoring and Evaluation Documentation	
Initial nutrition assessment with client	Patient/client's triene:tetraene ratio is 0.45, above the expected range (essential fatty acid deficiency). Will monitor change in triene:tetraene ratio at next encounter.
Reassessment after nutrition intervention	Significant progress toward the expect range. Patient/client's triene:tetraene ratio is 0.1.

Gastrointestinal Profile

Definition

Laboratory measures and medical tests associated with function of the gastrointestinal tract and related organs

Nutrition Assessment and Monitoring and Evaluation

Indicators

- Alkaline phosphatase (U/L)
- ALT (U/L)
- AST (U/L)
- Gamma glutamyl transferase (GGT) (U/L)
- Gastric residual volume (mL)
- Bilirubin, total (mg/dL or µmol/L)
- Ammonia, serum (µg/dL or µmol/L)
- Toxicology report, including alcohol (by report)
- Prothrombin time (PT) (seconds)
- Partial thromboplastin time (PTT) (seconds)
- INR ratio (ratio)
- Amylase (U/L)
- Lipase (U/L)
- Fecal fat, 24 hour (g/24 hours)
- Fecal fat, 72 hour (g/24 hours)
- Fecal fat, qualitative (by report)
- Fecal calprotectin (µg/g stool)
- Fecal lactoferrin (ordinal)
- Pancreatic elastase (µg/g stool)
- 5'-nucleotidase (U/L)
- D-xylose (mg/dL)
- Lactulose hydrogen breath test (ppm above baseline/by report)
- Lactose hydrogen breath test (ppm above baseline/by report)
- Fructose hydrogen breath test (ppm above baseline/by report)
- Glucose hydrogen breath test (ppm above baseline/by report)
- Urea hydrogen breath test (ppm above baseline/by report)
- Intestinal biopsy (by report)
- Stool culture (by report)
- Gastric emptying time (minutes)
- Small bowel transit time (minutes, hours)
- Abdominal x-ray (by report)
- Abdominal CT (computed tomography) (by report)
- Abdominal ultrasound (by report)
- Endoscopic ultrasound (by report)
- Pelvic CT (computed tomography) (by report)
- Modified barium swallow (by report)
- Barium swallow (by report)
- Esophagogastroduodenoscopy (by report)
- Endoscopic retrograde cholangiopancreatography (ERCP) (by report)
- Capsule endoscopy (by report)
- Esophageal manometry (by report)
- Esophageal pH test (pH)
- Gastroesophageal reflux monitoring (by report)
- Gastrointestinal sphincter monitoring (by report)
- Urate (mg/dL or µmol/L)

Examples of the measurement methods or data sources for these outcome indicators: Biochemical measurement, laboratory report

Typically used with the following domains of nutrition interventions: Food and/or nutrient delivery, nutrition education, nutrition counseling

Typically used to determine and monitor and evaluate change in the following nutrition diagnoses: Altered nutrition-related laboratory values, excess intake of protein or fat

Gastrointestinal Profile

Note: Judgment must be used to select indicators and determine the appropriate measurement techniques and reference standards for a given client population and setting. Once identified, these indicators, measurement techniques, and reference standards should be identified in policies and procedures or other documents for use in client records, quality or performance improvement, or in formal research projects.

Client Example

Example(s) of one or two of the nutrition care indicators (includes sample initial and reassessment documentation for one of the indicators)

Indicator(s) Selected

Ammonia, serum (µg/dL)

Criteria for Evaluation

Comparison to reference standard, recommendation, or goal

1. Reference standard: The client serum ammonia is 85 µg/dL which is above (above, below, or percent of) the expected range (11 to 35 µg/dL).
2. Recommendation: Not applicable
3. Goal: Not applicable

Sample Nutrition Assessment and Monitoring and Evaluation Documentation	
Initial nutrition assessment with client	Client's serum ammonia is 85 µg/dL, above the reference standard. Will monitor change in serum ammonia at next encounter.
Reassessment after nutrition intervention	Still above reference standard. Client's serum ammonia 45 µg/dL.

Glucose/Endocrine Profile

Definition

Laboratory measures associated with glycemic control and endocrine findings.

Nutrition Assessment and Monitoring and Evaluation

Indicators

- Glucose, fasting (mg/dL, mmol/L)
- Glucose, casual* (mg/dL, mmol/L)
- HgbA1c (%, mmol/mol)
- Preprandial capillary plasma glucose (mg/dL, mmol/L)
- Peak postprandial capillary plasma glucose (mg/dL, mmol/L)
- Glucose tolerance test (mg/dL, mmol/L)
- Cortisol level (μg/dL, mmol/L)
- IGF binding protein (ng/mL, mg/L)
- Thyroid stimulating hormone (μmol/mL, mIU/L)
- Thyroxine test or T4 (ng/dL, pmol/L)
- Triiodothyronine or T3 (ng/dL, pmol/L)
- Adrenocorticotropic hormone (pg/mL, pmol/L)
- Follicle stimulating hormone (mU/mL, IU/L)
- Growth hormone (ng/mL, μg/L)
- Luteinizing hormone (mU/mL, IU/L)

Examples of the measurement methods or data sources for these outcome indicators: Biochemical measurement, laboratory report

Typically used with the following domains of nutrition interventions: Biochemical measurement, laboratory report

Typically used to determine and monitor and evaluate change in the following nutrition diagnoses: Excessive or inadequate intake of carbohydrate, energy; intake of types of carbohydrate inconsistent with needs; inconsistent carbohydrate intake

Note: Judgment must be used to select indicators and determine the appropriate measurement techniques and reference standards for a given client population and setting. Once identified, these indicators, measurement techniques, and reference standards should be identified in policies and procedures or other documents for use in client records, quality or performance improvement, or in formal research projects.

Client Example

Example(s) of one or two of the nutrition care indicators (includes sample initial and reassessment documentation for one of the indicators)

Indicator(s) Selected

HgbA1c (%, mmol/mol)

---

* If a synonym for the term "glucose, casual" is helpful or needed, an approved alternative is "glucose, random."

Glucose/Endocrine Profile

Criteria for Evaluation

Comparison to goal or reference standard:

1. Goal: The client's HgbA1c is 7.8% (60 mmol/mol), which is above the expected limit, but is an acceptable goal in a pediatric patient.
   OR
2. Reference standard: The client's HgbA1c is 11% (97 mmol/mol), which is above (above, below, expected limit or range) the expected limit (< 6%, 42 mmol/mol).

Sample Nutrition Assessment and Monitoring and Evaluation Documentation	
Initial nutrition assessment with client	Client's HgbA1c is 9% (75 mmol/mol), which is above the expected limit. Will monitor change in HgbA1c at next encounter.
Reassessment after nutrition intervention	Regression from the expected limit. Patient/client's HgbA1c is 10% (86 mmol/mol).

Inflammatory Profile

Definition

Laboratory measures of inflammatory proteins.

Nutrition Assessment

Indicators

- C reactive protein, (mg/L) (cardiovascular disease)

Examples of the measurement methods or data sources for these outcome indicators: Direct measurement, medical record

Typically used with the following domains of nutrition interventions: Food and/or nutrient delivery

Typically used with the following domains of nutrition interventions: Increased nutrient need; less than optimal intake of types of fats inconsistent with needs; excessive physical activity

Note: Judgment must be used to select indicators and determine the appropriate measurement techniques and reference standards for a given client population and setting. Once identified, these indicators, measurement techniques, and reference standards should be identified in policies and procedures or other documents for use in client records, quality or performance improvement, or in formal research projects.

Client Example

Example(s) of one or two of the nutrition care indicators (includes sample initial and reassessment documentation for one of the indicators)

Indicator(s) Selected

C reactive protein (mg/L)

Criteria for Evaluation

Comparison to reference standard, recommendation, or goal:

1. Reference standard: A client has a C reactive protein level of 4.0 mg/L, which is above (above, below, within expected range) the reference standard of 1.0 to 3.0 mg/L.
2. Recommendation: Not applicable
3. Goal: Not applicable

Sample Nutrition Assessment and Monitoring and Evaluation Documentation	
Nutrition assessment	Client's C reactive protein level is 4.0 mg/L, which is above (above, below, within expected range) the reference standard of 1.0 to 3.0 mg/L.

Lipid Profile

Definition

Laboratory measures associated with lipid disorders.

Nutrition Assessment and Monitoring and Evaluation

Indicators

- Cholesterol, serum (mg/dL or mmol/L)
- Cholesterol, HDL (mg/dL or mmol/L)
- Cholesterol, LDL (mg/dL or mmol/L)
- Cholesterol, non-HDL (mg/dL or mmol/L)
- Total cholesterol:HDL cholesterol (ratio)
- LDL:HDL (ratio)
- Triglycerides, serum (mg/ dL or mmol/L)

Examples of the measurement methods or data sources for these outcome indicators: Biochemical measurement, laboratory report, patient/client report

Typically used with the following domains of nutrition interventions: Nutrition education, nutrition counseling

Typically used to determine and monitor and evaluate change in the following nutrition diagnoses: Excessive or inadequate intake of fat, energy

> *Note:* Judgment must be used to select indicators and determine the appropriate measurement techniques and reference standards for a given client population and setting. Once identified, these indicators, measurement techniques, and reference standards should be identified in policies and procedures or other documents for use in client records, quality or performance improvement, or in formal research projects.

Evaluation

Criteria for Evaluation

Comparison to goal or reference standard:

1. Goal (tailored to patient/client's needs)
   OR
2. Reference standard

Client Example

Example(s) of one or two of the nutrition care indicators (includes sample initial and reassessment documentation for one of the indicators)

Indicator(s) Selected

LDL cholesterol (mg/dL)

Lipid Profile

Criteria for Evaluation

Comparison to goal or reference standard:

1. Goal: The patient/client's LDL cholesterol is 200 mg/dL, compared to a goal of < 100 mg/dL. (Note: While reference standards are generally used for laboratory measures, a goal might be used in a special situation such as this example. The patient/client has a familial hypercholesterolemia where a normal reference standard may not be realistic.)
   OR
2. Reference standard: The patient/client's LDL cholesterol is 159 mg/dL, which is above the expected limit of the National Heart, Lung, and Blood Institute (NHLBI) recommendation of < 100 mg/dL.

Sample Nutrition Assessment and Monitoring and Evaluation Documentation	
Initial nutrition assessment with client	The patient/client LDL cholesterol is 159 mg/dL compared to the reference standard (eg, NHLBI) recommended level of < 100 mg/dL. Will monitor LDL cholesterol at next encounter.
Reassessment after nutrition intervention	Some progress toward goal/reference standard as patient/client's LDL cholesterol is 145 mg/dL.

Metabolic Rate Profile

Definition

Measures associated with or having implications for assessing metabolic rate.

Nutrition Assessment and Monitoring and Evaluation

Indicators

- RMR, measured (calories, kcal or kJ/day)
- Respiratory quotient, measured (RQ = CO2 produced/O2 consumed)

Note: Use of RQ is considered valid if respiratory factors (hyper- or hypoventilation), equipment failure, measurement protocol violations, or operator errors have not occurred.

Examples of the measurement methods or data sources for these outcome indicators: Direct measurement (indirect calorimetry), medical record

Typically used with the following domains of nutrition interventions: Food and/or nutrient delivery

Typically used to determine and monitor and evaluate change in the following nutrition diagnoses:- Excessive or inadequate intake of parenteral/enteral nutrition; enteral/parenteral nutrition composition or administration inconsistent with needs; excessive energy intake; excessive mineral intake; disordered eating pattern; excessive exercise, increased energy expenditure, increased nutrient needs (energy), inadequate protein-energy intake.

Note: Judgment must be used to select indicators and determine the appropriate measurement techniques and reference standards for a given client population and setting. Once identified, these indicators, measurement techniques, and reference standards should be identified in policies and procedures or other documents for use in client records, quality or performance improvement, or in formal research projects.

Client Example

Example of one (or more) of the nutrition care indicators (includes sample initial and reassessment documentation for one of the indicators)

Indicator(s) Selected

Respiratory quotient

Criteria for Evaluation

Comparison to reference standard, recommendation, or goal:

1. Reference standard: A client on parenteral nutrition support with an RQ of 1.04, which is above (above, below, within expected range) the expected range (0.7 to 1.0) with no apparent errors in the measurement
2. Recommendation: Not applicable
3. Goal: Not applicable

Metabolic Rate Profile

Sample Nutrition Assessment and Monitoring and Evaluation Documentation	
Initial encounter	Client's RQ is 1.04, with energy intake from parenteral nutrition 400 kcal (1,700 kJ) higher than measured metabolic rate. No apparent respiratory factors (hyper- or hypoventilation), equipment failure, measurement protocol violations, or operator errors. Will adjust content of parenteral nutrition and remeasure RQ.
Reassessment after nutrition intervention	RQ has dropped to 0.92 with no apparent measurement error. Metabolic rate and calorie/kcal/kJ intake are matched. Parenteral nutrition has been appropriately adjusted to equal client's energy requirement.

Mineral Profile

Definition

Laboratory measures associated with body mineral status.

Nutrition Assessment and Monitoring and Evaluation

Indicators

- Copper, serum or plasma (µg/dL or µmol/L)
- Iodine, urinary excretion (µg/24hr)
- Zinc, serum or plasma (µg/dL or µmol/L)
- Boron, serum or plasma (µg/L)
- Chromium, serum (ng/mL or nmol/L), urinary (µg/L)
- Fluoride, plasma (µmol/L)
- Manganese, urinary excretion (µg/L or nmol/L), blood (µg/L or nmol/L), plasma (µg/L or nmol/L
- Molybdenum, serum (ng/mL)
- Selenium, serum (µmol/L), urinary excretion (µg/L or µg/day)

Note: Other measures of body mineral status, such as urinary manganese excretion, are provided to offer complete information in the reference sheet. These are rarely used in practice but may be warranted in limited circumstances.

Serum calcium, magnesium, phosphorus, and potassium can be found on the Electrolyte and Renal Profile reference sheet on page 135.

Serum iron, serum ferritin, and transferrin saturation can be found on the Nutritional Anemia Profile reference sheet on page 150.

Thyroid stimulating hormone (↑ TSH as an indicator of excess iodine supplementation) can be found on the Glucose/Endocrine Profile reference sheet on page 141.

Examples of the measurement methods or data sources for these outcome indicators: Biochemical measurement, laboratory record

Typically used with the following domains of nutrition interventions: Food and/or nutrient delivery, nutrition education, nutrition counseling

Typically used to determine and monitor and evaluate change in the following nutrition diagnoses: Excessive or inadequate intake of minerals, parenteral nutrition

Note: Judgment must be used to select indicators and determine the appropriate measurement techniques and reference standards for a given client population and setting. Once identified, these indicators, measurement techniques, and reference standards should be identified in policies and procedures or other documents for use in client records, quality or performance improvement, or in formal research projects.

Mineral Profile

Evaluation

Criteria for Evaluation

Comparison to goal or reference standard:

1. Goal (tailored to patient/client's needs)
   OR
2. Reference standard

Client Example

Example(s) of one or two of the nutrition care indicators (includes sample initial and reassessment documentation for one of the indicators)

Indicator(s) Selected

Zinc, plasma (μg/dL)

Criteria for Evaluation

Comparison to goal or reference standard:

1. Goal: There is no goal generally associated with mineral status.
   OR
2. Reference standard: The patient/client's plasma zinc is 40 μg/dL, which is below (above, below, within expected range) the expected range (66 to 110 μg/dL) for adults.

Sample Nutrition Assessment and Monitoring and Evaluation Documentation	
Initial nutrition assessment with client	Patient/client's plasma zinc is 40 μg/dL, which is below the expected range for adults. Will monitor change in plasma zinc at next encounter.
Reassessment after nutrition intervention	Goal/reference standard achieved as patient/client's plasma zinc is 90 μg/dL.

Nutritional Anemia Profile

Definition

Laboratory measures associated with nutritional anemias

Nutrition Assessment and Monitoring and Evaluation

Indicators

- Hemoglobin (g/dL g/L or mmol/L)
- Hematocrit (% or proportion of 1)
- Mean corpuscular volume (MCV) (fL)
- Red blood cell (RBC) folate (ng/mL or nmol/L)
- Red cell distribution width (RDW) (%)
- Serum B12 (pg/mL or pmol/L)
- Methylmalonic acid, serum (nmol/L)
- Serum folate (ng/mL or nmol/L)
- Serum homocysteine (μmol/L)
- Serum ferritin (ng/mL or pmol/L
- Serum iron (μg/dL or μmol/L)
- Total iron-binding capacity (TIBC) (μg/dL or μmol/L)
- Transferrin saturation (%)

Examples of the measurement methods or data sources for these outcome indicators: Biochemical measurement, patient/client laboratory record; national/state/local nutrition monitoring and surveillance data

Typically used with the following domains of nutrition interventions: Food and/or nutrient delivery, nutrition education, nutrition counseling, coordination of nutrition care by nutrition professional

Typically used to determine and monitor and evaluate change in the following nutrition diagnoses: Excessive or inadequate intake of vitamins or minerals (eg, iron, B12, folate); altered nutrition-related laboratory values; impaired nutrient utilization

Note: Judgment must be used to select indicators and determine the appropriate measurement techniques and reference standards for a given client population and setting. Once identified, these indicators, measurement techniques, and reference standards should be identified in policies and procedures or other documents for use in client records, quality or performance improvement, or in formal research projects.

Evaluation

Criteria for Evaluation

Comparison to goal or reference standard:

1. Goal (tailored to patient/client's needs)
   OR
2. Reference standard

Nutritional Anemia Profile

Client Example

Example(s) of one or two of the nutrition care indicators (includes sample initial and reassessment documentation for one of the indicators)

Indicator(s) Selected

Hemoglobin (gm/dL)
Serum ferritin (ng/mL)

Criteria for Evaluation

Comparison to goal or reference standard

1. Goal: The patient/client's hemoglobin and hematocrit are below the expected limits for adult males but are within the goal range for a patient/client receiving hemodialysis.
   OR
2. Reference standard: The patient/client's serum ferritin is 8 ng/mL, which is below (above, below, or within expected range) the expected range for adult females.

Sample Nutrition Assessment and Monitoring and Evaluation Documentation	
Initial nutrition assessment with client	Patient/client's serum ferritin is 8 ng/mL, which is below the expected range for adult females. Will monitor change in serum ferritin at next encounter.
Reassessment after nutrition intervention	Patient/client's serum ferritin is 10.9 ng/mL, within the expected range.

Protein Profile

Definition

Laboratory measures associated with hepatic and circulating proteins and protein metabolism.

Nutrition Assessment and Monitoring and Evaluation

- Albumin (g/dL or g/L)
- Prealbumin (mg/dL or mg/L)
- Transferrin (mg/dL or g/L)
- Phenylalanine, plasma (mg/dL or µmol/L)
- Tyrosine, plasma (mg/dL or µmol/L)
- Amino acid panel (by report)
- Phenylalanine, dried blood spot (ordinal)
- Tyrosine, dried blood spot (ordinal)
- Phenylalanine:tyrosine ratio (ratio)
- Hydroxyproline (mg/dL or µmol/L)
- Threonine (mg/dL or µmol/L)
- Serine (mg/dL or µmol/L)
- Asparagine (mg/dL or µmol/L)
- Glutamate (mg/dL or µmol/L)
- Glutamine (mg/dL or µmol/L)
- Proline (mg/dL or µmol/L)
- Glycine (mg/dL or µmol/L)
- Alanine (mg/dL or µmol/L)
- Citrulline (mg/dL or µmol/L)
- Valine (mg/dL or µmol/L)
- Cysteine (mg/dL or µmol/L)
- Methionine (mg/dL or µmol/L)
- Isoleucine (mg/dL or µmol/L)
- Leucine (mg/dL or µmol/L)
- Ornithine (mg/dL or µmol/L)
- Lysine (mg/dL or µmol/L)
- Histidine (mg/dL or µmol/L)
- Arginine (mg/dL or µmol/L)
- Lysine:arginine ratio (ratio)
- Tryptophan, plasma or serum
- Plasma organic acid panel (by report)
- Organic acids/creatinine (mmol/mol creatinine)
- 3 hydroxybutyrate (mg/dL or µmol/L)
- 3 hydroxyisovalerate (mg/dL or µmol/L)
- Acetoacetate (mg/dL or µmol/L)
- Ethylmalonate (mg/dL or µmol/L)
- Succinate (mg/dL or µmol/L)
- Fumarate (mg/dL or µmol/L)
- Glutarate (ng/dL or nmol/L)
- 3 methylglutarate (mg/dL or µmol/L)
- Adipate (mg/dL or µmol/L)
- 2 hydroxyglutarate (mg/dL or µmol/L)
- 3 hydroxypheylacetate (mg/dL or µmol/L)
- 2 ketoglutarate (mg/dL or µmol/L)
- Citrate (mg/dL or µmol/L)
- Propionate (mg/dL or µmol/L)
- Methylcitrate (mg/dL or µmol/L)
- 3 hydroxy propionate (mg/dL or µmol/L)
- Beta hydroxy butyrate (mg/dL or µmol/L)
- Creatine kinase (U/L)
- Troponin I. cardiac (ng/mL)
- Troponin T.cardiac (ng/mL)
- B type natriuretic peptide (pg/mL)
- Succinylacetone (mg/dL or µmol/L)
- Total serum immunoglobulin A (IgA) (mg/dL or µmol/L)
- Tissue transglutaminase antibodies (IgA) (U/mL)
- Tissue transglutaminase antibodies (immunoglobulin G [IgG]) (U/mL)
- Deamidated gliadin peptide antibodies (IgG) (U/mL)
- Endomysial antibodies (ordinal)
- Carbohydrate deficient transferrin (mg/dL or %)

Protein Profile

Note: Methylmalonic acid can be found on the Nutritional Anemia Profile reference sheet on page 150. Also, in the past, hepatic transport protein measures (eg, albumin and prealbumin) were used as indicators of malnutrition. See the Evidence Analysis Library questions on this topic at: www.andevidencelibrary.com/topic.cfm?cat=4302

Examples of the measurement methods or data sources for these outcome indicators: Biochemical measurement, laboratory report

Typically used with the following domains of nutrition interventions: Food and/or nutrient delivery, nutrition education, nutrition counseling, coordination of nutrition care by nutrition professional

Typically used to determine and monitor and evaluate change in the following nutrition diagnoses: Increased nutrient needs, malnutrition, inadequate enteral/parenteral nutrition infusion

Note: Judgment must be used to select indicators and determine the appropriate measurement techniques and reference standards for a given client population and setting. Once identified, these indicators, measurement techniques, and reference standards should be identified in policies and procedures or other documents for use in client records, quality or performance improvement, or in formal research projects.

Client Example

Example(s) of one or two of the nutrition care indicators (includes sample initial and reassessment documentation for one of the indicators)

Indicator(s) Selected]

Prealbumin (mg/dL)

Criteria for Evaluation

Comparison to reference standard, recommendation, or goal:

1. Reference standard: The client's prealbumin is 7 mg/dL, which is below (above, below, or within the expected range) the reference standard (16 to 40 mg/dL) for adults.
2. Recommendation: Not applicable
3. Goal: Not applicable

Sample Nutrition Assessment and Monitoring and Evaluation Documentation	
Initial nutrition assessment	Client's prealbumin is 7.0 mg/dL, below the reference standard (16 to 40 mg/dL) for adults. Will monitor change in prealbumin at next encounter.
Reassessment after nutrition intervention	Significant progress toward expected range as client's serum prealbumin is 13.0 mg/dL.

Urine Profile

Definition

Physical and/or chemical properties of urine.

Nutrition Assessment and Monitoring and Evaluation

Indicators

- Urine color (by visualization)
- Urine osmolality (mOsm/kg H2O)
- Urine specific gravity (number)
- Urine volume (mL/24 hours; however, in certain populations, eg, infants, this indicator may be reported in number of wet diapers/day)
- Urine calcium, 24 hour (mg/24 hours or mmol/24hours)
- Urine d-xylose (mg/dL or mmol/L)
- Urine glucose (ordinal)
- Urine ketones (ordinal)
- Urine sodium (mg/dL or mmol/L)
- Urine microalbumin (mg/dL or mmol/L)
- Urine protein, random (mg/dL or mmol/L)
- Urine protein, 24-hour (mg/24 hours or mmol/24 hours)
- Urine uric acid, random (mg/dL or µmol/L)
- Urine uric acid, 24 hour (mg/24 hours or mmol/24 hours)
- Urine organic acid panel (by report)
- Urine glutarate (ordinal)
- Urine methylmalonate (µg/dL)
- Urine acylglycines/creatinine (mg/g creatinine or mmol/mol creatinine)
- Urine argininosuccinate (mmol/L)
- Urine succinylacetone/creatinine (µmol/mmol creatinine)
- Urine orotate (µmol/L)
- Urine orotate/creatinine (µmol/mmol creatinine)
- Urine 2-hydroxyisovalerate (ordinal)
- Urine 2-oxoisovalerate (ordinal)
- Urine galactitol (ordinal)
- Urine reducing substances (ordinal)
- Urine porphyrins (ordinal)
- Urine creatinine, 24 hour (mg/24hours or mmol/24hours)
- Urine citrate, 24 hour (mg/24 hours or mmol/24 hours)
- Urine phosphorus, 24 hour (mg/24 hours or mmol/24 hours)
- Urine pH, random (number)
- Urine pH, 24 hour (number)
- Urine sodium, 24 hour (mEq/24 hours or mmol/24 hours)
- Urine urea nitrogen, 24 hour (mg/24 hours or mmol/24 hours)
- Urine oxalate, 24 hour (mg/24 hours or mmol/24 hours)
- Urine chloride, 24 hour (mEq/24 hours or mmol/24 hours)
- Urine ammonium, 24 hour (mg/24 hours or mmol/24 hours)
- Urine magnesium, 24 hour (mg/24 hours or mmol/24 hours)
- Urine potassium, 24 hour (mEq/24 hours or mmol/24 hours)
- Urine sulfate, 24 hour (mg/24 hours or mmol/24 hours)
- Urine cystine, 24 hour (mg/24 hours or µmol/24 hours)
- Calcium oxalate supersaturation in 24 hour urine (number)
- Calcium phosphate supersaturation in 24 hour urine (number)
- Brushite supersaturation in 24 hour urine (number)
- Uric acid supersaturation in 24 hour urine (number)

Urine Profile

Examples of the measurement methods or data sources for these outcome indicators: Observation, biochemical measurement, laboratory report, client report

Typically used with the following domains of nutrition interventions: Food and/or nutrient delivery, nutrition education, nutrition counseling, coordination of nutrition care by nutrition professional

Typically used to determine and monitor and evaluate change in the following nutrition diagnoses: Inadequate or excessive fluid intake; inadequate or excessive enteral/parenteral nutrition infusion; inadequate or excessive mineral intake; inadequate or excessive bioactive substance intake

Note: Judgment must be used to select indicators and determine the appropriate measurement techniques and reference standards for a given client population and setting. Once identified, these indicators, measurement techniques, and reference standards should be identified in policies and procedures or other documents for use in client records, quality or performance improvement, or in formal research projects.

Client Example

Example(s) of one (or more) of the nutrition care indicators (includes sample initial and reassessment documentation for one of the indicators)

Indicator(s) Selected

Urine specific gravity (number)

Criteria for Evaluation

Comparison to reference standard, recommendation, or goal:

1. Reference standard: The client's urine specific gravity is 1.050, which is above (above, below, within expected range) the expected range (1.003 to 1.030).
2. Recommendation: Not applicable
3. Goal: Not applicable

Sample Nutrition Assessment and Monitoring and Evaluation Documentation	
Initial encounter	Client's urine specific gravity is 1.050, which is above the expected range. Will monitor change in urine specific gravity at next encounter.
Reassessment after nutrition intervention	Significant progress toward goal, client's urine specific gravity is 1.035, which is within the expected range.

Vitamin Profile

Definition

Laboratory measures associated with body vitamin status.

Nutrition Assessment and Monitoring and Evaluation

Indicators

- Vitamin A, serum or plasma retinol (µg/dL or µmol/L)
- Vitamin C, plasma or serum (mg/dL or µmol/L)
- Vitamin D, 25 hydroxy (ng/mL or nmol/L)
- Vitamin E plasma alpha-tocopherol (mg/dL or µmol/L)
- Thiamin, activity coefficient for erythrocyte transketolase activity (µg/mL/hr)
- Riboflavin, activity coefficient for erythrocyte glutathione reductase activity (IU/g hemoglobin)
- Niacin, urinary N'methyl nicotinamide concentration (µmol/day)
- Vitamin B6, plasma or serum pyridoxal 5'-phosphate concentration (ng/mL or nmol/L)
- Pantothenic acid, urinary pantothenate excretion (mg/day), plasma (ng/mL or nmol/L)
- Biotin, urinary 3 hydroxyisovaleric acid excretion (mmol/mmol creatinine)
- Biotin, lymphocyte propionyl CoA carboxylase in pregnancy [pmol/(min × mg)], serum (ng/mL or nmol/L)
- Biotinidase (U/L)
- Protein induced by vitamin K absence or antagonist II ng/mL or nmol/L)

Note: Other measures of body vitamin status, such as urinary pantothenate excretion, are provided to offer complete information in the reference sheet. These are rarely used in practice but may be warranted in limited circumstances.

Measures for folate and vitamin B12 can be found on the Nutritional Anemia Profile reference sheet on page 150.

Measures related to vitamin K (PT, PTT, INR) can be found on the Gastrointestinal Profile reference sheet on page 139.

A test for choline is not available. According to the Dietary DRIs, it should be evaluated in light of serum alanine amino transferase (ALT) levels which can be found on the Gastrointestinal Profile.

Examples of the measurement methods or data sources for these outcome indicators: Biochemical measurement, client record

Typically used with the following domains of nutrition interventions: Food and/or nutrient delivery, coordination of nutrition care by nutrition professional

Typically used to determine and monitor and evaluate change in the following nutrition diagnoses: Excessive or inadequate intake of vitamins

Note: Judgment must be used to select indicators and determine the appropriate measurement techniques and reference standards for a given client population and setting. Once identified, these indicators, measurement techniques, and reference standards should be identified in policies and procedures or other documents for use in client records, quality or performance improvement, or in formal research projects.

Vitamin Profile

Client Example

Example(s) of one or two of the nutrition care indicators (includes sample initial and reassessment documentation for one of the indicators)

Indicator(s) Selected

Vitamin A, serum retinol (μg/dL)

Criteria for Evaluation

Comparison to reference standard, recommendation, or goal:

1. Reference standard: The client's serum retinol is 95 μg/dL which is above (above, below, within expected range) the reference standard (10 to 60 μg/dL).
2. Recommendation: Not applicable
3. Goal: Not applicable

Sample Nutrition Assessment and Monitoring and Evaluation Documentation	
Initial nutrition assessment	Client's vitamin A, serum retinol is 95 μg/dL, which is above the expected range. Will monitor change in vitamin A, serum retinol at next encounter, along with vitamin A and beta-carotene intake.
Reassessment after nutrition intervention	Significant progress toward reference standard. Client's vitamin A, serum retinol is 70 μg/dL.

Carbohydrate Metabolism Profile

Definition

Laboratory measures associated with carbohydrate metabolism

Nutrition Assessment and Monitoring and Evaluation

Indicators

- Galactose 1 phosphate in red blood cells (mg/dL or μmol/L)
- Galactose 1 phosphate uridyl transferase (U/g Hgb)
- Fructose (mg/dL or μmol/L)
- Lactate (mg/dL or μmol/L)
- Pyruvate (mg/dL or μmol/L)
- Lactate/pyruvate (ratio)

Note: Other measures of metabolic conditions, such as pyruvate, are listed on the Protein Profile reference sheet on page 152.

Examples of the measurement methods or data sources for these outcome indicators: Biochemical measurement, laboratory report, patient/client report

Typically used with the following domains of nutrition interventions: Food and/or nutrient delivery, Nutrition education, Nutrition counseling

Typically used to determine and monitor and evaluate change in the following nutrition diagnoses: Intake of types of carbohydrate inconsistent with needs, Inadequate energy intake

Note: Judgment must be used to select indicators and determine the appropriate measurement techniques and reference standards for a given client population and setting. Once identified, these indicators, measurement techniques, and reference standards should be identified in policies and procedures or other documents for use in client records, quality or performance improvement, or in formal research projects.

Evaluation

Criteria for Evaluation

Comparison to goal or reference standard:

1. Goal (tailored to patient/client's needs)
   OR
2. Reference standard

Client Example

Example(s) of one or two of the nutrition care indicators (includes sample initial and reassessment documentation for one of the indicators)

Indicator(s) Selected

Galactose 1 phosphate in red blood cells (RBC) (mg/dL or μmol/L)

Carbohydrate Metabolism Profile

Criteria for Evaluation

Comparison to goal or reference standard:

1. Goal: The patient/client's galactose-1-phosphate in RBCs is 165 mg/dL, which is above the goal for patients with galactosemia on diet (> 125 mg/dL). (Note: While reference standards are generally used for laboratory measures, a goal might be used in a special situation such as this example where a population reference standard may not be realistic.) OR
2. Reference standard: The patient/client's galactose-1-phosphate in RBCs is 165 mg/dL, which is above the upper limit for patients with galactosemia on diet (>125 mg/dL).

Sample Nutrition Assessment and Monitoring and Evaluation Documentation	
Initial nutrition assessment with client	The patient/client's galactose-1-phosphate in RBCs is 165 mg/dL, which is above the goal for patients with galactosemia on diet (> 125 mg/dL). Will monitor at next encounter.
Reassessment after nutrition intervention	Significant progress toward expected range. Patient/client's galactose-1-phosphate in RBCs is 135 mg/dL

Fatty Acid Profile

Definition

Laboratory measures associated with fatty acid metabolism

Nutrition Assessment and Monitoring and Evaluation

Indicators

- Acylcarnitine panel (μmol/L)
- Acylcarnitine, plasma (μmol/L)
- Free carnitine, plasma (μmol/L)
- Total carnitine, plasma (μmol/L)
- Free carnitine: total carnitine (ratio)
- Fatty acid panel mitochondrial C8-C18, serum or plasma (μmol/L)
- Fatty acid panel essential C12-C22, serum or plasma (μmol/L)
- Fatty acid panel peroxisomal C22-C26, serum or plasma (μmol/L)
- MCAD enzyme assay in fibroblasts or other tissues (confirmatory)
- Fatty acid beta oxidation in fibroblasts (confirmatory)

Examples of the measurement methods or data sources for these outcome indicators: Biochemical measurement, laboratory report, patient/client report

Typically used with the following domains of nutrition interventions: Food and/or nutrient delivery, Nutrition education, Nutrition counseling

Typically used to determine and monitor and evaluate change in the following nutrition diagnoses: Intake of types of fat inconsistent with needs, Inadequate energy intake

> *Note:* Judgment must be used to select indicators and determine the appropriate measurement techniques and reference standards for a given client population and setting. Once identified, these indicators, measurement techniques, and reference standards should be identified in policies and procedures or other documents for use in client records, quality or performance improvement, or in formal research projects.

Evaluation

Criteria for Evaluation

Comparison to goal or reference standard:

1. Goal (tailored to patient/client's needs)
   OR
2. Reference standard

Client Example

Example(s) of one or two of the nutrition care indicators (includes sample initial and reassessment documentation for one of the indicators)

Fatty Acid Profile

Indicator(s) Selected

Fatty acid panel mitochondrial C8-C18 (specifically octanoylcarnitine [C8] and octanoylcarnitine [C8]:decanoylcarnitine [C10] ratio)

Criteria for Evaluation

Comparison to goal or reference standard:

1. Goal: The patient/client's octanoylcarnitine is 0.8 μmol/L, which is above the goal of 0.3 μmol/L and a ratio of octanoylcarnitine:decanoylcarnitine is 10, which is above the goal of 5 for this patient/client with MCAD. (Note: While reference standards are generally used for laboratory measures, a goal might be used in a special situation such as this example where a population reference standard may not be realistic.) OR
2. Reference standard: The patient/client's octanoylcarnitine is 0.8 μmol/L, which is above the expected upper limit (>0.3μmol/L) and ratio of octanoylcarnitine:decanoylcarnitine is 10, which is above the upper limit (>5).

Sample Nutrition Assessment and Monitoring and Evaluation Documentation	
Initial nutrition assessment with client	The patient/client's octanoylcarnitine is 0.8 μmol/L, which is above the reference standard upper limit (>0.3μmol/L) and ratio of octanoylcarnitine:-decanoylcarnitine is 10, which is above the upper limit (>5). Will monitor at next encounter.
Reassessment after nutrition intervention	Significant progress toward expected range. Patient/client's octanoylcarnitine concentration is 0.4, ratio of octanoylcarnitine:decanoylcarnitine is 7.

Nutrition Focused Physical Findings

Definition

Nutrition-related physical signs or symptoms associated with pathophysiological states derived from a nutrition focused physical exam, interview, and/or the health record.

Nutrition Assessment and Monitoring and Evaluation

Indicators

Note: Presence or absence unless otherwise specified.

- Overall finding
  - Asthenia (weakness)
  - Buffalo hump
  - Cachexia
  - Cushingoid appearance
  - Ectomorph
  - Endomorph
  - Lethargic
  - Mesomorph
  - Neglect of personal hygiene
  - Obese
  - Short stature for age
  - Tall stature
  - Body language that may suggest discomfort with interaction (eg, frowning, crossed arms, limited eye contact)
- Adipose finding
  - Atrophy of orbital fat
  - Excess subcutaneous fat
  - Loss of subcutaneous fat
  - Central adiposity
  - Loss of subcutaneous triceps fat
  - Loss of subcutaneous biceps fat
  - Loss of subcutaneous fat overlying the ribs
  - Lipodystrophy
- Bone finding
  - Bowlegs
  - Frontal bossing
  - Harrison's sulcus
  - Rachitic rosary
  - Rickets
  - Scoliosis
  - Acromion abnormal prominence
  - Bone widening at ends
  - Clavicle abnormal prominence
  - Rib abnormal prominence
  - Scapula abnormal prominence
  - Spine abnormal prominence
  - Iliac crest abnormal prominence
  - Patella abnormal prominence
  - Lordosis
- Cardiovascular-pulmonary system finding
  - Absent breath sounds
  - Bradycardia
  - Bradypnea (slow respiration)
  - Decreased breath sounds
  - Dyspnea (shortness of breath)
  - Increased breath sounds
  - Normal breath sounds
  - Tachypnea
  - Tachycardia
  - Respiratory crackles (rales)
  - Decreased functional residual capacity
  - Diaphragmatic weakness (also called diaphragmatic muscle weakness, diaphragmatic paresis)
- Digestive system finding
  - Abdominal bloating
  - Abdominal cramping
  - Abdominal distension
  - Abdominal pain
  - Absence of bowel sounds

Nutrition Focused Physical Findings

  - Mucosal edema
  - Sacral edema
- Extremity finding
  - Amputated foot
  - Amputated hand
  - Amputated leg
  - Athetoid movement
  - Decreased range of ankle movement
  - Decreased range of cervical spine movement
  - Decreased range of elbow movement
  - Decreased range of finger movement
  - Decreased range of foot movement
  - Decreased range of hip movement
  - Decreased range of knee movement
  - Decreased range of lumbar spine movement
  - Decreased range of shoulder movement
  - Decreased range of subtalar movement
  - Decreased range of thumb movement
  - Decreased range of toe movement
  - Decreased range of thoracic spine movement
  - Decreased range of wrist movement
  - Hypertonia
  - Hypotonia
  - Joint arthralgia (joint pain)
  - Lower limb spasticity
  - Peripheral cyanosis
  - Spasticity
  - Tetany
  - Upper limb spasticity
  - Talipes planus
- Eye finding
  - Abnormal vision
  - Angular blepharitis
  - Bitot's spots
  - Circles under eyes
  - Corneal arcus
  - Conjunctival discoloration
  - Conjunctival hemorrhage
  - Conjunctival keratinization
  - Excessive tear production
  - Keratomalacia
  - Jaundiced sclera
  - Night blindness
  - Ophthalmoplegia
  - Sunken eyes
  - Xerophthalmia
  - Xanthelasma
  - Pale conjunctiva
- Genitourinary finding
  - Amenorrhea
  - Anuria
  - Delay in sexual development and/or puberty
  - Menorrhagia
  - Oliguria
  - Polyuria
- Hair finding
  - Abnormal keratinization of hair follicle
  - Alopecia
  - Brittle hair
  - Corkscrew hairs
  - Dry hair
  - Fine hair
  - Follicular hyperkeratosis
  - Hair changes due to malnutrition
  - Hair lacks luster
  - Hypertrichosis
  - Increased loss of hair
  - Nutritional hair color change
  - White hair
  - Easily pluckable hair
  - Lanugo hair formation
- Head finding
  - Altered olfactory sense
  - Anosmia (loss of sense of smell)
  - Bulging fontanelle
  - Epistaxis
  - Headache
  - Hyposmia (decreased sense of smell)

Nutrition Focused Physical Findings

  - Macrocephaly
  - Microcephaly
  - Nasal mucosa dry
  - Sunken fontanelle
- Hand and nail finding
  - Beau's lines
  - Clubbing of nail
  - Flaking of nails
  - Koilonychia (spoon shaped nails)
  - Leukonychia
  - Longitudinal grooving of nails
  - Muehrcke's lines
  - Nail changes
  - Palmar erythema
  - Ridged nails
  - Splits in nails
  - Thin nails
  - Trachyonychia (brittle nails)
  - Splinter hemorrhages under nail
  - White flecks in nails
  - Blue nail bed
  - Pale nail bed
  - Russell's sign
- Mouth finding
  - Ageusia (loss of taste)
  - Angular stomatitis
  - Aphthous ulcer of mouth
  - Aptyalism (xerostomia)
  - Blue lips
  - Blue line on gingiva
  - Candidiasis of the mouth
  - Cheilosis (dry lips)
  - Cheilitis
  - Cleft palate
  - Cracked lips
  - Drooling
  - Dry mucous membranes
  - Dysgeusia
  - Excessive salivation
  - Excessive thirst
  - Gingival hypertrophy
  - Gingivitis
  - Halitosis (breath smells unpleasant)
  - Hemorrhagic gingivitis (bleeding gums)
  - Hypogeusia
  - Ketotic breath
  - Micrognathia
  - Swollen gums
  - Oral candidiasis
  - Oral lesion
  - Parotid swelling
  - Poor oral hygiene
  - Retains food in mouth
  - Stomatitis
  - Uremic breath
  - Pale gums
  - Cleft lip
- Muscle finding
  - Muscle atrophy
  - Muscle contracture
  - Muscle cramp
  - Muscle pain
  - Muscle weakness
  - Quadricep muscle atrophy
  - Deltoid muscle atrophy
  - Gastrocnemius (calf) muscle atrophy
  - Gluteal muscle atrophy
  - Interosseous hand muscle atrophy
  - Pectoral muscle atrophy
  - Temporalis muscle atrophy
  - Trapezius muscle atrophy
  - Latissimus dorsi muscle atrophy
  - Abnormal muscle function—defined as altered muscle activity, independent of muscle mass, where muscle activity is inconsistent with expected physiologic capability (eg, swallowing coordination, diaphragmatic capacity)
  - Loss of muscle function—defined as muscle activity that is reduced compared to a previous assessment and/or a previous functional state

Nutrition Focused Physical Findings

   - Low muscle function—defined as quantitative and qualitative muscle changes that result in functional muscle outcomes that are less than expected
   - Loss of physical performance—defined as muscle power and/or coordination that is reduced compared to a previous ability level
   - Skeletal muscle problem
   - Skeletal muscle power problem
- Neck finding
   - Goiter (thyroid enlargement)
- Nerves, cognition, and feeling finding
   - Abnormal gait
   - Absent reflex
   - Asterixis
   - Ataxia
   - Clouded consciousness (confusion)
   - Cranial nerve finding
   - Decreased vibratory sense
   - Delirious
   - Dementia
   - Depressed mood
   - Disoriented
   - Dizziness
   - Feels cold
   - Flat affect
   - Hyperreflexia (exaggeration of deep reflexes)
   - Hyporeflexia (diminished reflexes)
   - Inappropriate affect
   - Many seizures a day
   - Numbness of foot
   - Numbness of hand
   - Peripheral nerve disease
   - Tremor of outstretched hand
   - Tingling of foot
   - Tingling of hand
- Skin finding
   - Acanthosis nigricans
   - Calcinosis
   - Carotenemia
   - Cutaneous xanthoma
   - Decreased skin turgor
   - Dermatitis
   - Diaper rash
   - Dry skin
   - Ecchymosis
   - Erythema
   - Eczema
   - Flushing
   - Hirsutism
   - Hyperpigmentation of skin
   - Impaired skin integrity
   - Jaundice
   - Keratinization of skin
   - Pale complexion
   - Peeling skin
   - Petechiae
   - Impaired wound healing
   - Pressure injury of ankles
   - Pressure injury of back
   - Pressure injury of breast
   - Pressure injury of buttock
   - Pressure injury of dorsum of foot
   - Pressure injury of elbow
   - Pressure injury of head
   - Pressure injury of heel
   - Pressure injury of hip
   - Pressure injury of knee
   - Pressure injury of natal cleft
   - Pressure injury of shoulder
   - Pressure injury stage 1
   - Pressure injury stage 2
   - Pressure injury stage 3
   - Pressure injury stage 4
   - Pruritus of the skin
   - Psoriasis
   - Scaly skin
   - Seborrheic dermatitis
   - Skin rash

Nutrition Focused Physical Findings

  - Venous stasis ulcer of leg
  - Yellow skin
  - Perifollicular hemorrhages
  - Pressure injury of the coccyx
  - Pressure injury of the sacrum
  - Vesiculobullous rash
  - Acne
  - Intertrigo
  - Excess panniculus of abdomen
  - Skin striae
- Teeth finding
  - Baby bottle tooth decay
  - Broken denture
  - Broken teeth
  - Dental caries
  - Dental fluorosis
  - Dental plaque
  - Denture loose
  - Denture lost
  - Denture present
  - Edentulous
  - Erosion of teeth
  - Impaired dentition
  - Ill fitting denture
  - Mottling of enamel
  - Partially edentulous mandible
  - Partially edentulous maxilla
  - Rampant dental caries
- Throat and swallowing finding
  - Choking during swallowing
  - Cough
  - Dysphagia
  - Esophageal lesion
  - Food sticks on swallowing
  - Gagging
  - Hoarse voice
  - Hypoactive gag reflex
  - Odynophagia (painful swallowing)
  - Swallow impairment
  - Suck/swallow incoordination (infants)
  - Wet voice
- Tongue finding
  - Atrophy of tongue papillae
  - Beefy red tongue
  - Difficulty moving tongue
  - Dry tongue
  - Glossitis
  - Glossodynia (painful tongue)
  - Hypertrophy of tongue papillae
  - Lesion of the tongue
  - Macroglossia
  - Strawberry tongue
  - Short frenulum of tongue
  - Split frenulum of tongue
  - Blue tongue
  - Cracked tongue
  - Magenta tongue
  - Pale tongue
- Vital signs
  - Blood pressure, systolic
  - Blood pressure, diastolic
  - Blood pressure, systolic, reported
  - Blood pressure, diastolic, reported
  - Heart rate
  - Jugular venous pressure
  - Mean arterial pressure
  - Pulse rate
  - Respiratory rate
  - Body temperature

Nutrition Focused Physical Findings

Examples of the measurement methods or data sources for these outcome indicators: Direct observation, client report, health record, physician referral

Typically used with the following domains of nutrition interventions: Food and nutrient delivery, nutrition education, nutrition counseling, coordination of care, population based nutrition action

Typically used to determine and monitor and evaluate change in the following nutrition diagnoses: Excessive or inadequate intake of vitamins/minerals, fiber, fluid, parenteral/enteral nutrition; overweight/obesity, underweight, unintended weight loss, malnutrition (undernutrition), sarcopenia

Note: Judgment must be used to select indicators and determine the appropriate measurement techniques and reference standards for a given client population and setting. Once identified, these indicators, measurement techniques, and reference standards should be identified in policies and procedures or other documents for use in client records, quality or performance improvement, or in formal research projects.

Client Example

Example(s) of one (or more) of the nutrition care indicators (includes sample initial and reassessment documentation for one of the indicators)

Indicator(s) Selected

Muscle atrophy, loss of subcutaneous fat

Criteria for Evaluation

Comparison to goal or reference standard:

1. Reference standard: The client's muscle atrophy and subcutaneous fat loss are consistent with mild undernutrition in the context of acute illness or injury, which is consistent with the nutrition diagnosis of non-severe (moderate) malnutrition. Normal reference standard is no muscle atrophy and fat pads slightly bulged.
2. Recommendation: The client maintains or gains muscle and subcutaneous fat (as appropriate) as determined by a nutrition focused physical exam.
3. Goal: Client establishes goal to consume a mid-afternoon snack of whole milk yogurt on 5 of 7 days per week.

Sample Nutrition Assessment and Monitoring and Evaluation Documentation	
Initial encounter	Client's muscle atrophy and subcutaneous fat loss is mild, which is consistent with non-severe (moderate) malnutrition. Client establishes goal to consume a mid-afternoon snack of whole milk yogurt on 5 of 7 days per week. Will review client intake log. Will monitor changes in muscle and subcutaneous fat status in 3 months.
Reassessment after nutrition intervention	Progress toward maintaining or gaining of muscle mass and (as appropriate) subcutaneous fat. Nutrition focused physical exam reveals client's muscle and subcutaneous fat status is improved over the last 3 months.

Personal Data

Definition

General client information such as age, gender, sex, race, ethnicity, occupation, tobacco use, and physical disability.

Nutrition Assessment

Indicators

Note: The examples may vary from those listed below to meet population needs. Additional and/or alternative options may be warranted.

- Age*
- Corrected age*† (weeks and/or months)—defined as the chronological age in weeks and/or months minus the number of weeks and/or months premature
  Examples:
  - Age in days (neonates)*
  - Age in months (up to 36 months)*
  - Age in years*
- Gender* (as the behavioral, cultural, or psychological traits)
  Examples:
  - Female*
  - Male*
- Sex* (as female or male based upon reproductive organs and structures)
  Examples:
  - Female*
  - Male*
- Race* (A group of people connected by common descent or origin)
  Examples:
  - American Indian or Alaska Native*
  - Asian*
  - Black or African American*
  - Native Hawaiian or Other Pacific Islander*
  - White*
- Ethnicity* (pertaining to or having common racial, cultural, religious, or linguistic characteristics)
  Examples:
  - Hispanic or Latino*
  - Not Hispanic or Latino*
- Language*
  Examples:
  - English*
  - Spanish*
- Literacy factors*
  Examples:
  - Language barrier*
  - Low literacy*
- Education*
  Example:
  - Years of education (Year of education)*
- Role in family* (client's reported role, eg, mother, cousin, in the description of his/her family)
- Tobacco use*
  Examples:
  - Yes*
  - Average number cigarettes smoked per day (number/day)*
  - Total number of other tobacco products used/day (number/day)*
  - Number years tobacco products used on a regular basis (years)*
  - No*
- Physical ability difference*
  Examples:
  - Eyesight impaired*
  - Hearing impaired*
- Mobility*
  Examples:
  - House bound*
  - Bed or chair bound*
  - Tremors (Parkinson)*

---

* Denotes indicator is used for nutrition assessment only. Other indicators are used for both nutrition assessment and nutrition monitoring and evaluation.

† If a synonym for the term "corrected age" is helpful or needed, an approved alternate is "adjusted age."

Personal Data

Examples of the measurement methods or data sources for these outcome indicators: Client report, health record, referring health care provider or agency, surveys, administrative data sets

Typically used with the following domains of nutrition interventions: Food and/or nutrient delivery, nutrition education, nutrition counseling, coordination of nutrition care by nutrition professional, population based nutrition action

Typically used to determine and monitor and evaluate change in the following nutrition diagnoses: Not applicable

Note: Judgment must be used to select indicators and determine the appropriate measurement techniques and reference standards for a given client population and setting. Once identified, these indicators, measurement techniques, and reference standards should be identified in policies and procedures or other documents for use in client records, quality or performance improvement, or in formal research projects.

Client Example

Example(s) of one or more of the nutrition care indicators (includes sample initial assessment documentation for one of the indicators)

Indicator(s) Selected

Corrected age (weeks and/or months)

Criteria for Evaluation

Comparison to reference standard, recommendation, or goal:

1. Reference standard: Not applicable
2. Recommendation: Not applicable
3. Goal: Not applicable

Sample Nutrition Assessment and Monitoring and Evaluation Documentation	
Initial nutrition assessment	Client born 1 month premature, so the corrected age is 36 weeks (9 months)

Individual Client and/or Family Nutrition Related Health History

Definition

Individual client and/or family member health states, conditions, and illnesses that may impact nutritional status.

Nutrition Assessment

Indicators

Note: The examples may vary from those listed below to meet population needs. Additional and/or alternative options may be warranted.

Individual

- Individual client nutrition related health history*
- Cancer history*
- Cardiovascular disease history*
  Examples:
  - Heart failure*
  - Hyperlipidemia*
  - Hypertension*
  - Stroke*
- Endocrine disease history*
  Examples:
  - Diabetes mellitus*
  - Gestational diabetes*
  - Failure to thrive*
  - Obesity*
  - Overweight*
- Excretory disease history*
  Examples:
  - Dehydration*
  - Kidney disease*
- Gastrointestinal disease history*
  Examples:
  - Crohn's disease*
  - Diverticulitis*
  - Diverticulosis*
  - Dyspepsia*
  - Inflammatory bowel disease*

Family

- Family nutrition related health history*
- Family history of cancer*
- Family history of cardiovascular disease*
  Examples:
  - Family history of heart failure*
  - Family history of hyperlipidemia*
  - Family history of hypertension*
  - Family history of stroke*
- Family history of endocrine disease*
  Examples:
  - Family history of diabetes mellitus*
  - Family history of gestational diabetes*
  - Family history of failure to thrive*
  - Family history of obesity*
  - Family history of overweight*
- Family history of excretory disease*
  Example:
  - Family history of kidney disease*
- Family history of gastrointestinal disease*
  Examples:
  - Family history of Crohn's disease*
  - Family history of diverticulitis*
  - Family history of diverticulosis*
  - Family history of dyspepsia
  - Family history of inflammatory bowel disease*

* Denotes indicator is used for nutrition assessment only. Other indicators are used for both nutrition assessment and nutrition monitoring and evaluation.

Individual Client and/or Family Nutrition Related Health History

Individual

Gastrointestinal disease history examples, continued

- Lactase deficiency*
- Liver disease*
- Pancreatic disease*
- Celiac disease*

- Gynecological history*
  Examples:
  - Amenorrhea*
  - Lactating*
  - Mastitis*
  - Perimenopausal*
  - Polycystic ovary syndrome*
- Postmenopausal*
- Pregnant*
  - Gestational age (weeks)*
  - Single fetus pregnancy*
  - Multiple fetus pregnancy*
- Hematologic disease history*
  Example:
  - Anemia
- Immune disease history*
  Examples:
  - AIDS*
  - HIV*
  - Food allergies*
  - Sepsis*
- Integumentary disease history*
  Examples:
  - Burns*
  - Eczema*
- Metabolic disease history*
  Examples:
  - Cystic fibrosis*
  - Inborn errors of metabolism*
  - Metabolic syndrome*

Family

Family history of gastrointestinal disease examples, continued

- Family history of lactase deficiency*
- Family history of liver disease*
- Family history of pancreatic disease*
- Family history of celiac disease*

- Family history of gynecological disorder*
  Examples:
  - Family history of amenorrhea*
  - Family history of polycystic ovary syndrome*
  - Family history of early menopause*
  - Family history of premature delivery*
  - Family history of premature delivery of single fetus*
  - Family history of premature delivery of multiple fetuses*
- Family history of hematologic disease*
  Example:
  - Family history of anemia*
- Family history of immune disease*
  Example:
  - Family history of food allergies*
- Family history of integumentary disease*
  Example:
  - Family history of eczema*
- Family history of malnutrition*
- Family history of metabolic disease*
  Examples:
  - Family history of cystic fibrosis*
  - Family history of inborn errors of metabolism*
  - Family history of metabolic syndrome*
- Family history of musculoskeletal disease*
  Example:
  - Family history of osteoporosis*

---

* Denotes indicator is used for nutrition assessment only. Other indicators are used for both nutrition assessment and nutrition monitoring and evaluation.

Individual Client and/or Family Nutrition Related Health History

Individual

- Musculoskeletal disease history*
  Examples:
  - Trauma*
  - Osteoporosis*
- Neurological disease history*
  Examples:
  - Developmental delay*
  - Alzheimer disease*
  - Parkinson disease*
- Psychological disease history*
  Examples:
  - Alcoholism*
  - Cognitive impairment*
  - Dementia*
  - Depression*
  - Eating disorder*
  - Psychosis*
- Respiratory disease history*
  Example:
  - Chronic obstructive pulmonary disease*

Family

- Family history of neurological disease*
  Examples:
  - Family history of developmental delay*
  - Family history of Parkinson disease*
  - Family history of Alzheimer disease*
- Family history of psychological disease*
  Examples:
  - Family history of alcoholism*
  - Family history of cognitive impairment*
  - Family history of dementia*
  - Family history of depression*
  - Family history of eating disorder*
  - Family history of psychosis*
- Family history of respiratory disease*
  Example:
  - Family history of chronic obstructive pulmonary disease*

Examples of the measurement methods or data sources for these outcome indicators: Health record, referring health care provider or agency, client survey.

Typically used with the following domains of nutrition interventions: Nutrition education, nutrition counseling, food and/or nutrient delivery, population based nutrition action.

Typically used to determine and monitor and evaluate change in the following nutrition diagnoses: All

Note: Judgment must be used to select indicators and determine the appropriate measurement techniques and reference standards for a given client population and setting. Once identified, these indicators, measurement techniques, and reference standards should be identified in policies and procedures or other documents for use in client records, quality or performance improvement, or in formal research projects.

Client Example

Example(s) of one of the nutrition care indicators (includes sample initial assessment documentation for one of the indicators)

* Denotes indicator is used for nutrition assessment only. Other indicators are used for both nutrition assessment and nutrition monitoring and evaluation.

Individual Client and/or Family Nutrition Related Health History

Indicator(s) Selected

Obesity

Criteria for Evaluation

Comparison to reference standard, recommendation, or goal:

1. Reference standard: Evidence-based guideline for obesity.
2. Recommendation: Not applicable
3. Goal: Change to overweight or weight within guideline.

Sample Nutrition Assessment Documentation	
Initial Nutrition Assessment	Client referred with diagnosis of obesity and family history (both parents) of obesity.

Treatments/Therapy

Definition

Documented medical or surgical treatments that may impact nutritional status of the client.

Nutrition Assessment

Indicators

Note: The examples may vary from those listed below to meet population needs. Additional and/or alternative options may be warranted.

- Medical treatment/therapy*
  Examples:
  - Chemotherapy*
  - Dialysis*
  - Mechanical ventilation/oxygen therapy*
  - Ostomy*
  - Radiation therapy*
- Surgical treatment*
  Examples:
  - Coronary artery bypass graft (CABG)*
  - Gastric bypass*
  - Intestinal resection*
  - Joint/orthopedic surgery/replacement*
  - Limb amputation*
  - Organ transplant*
  - Total gastrectomy*
  - Palliative/end-of-life care (care of client with terminal or life-threatening conditions)*

Examples of the measurement methods or data sources for these outcome indicators: Client interview, health record, referring health care provider or agency

Typically used with the following domains of nutrition interventions: Food and/or nutrient delivery, nutrition education, nutrition counseling, coordination of nutrition care by nutrition professional

Typically used to determine and monitor and evaluate change in the following nutrition diagnoses: Impaired nutrient utilization, increased nutrient needs, altered gastrointestinal function, chewing difficulty, unintended weight loss

Note: Judgment must be used to select indicators and determine the appropriate measurement techniques and reference standards for a given client population and setting. Once identified, these indicators, measurement techniques, and reference standards should be identified in policies and procedures or other documents for use in client records, quality or performance improvement, or in formal research projects.

---

* Denotes indicator is used for nutrition assessment only. Other indicators are used for both nutrition assessment and nutrition monitoring and evaluation.

Treatments/Therapy

Client Example

Example(s) of one of the nutrition care indicators (includes sample initial assessment documentation for one of the indicators)

Indicator(s) Selected

Radiation therapy

Criteria for Evaluation

Comparison to reference standard, recommendation, or goal:

1. Reference standard: Not applicable
2. Recommendation: Not applicable
3. Goal: Client receiving radiation therapy for lung cancer, experiencing decreased appetite and pain with eating. Goal is to optimize nutrition during radiation therapy.

Sample Nutrition Assessment Documentation	
Initial nutrition assessment	Client receiving radiation therapy for lung cancer, experiencing decreased appetite due to fatigue and pain with eating.

Social History

Definition

Client socioeconomic status, housing situation, medical support, and involvement in social groups.

Nutrition Assessment

Indicators

Note: The examples may vary from those listed below to meet population needs. Additional and/or alternative options may be warranted.

- Socioeconomic factors*
  Examples:
  - Economic constraints*
  - Access to medical care (full/limited/none)*
  - Diverts food money to other needs*
- Living/housing situation*
  Examples:
  - Lives alone*
  - Lives with family member/caregiver*
  - Homeless*
- Domestic issues*
- Social and medical support*
  Examples:
  - Family members*
  - Caregivers*
  - Community group/senior center/church*
  - Support group attendance (eg, weight control, substance abuse, etc)*
- Geographic location of home*
  Examples:
  - Urban*
  - Rural*
  - Limited exposure to sunlight (vitamin D)*
- Occupation*
  Examples:
  - Stay-at-home parent*
  - Student*
  - Retired*
- Religion*
  Examples:
  - Catholic*
  - Jewish*
  - Protestant*
  - Islam*
- History of recent crisis*
  Examples:
  - Job loss*
  - Family member death*
  - Trauma, surgery*
- Daily stress level (high, moderate, low bodily or mental tension)*

Examples of the measurement methods or data sources for these outcome indicators: Client report, health record, referring health care provider or agency

Typically used with the following domains of nutrition interventions: Food and/or nutrient delivery, nutrition education, nutrition counseling, coordination of nutrition care by nutrition professional

Typically used to determine and monitor and evaluate change in the following nutrition diagnoses: All

---

* Denotes indicator is used for nutrition assessment only. Other indicators are used for both nutrition assessment and nutrition monitoring and evaluation.

Social History

Note: Judgment must be used to select indicators and determine the appropriate measurement techniques and reference standards for a given client population and setting. Once identified, these indicators, measurement techniques, and reference standards should be identified in policies and procedures or other documents for use in client records, quality or performance improvement, or in formal research projects.

Client Example

Example(s) of one or two of the nutrition care indicators (includes sample initial assessment documentation for one of the indicators)

Indicator(s) Selected

Living/housing situation and geographic location of home

Criteria for Evaluation

Comparison to goal or reference standard, recommendation, or goal:

1. Reference standard: Not applicable
2. Recommendation: Not applicable
3. Goal: Not applicable

Sample Nutrition Assessment Documentation	
Initial nutrition assessment	Client is house bound, lives in a rural area, and receives one meal/day from home delivery program.

Nutrition Assessment, Monitoring and Evaluation Tool Ratings

Definition

Validated tool ratings or scores that provide data for the purpose of evaluating nutrition status.

Nutrition Assessment and Monitoring and Evaluation

Indicators

- Subjective Global Assessment (SGA) rating (Stage A: well-nourished; Stage B: moderately [or suspected of being] malnourished; Stage C: severely malnourished)—defined as a nutrition assessment rating reflecting a valid assessment of overall nutrition status and the risk of or presence of malnutrition in adults of all ages based upon recent change in intake, weight change, gastrointestinal symptoms, functional status, metabolic demand of disease, and physical exam parameters, related to fat and muscle mass loss and fluid retention
- Subjective global assessment (SGA) score (number)—defined as an additive numerical score reflecting a valid assessment of overall nutrition status and the risk of or presence of malnutrition in adults of all ages based upon recent change in intake, weight change, gastrointestinal symptoms, functional status, metabolic demand of disease, and physical exam parameters, related to fat and muscle mass loss and fluid retention
- Scored Patient-Generated Subjective Global Assessment (PG-SGA) rating (Stage A: well-nourished; Stage B: moderate/suspected malnutrition; Stage C: severely malnourished)—defined as a nutrition assessment rating reflecting a valid assessment of overall nutrition status and the risk of or presence of malnutrition in adults of all ages based upon recent change in intake, weight change, gastrointestinal symptoms, functional status, clinical symptoms, metabolic demand of disease, and physical exam parameters; includes both client and practitioner components
- The scored patient generated subjective global assessment (PG-SGA) score (number)—defined as an additive numerical score based on intake, weight change, gastrointestinal symptoms, functional status, clinical symptoms, metabolic demand of disease, and physical exam parameters that are used for triaging nutrition intervention rather than determining the PG-SGA rating
- Mini Nutritional Assessment Long Form (MNA-LF) rating (normal nutritional status, at risk of malnutrition, malnourished)—defined as a nutrition assessment rating reflecting a valid assessment of overall nutrition status and the risk of or presence of malnutrition in adults aged > 65 years based upon weight change, intake, functional status, psychological stressors or problems, and clinical exam parameters
- Mini nutritional assessment long form (MNA-LF) score (number)—defined as an additive numerical score reflecting a valid assessment of overall nutrition status and the risk of or presence of malnutrition in adults aged > 65 years based upon weight change, intake, functional status, psychological stressors or problems, and clinical exam parameters
- Subjective Global Nutritional Assessment (SGNA) for children rating (normal nutrition, moderate malnutrition, severe malnutrition)—defined as a nutrition assessment rating reflecting a valid assessment of nutritional status of children*
- Subjective global nutritional assessment (SGNA) for children score (number)—defined as an additive numerical score reflecting a valid assessment of nutritional status of children*

* Alternate approaches to interpretation of anthropometric measurements are recommended for children. Therefore, this tool should be used in conjunction with the evidence-based anthropometric measurement assessment criteria.

Nutrition Assessment, Monitoring and Evaluation Tool Ratings

Note: Assessment tool terms, depending on the use, may require the permission of the author.

Examples of the measurement methods or data sources for these outcome indicators: Client report, health records, practitioner observation, nutrition focused physical findings, self-monitoring records, survey data
Typically used with the following domains of nutrition interventions: Food and/or nutrient delivery, nutrition education, nutrition counseling, coordination of nutrition care by nutrition professional
Typically used to determine and to monitor and evaluate change in the following nutrition diagnoses: Acute disease or injury related malnutrition, chronic disease or injury related malnutrition, starvation related malnutrition, unintended weight loss, disordered eating pattern, inadequate intake diagnoses

Note: Judgment must be used to select indicators and determine the appropriate measurement techniques and reference standards for a given client population and setting. Once identified, these indicators, measurement techniques, and reference standards should be identified in policies and procedures or other documents for use in client records, quality or performance improvement, or in formal research projects.

Client Example(s)

Example of one (or more) of the nutrition care indicators (includes sample initial and reassessment of documentation for one of the indicators)

Indicator(s) Selected

Patient generated subjective global assessment (PG-SGA) rating and Patient generated subjective global assessment (PG-SGA) score

Criteria for Evaluation

Comparison to reference standard, recommendation, or goal:

1. Reference standard: Refer to specific tool.
2. Recommendation: Not applicable
3. Goal: Not applicable

Sample Nutrition Assessment and Monitoring and Evaluation Documentation	
Initial encounter	Oncology client Patient generated subjective global assessment (PG-SGA) rating B and Patient generated subjective global assessment (PG-SGA) score 9.
Reassessment after nutrition intervention	Client Patient generated subjective global assessment (PG-SGA) rating B and Patient generated subjective global assessment (PG-SGA) score 5 with improvement in some parameters.

Household Food Security Assessment Tool Scores

Definition

Tool scores that provide data for the purpose of evaluating household food security.

Nutrition Assessment and Monitoring and Evaluation

Indicators

- US household food security module six item short form raw score (0-6)—defined as the sum of affirmative household responses to the six questions in the module
- US household food security module six item short form scale score (0 = NA, 1 = 2.86, 2 = 4.19, 3 = 5.27, 4 = 6.30, 5 = 7.54, 6 [evaluated at 5.5] = 8.48)—defined as the degree to which a client is food secure based on the overall pattern of responses to the set of indicator questions
- Food insecurity experience scale (FIES) raw score (numerical score)—defined as an interval measure of the severity of food insecurity and makes it possible to produce measures of food insecurity at the individual or household level that are comparable across countries and contexts

Examples of the measurement methods or data sources for these outcome indicators: Survey data, program records

Typically used with the following domains of nutrition interventions: Food and/or nutrient delivery, nutrition education, nutrition counseling, coordination and referral of nutrition care, population based nutrition action

Typically used to determine and to monitor and evaluate change in the following nutrition diagnoses: Underweight, overweight/obesity, growth rate below expected, limited food acceptance, undesirable food choices, intake of unsafe food, limited access to food

Note: Judgment must be used to select indicators and determine the appropriate measurement techniques and reference standards for a given client population and setting. Once identified, these indicators, measurement techniques, and reference standards should be identified in policies and procedures or other documents for use in client records, quality or performance improvement, or in formal research projects.

Client Example(s)

Example of one (or more) of the nutrition care indicators (includes sample initial and reassessment of documentation for one of the indicators)

Indicator(s) Selected

US household food security module six item short form raw score (0-6)

Criteria for Evaluation

Comparison to reference standard, recommendation, or goal:

1. Reference standard: Refer to specific tool.
2. Recommendation: Not applicable
3. Goal: Not applicable

Household Food Security Assessment Tool Scores

Sample Nutrition Assessment and Monitoring and Evaluation Documentation	
Initial encounter	US household food security module six item short form raw score of 2, low food security. Tool was administered to client at public health center.
Reassessment after nutrition intervention	US household food security module six item short form raw score of 1, marginal food security. Tool was administered to client at public health center. Client's food security has improved.

Food Variety Assessment Tool Scores

Definition

Tool scores that provide data for the purpose of evaluating food variety for an individual, household, or population.

Nutrition Assessment and Monitoring and Evaluation

Indicators

- Minimum dietary diversity for women (MDD-W) indicator score (0-10)—defined as a dichotomous indicator of whether or not women of reproductive age (15-49) years have consumed at least five out of ten defined food groups the previous day or night. The proportion of women in a population who reach this minimum can be used as a proxy indicator for micronutrient adequacy. Scores are aggregated for a population of women rather than used as measures for an individual

Examples of the measurement methods or data sources for these outcome indicators: Survey data, program records, client report

Typically used with the following domains of nutrition interventions: Food and/or nutrient delivery, nutrition education, nutrition counseling, coordination and referral of nutrition care, population based nutrition action

Typically used to determine and to monitor and evaluate change in the following nutrition diagnoses: Underweight, overweight/obesity, growth rate below expected, food and nutrition related knowledge deficit, limited food acceptance, undesirable food choices, intake of unsafe food, limited access to food

Note: Judgment must be used to select indicators and determine the appropriate measurement techniques and reference standards for a given client population and setting. Once identified, these indicators, measurement techniques, and reference standards should be identified in policies and procedures or other documents for use in client records, quality or performance improvement, or in formal research projects.

Client Example(s)

Example of one of the nutrition care indicators (includes sample initial and reassessment of documentation for one of the indicators)

Indicator(s) Selected

MDD-W indicator score

Criteria for Evaluation

Comparison to reference standard, recommendation, or goal:

1. Reference standard: Refer to specific tool.
2. Recommendation: Not applicable
3. Goal: Not applicable

Sample Nutrition Assessment and Monitoring and Evaluation Documentation	
Initial encounter	Client (population) survey responses MDD-W indicator score 4, diversity not achieved.
Reassessment after nutrition intervention	Client (population) survey responses MDD-W indicator score 6, diversity achieved. Client has shown improvement in dietary diversity indicator.

Dysphagia Assessment, Monitoring and Evaluation Tool Scores

Definition

Validated tool scores that provide data regarding functional swallowing findings.

Nutrition Assessment and Monitoring and Evaluation

Indicators

- International Dysphagia Diet Standardisation Initiative (IDDSI) Framework drinks level (number, 0-4)—defined as the clinician-recommended drinks thickness for a person based on their comprehensive clinical assessment and represented by IDDSI Framework level*
- IDDSI Framework food level (number, 3-7)—defined as the clinician-recommended food textures for a person based on their comprehensive clinical assessment and represented by the IDDSI Framework level*
- IDDSI Functional Diet Scale score (number, 0-8)—defined as the number in the intersecting cell of the column showing the food level score and the row showing the drink level score and recommended for the person*

Note: The original IDDSI definitions use the word "patient," which has been changed in this publication to "person" to be more person-centered.

Examples of the measurement methods or data sources for these outcome indicators: Client report, health records, professional observation, self-monitoring records, survey data

Typically used with the following domains of nutrition interventions: Food and/or nutrient delivery, nutrition education, nutrition counseling, coordination of nutrition care by nutrition professional

Typically used to determine and to monitor and evaluate change in the following nutrition diagnoses: Swallowing difficulty, difficulty chewing, malnutrition, sarcopenia, unintended weight loss, growth rate below expected

Note: Judgment must be used to select indicators and determine the appropriate measurement techniques and reference standards for a given client population and setting. Once identified, these indicators, measurement techniques, and reference standards should be identified in policies and procedures or other documents for use in client records, quality or performance improvement, or in formal research projects.

Client Example(s)

Example of one (or more) of the nutrition care indicators (includes sample initial and reassessment of documentation for one of the indicators)

Indicator(s) Selected

IDDSI Framework food level (number, 3-7)

* These terms are included in NCPT with IDDSI's permission.

Dysphagia Assessment, Monitoring and Evaluation Tool Scores

Criteria for Evaluation

Comparison to reference standard, recommendation, or goal:

1. Reference standard: Refer to framework tool.
2. Recommendation: Not applicable
3. Goal: Not applicable

Sample Nutrition Assessment and Monitoring and Evaluation Documentation	
Initial encounter	IDDSI Initiative Framework food level 7. IDDSI Framework—easy to chew/level 7 diet recommended.
Reassessment after nutrition intervention	IDDSI Framework food level 7. However, client now able to consume IDDSI Framework—regular level 7 diet.

Nutrition Diagnosis Etiology Category Identification

Definition

Assessing the etiology category to communicate the cause or contributing factor of a nutrition diagnosis (problem).

Purpose

To ensure clear communication of the known root cause of a nutrition diagnosis and to link an effective nutrition intervention resolve or mitigate the problem

Indicators

- Beliefs attitudes etiology—defined as a cause or contributing risk factors related to the conviction of the truth of some nutrition-related statement or phenomenon; feelings or emotions toward that truth or phenomenon and activities
- Cultural etiology—defined as a cause or contributing risk factors related to the client's values, social norms, customs, religious beliefs, and/or political systems
- Knowledge etiology—defined as a cause or contributing risk factors impacting the level of understanding about food, nutrition and health, or nutrition-related information and guidelines
- Physical function etiology—defined as a cause or contributing risk factors related to physical ability to engage in specific tasks; may be cognitive in nature
- Physiologic metabolic etiology—defined as a cause or contributing risk factors related to medical/health status that may have a nutritional impact (excludes psychological etiologies—see separate category)
- Psychological etiology—defined as a cause or contributing risk factors related to a diagnosed or suspected mental health/psychological problem (*Diagnostic and Statistical Manual of Mental Disorders* [*DSM*])
- Social personal etiology—defined as a cause or contributing risk factors associated with the client's personal and/or social history
- Treatment etiology—defined as a cause or contributing risk factors related to medical or surgical treatment or other therapies and management or care
- Access etiology—defined as a cause or contributing risk factors that affect intake and the availability of safe, healthful food, water, and food/nutrition-related supplies. A more specific root cause of Access Etiologies may not be known but may eventually reveal Beliefs-Attitudes, Cultural, Knowledge, Physical Function, Psychological, Social–Personal, or Treatment Etiologies
- Behavior etiology—defined as a cause or contributing risk factors related to actions which influence achievement of nutrition-related goals. A more specific root cause of Behavior Etiologies may not be known but may eventually reveal Beliefs-Attitudes, Cultural, Knowledge, Physical Function, Psychological, Social-Personal, or Treatment Etiologies

Examples of the measurement methods or data sources for these outcome indicators: Client report, survey data

Typically used with the following domains of nutrition interventions: Food and/or nutrient delivery, education, counseling, coordination of nutrition care by nutrition professional, population based nutrition action

Typically used to determine and to monitor and evaluate change in the following nutrition diagnoses: all nutrition diagnoses

Nutrition Diagnosis Etiology Category Identification

Note: Judgment must be used to select indicators and determine the appropriate measurement techniques and reference standards for a given client population and setting. Once identified, these indicators, measurement techniques, and reference standards should be identified in policies and procedures or other documents for use in client records, quality or performance improvement, or in formal research projects.

Client Example(s)

Note: Accompanying nutrition diagnoses should be assessment and communication of the etiology category. This aids in evaluating the appropriateness of the nutrition intervention planned and executed. Examples below show the etiology category clearly associated with the PES (problem, etiology, and signs and symptoms) statement or included in the PES statement. Either approach is acceptable.

Inadequate oral intake *related to* reduced appetite, altered taste, pain, and sore mucosa due to radiotherapy treatment *as evidenced by 4% weight loss in 3 weeks and consuming < ½ of meals.*

*Please indicate the etiol*ogy category: Treatment etiology

Self monitoring deficit *related to* limited adherence with insulin regimen and blood glucose readings **[behavior etiology]** *as evidenced by* skipping mealtime insulin and no blood glucose values/readings documented.

Food and nutrition related knowledge deficit *related to* recent relocation **[knowledge etiology]** *as evidenced by* community survey revealing 40% of population reports not knowing where to purchase fresh fruits and vegetables.

Estimated Energy Needs

Definition

Estimated quantity of total energy needed for nutritional adequacy.

Purpose

Identify appropriate reference standard of energy intake needs for clients. Utilized as a basis of comparison to assess adequacy or excessiveness of client's estimated total energy intake as compared to estimated needs and for development of the nutrition prescription.

Indicators

- Total energy estimated needs in 24 hours (calories, kcal, or kJ/day)—defined as the estimated quantity of total energy needed for nutritional adequacy in one day
- Method for estimating 24 hour energy needs defined as the approach for estimating total energy needs for one day.
- Energy estimated needs per kg body weight in 24 hours (calories, kcal or kJ/kg/day)—defined as the estimated quantity of total energy needed for nutritional adequacy for each kg of body weight in one day

Reference

Dietary Reference Intakes for Energy, National Library of Medicine. https://www.ncbi.nlm.nih.gov/books/NBK591034

Estimated Fat Needs

Definition

Estimated quantity of total and/or type fat intake needed for nutritional adequacy.

Purpose

Identify appropriate reference standard of fat intake needs for clients. Utilized as a basis of comparison to assess adequacy or excessiveness of client's estimated total fat intake as compared to needs and for development of the nutrition prescription.

Indicators

- Total fat estimated needs in 24 hours (g/day)—defined as the total fat needed for nutritional adequacy in one day

Macronutrients*	EAR	RDA	AI	UL	Other
Fat			X		AMDR (children and adults)
n-6 polyunsaturated fatty acids (linoleic acid)			X (All ages)		AMDR (children and adults)
n-3 polyunsaturated fatty acids (alpha linolenic acid)			X (All ages)		AMDR (children and adults)
Dietary cholesterol *Trans* fatty acids Saturated fatty acids					As low as possible while consuming a nutritionally adequate diet

See Appendix: DRI Interpretation on page 524.

- Fat estimated needs per kg body weight in 24 hours (calories, kcal, or kJ/kg/day)—defined as the estimated quantity of total fat needed for nutrition adequacy for each kg of body weight in one day
- Method for estimating 24 hour fat needs defined as the approach for estimating total fat needs for one day
- Proportion of energy needs from fat in 24 hours (specify, percent)—defined as the portion of total estimated energy needs to be derived from fat

Note: Comparison to the DRIs is assumed, but other reference intake standards may be used.

Estimated Protein Needs

Definition

Estimated quantity and/or type of protein needed for nutritional adequacy.

Purpose

Identify appropriate reference standard of protein intake needs for clients. Utilized as a basis of comparison to assess adequacy or excessiveness of client's estimated total protein intake as compared to estimated needs and for development of the nutrition prescription.

Indicators

- Total protein estimated needs in 24 hours (day)—defined as the estimated quantity of total protein needed for nutritional adequacy in one day

Macronutrients*	EAR	RDA	AI	UL	Other
Protein	X All except infants 0 to 6 months	X All except infants 0 to 6 months	X Infants 0 to 6 months		AMDR (children and adults)

*See Appendix: DRI Interpretation on page 524.

- Protein estimated needs per kg body weight in 24 hours (g/kg/day)—defined as the estimated quantity of total protein needed for nutritional adequacy for each kg of body weight in one day
- Method for estimating 24 hour protein needs defined as the approach for estimating total protein needs for one day
- Proportion of energy needs from protein in 24 hours (percent/day)—defined as the portion of total estimated energy needs in one day to be derived from protein

Note: Comparison to the DRIs is assumed, but other reference intake standards may be used.

Estimated Carbohydrate Needs

Definition

Estimated quantity of total and/or type of carbohydrates needed for nutritional adequacy.

Purpose

Identify appropriate reference standard of carbohydrate intake needs for individual clients. Utilized for assessing the adequacy or excessiveness of client's estimated total carbohydrate intake as compared to estimated needs and for development of the nutrition prescription.

Indicators

- Total carbohydrate estimated needs in 24 hours (day)—defined as the estimated quantity of total carbohydrate needed for nutritional adequacy in one day

Macronutrients*	EAR	RDA	AI	UL	Other
Carbohydrates		X	X infants		AMDR (children and adults) Added sugars: limit to no more than 25% of total energy (all ages)

*See Appendix: DRI Interpretation on page 524.

- Carbohydrate estimated needs per kg body weight in 24 hours (g/kg/day)—defined as the estimated quantity of carbohydrate needed for nutritional adequacy for each kg of body weight in one day
- Method for estimating 24 hour carbohydrate needs defined as the approach for estimating total carbohydrate needs for one day
- Proportion of energy needs from carbohydrate in 24 hours (specify, percent)—defined as the portion of estimated energy needs in one day to be derived from carbohydrate

Note: Comparison to the DRIs is assumed, but other reference intake standards may be used.

Estimated Fiber Needs

Definition

Estimated quantity of total and/or type of fiber needed for nutritional adequacy.

Purpose

Identify appropriate reference standard of fiber intake needs for clients. Utilized as a basis of comparison to assess adequacy or excessiveness of client's estimated total fiber intake as compared to estimated needs and for development of the nutrition prescription.

Indicators

- Total fiber estimated needs in 24 hours (g/day)—defined as the estimated quantity of total fiber needed for nutritional adequacy in one day

Macronutrients*	EAR	RDA	AI	UL	Other
Fiber			X Children and adults		

*See Appendix: DRI Interpretation on page 524.

- Method for estimating 24 hour fiber needs (specify, eg, client goal or nutrition prescription, disease/condition-based reference standard, DRI)—defined as the approach for estimating total fiber needs for one day

Note: Comparison to the DRIs is assumed, but other reference intake standards may be used.

Estimated Fluid Needs

Definition

Estimated quantity of fluid needed for nutritional adequacy.

Purpose

Identify appropriate reference standard of fluid intake needs for clients. Utilized as a basis of comparison to assess adequacy or excessiveness of client's estimated total fluid intake as compared to estimated need and for development of the nutrition prescription.

Indicators

- Total fluid estimated needs in 24 hours (mL/day)—defined as the estimated quantity of total fluid needed for hydration adequacy in one day

Macronutrients*	EAR	RDA	AI	UL	Other
Total Water			X		

**See Appendix: DRI Interpretation on page 524.*

- Method for estimating 24 hour fluid needs—defined as the approach for estimating total fluid needs for one day (specify, eg, client goal or nutrition prescription, disease/condition-based reference standard, and DRI, and adjustments for fever, sweating, hyperventilation, renal or liver disease)

Note: Comparison to the DRIs is assumed, but other reference intake standards may be used.

Estimated Vitamin Needs

Definition

Estimated quantity of one or more vitamins needed for nutritional adequacy and avoidance of toxicity.

Purpose

Identify appropriate reference standard of vitamin intake needs for clients. Utilized as a basis of comparison to assess adequacy or excessiveness of client's estimated total vitamin intake as compared to estimated needs and for development of the nutrition prescription.

Indicators

Estimated vitamin needs:

Micronutrients: vitamins*	EAR	RDA	AI	UL
Estimated vitamin A needs in 24 hours (μg/day)—defined as the estimated quantity of vitamin A needed for nutritional adequacy in one day	X	X	X Infants	X
Estimated vitamin C needs in 24 hours (mg/day)—defined as the estimated quantity of vitamin C needed for nutritional adequacy in one day	X	X	X Infants	X Children and adults
Estimated vitamin D needs in 24 hours (μg/day)—defined as the estimated quantity of vitamin D needed for nutritional adequacy in one day	X	X	X Infants	X
Estimated vitamin E needs in 24 hours (mg/day)—defined as the estimated quantity of vitamin E needed for nutritional adequacy in one day	X	X	X Infants	X Children and adults
Estimated vitamin K needs in 24 hours (μg/day)—defined as the estimated quantity of vitamin K needed for nutritional adequacy in one day			X	
Estimated thiamin needs in 24 hours (mg/day)—defined as the estimated quantity of thiamin needed for nutritional adequacy in one day	X	X	X Infants	
Estimated riboflavin needs in 24 hours (mg/day)—defined as the estimated quantity of riboflavin needed for nutritional adequacy in one day	X	X	X Infants	

Estimated Vitamin Needs

Micronutrients: vitamins*	EAR	RDA	AI	UL
Estimated niacin needs in 24 hours (mg/day)—defined as the estimated quantity of niacin needed for nutritional adequacy in one day	X	X	X Infants	X Children and adults
Estimated vitamin B6 needs in 24 hours (mg/day)—defined as the estimated quantity of vitamin B6 needed for nutritional adequacy in one day	X	X	X Infants	X Children and adults
Estimated folate needs in 24 hours (µg/day)—defined as the estimated quantity of folate needed for nutritional adequacy in one day	X	X	X Infants	X Children and adults
Estimated vitamin B12 needs in 24 hours (µg/day)—defined as the estimated quantity of vitamin B12 needed for nutritional adequacy in one day	X	X	X Infants	
Estimated pantothenic acid needs in 24 hours (mg/day)—defined as the estimated quantity of pantothenic acid needed for nutritional adequacy in one day			X	
Estimated biotin needs in 24 hours (µg/day)—defined as the estimated quantity of biotin needed for nutritional adequacy in one day			X	
Estimated choline needs in 24 hours (mg/day)—defined as the estimated quantity of choline needed for nutritional adequacy in one day			X	X Children and adults

*See Appendix: DRI Interpretation on page 524.

- Method for estimating 24 hour vitamin needs-defined as the approach for estimating vitamin needs for one day (specify, eg, client goal or nutrition prescription, disease/condition-based reference standard, any adjustments for special conditions or situations, DRI)

Note: Comparison to the DRIs is assumed, but other reference intake standards may be used.

Estimated Mineral Needs

Definition

Estimated quantity of one or more minerals needed for nutritional adequacy and avoidance of toxicity.

Purpose

Identify appropriate reference standard of mineral intake needs for clients. Utilized as a basis of comparison to assess adequacy or excessiveness of client's estimated mineral intake as compared to estimated needs and for development of the nutrition prescription.

Indicators

Estimated mineral needs

Micronutrients: minerals/elements*	EAR	RDA	AI	UL	Other
Estimated calcium needs in 24 hours (mg/day)—defined as the calcium needed for nutritional adequacy in one day	X	X	X Infants	X Children and adults	
Estimated chloride needs in 24 hours (g/day)—defined as the chloride needed for nutritional adequacy in one day			X	X Children and adults	
Estimated iron needs in 24 hours (mg/day)—defined as the iron needed for nutritional adequacy in one day	X	X	X Infants 0-6 mo	X	
Estimated magnesium needs in 24 hours (mg/day)—defined as the magnesium needed for nutritional adequacy in one day	X	X	X Infants	X Children and adults	
Estimated potassium needs in 24 hours (g/day)—defined as the potassium needed for nutritional adequacy in one day			X		
Estimated phosphorus needs in 24 hours (mg/day)—defined as the phosphorus needed for nutritional adequacy in one day	X	X	X Infants	X Children and adults	
Estimated sodium needs in 24 hours (g/day)—defined as the sodium needed for nutritional adequacy in one day			X	X Children and adults	
Estimated zinc needs in 24 hours (mg/day)—defined as the zinc needed for nutritional adequacy in one day	X	X	X Infants 0-6 mos.	X	

Estimated Mineral Needs

Micronutrients: minerals/elements*	EAR	RDA	AI	UL	Other
Estimated sulfate needs in 24 hours (g/day)—defined as the sulfate needed for nutritional adequacy in one day	X	X	X Infants	X	
Estimated fluoride needs in 24 hours (mg/day)—defined as the fluoride needed for nutritional adequacy in one day			X	X	
Estimated copper needs in 24 hours (µg/day)—defined as the copper needed for nutritional adequacy in one day	X	X	X Infants	X Children and adults	
Estimated iodine needs in 24 hours (µg/day)—defined as the iodine needed for nutritional adequacy in one day	X	X	X Infants	X Children and adults	
Estimated selenium needs in 24 hours (µg/day)—defined as the selenium needed for nutritional adequacy in one day	X	X	X Infants	X	
Estimated manganese needs in 24 hours (µg/day)—defined as the manganese needed for nutritional adequacy in one day			X	X Children and adults	
Estimated chromium needs in 24 hours (µg/day)—defined as the chromium needed for nutritional adequacy in one day			X		
Estimated molybdenum needs in 24 hours (mg/day)—defined as the molybdenum needed for nutritional adequacy in one day	X Children and adults	X Children and adults	X Infants	X Children and adults	
Estimated boron needs in 24 hours (mg/day)—defined as the boron needed for nutritional adequacy in one day				X Children and adults	
Estimated cobalt needs in 24 hours (µg/day)—defined as the cobalt needed for nutritional adequacy in one day					Not addressed in the DRIs

See Appendix: DRI Interpretation on page 524.

- Method for estimating 24 hour mineral needs (specify, eg, client goal or nutrition prescription, disease/condition-based reference standard, any adjustments for special conditions or situations, DRI)—defined as the approach for estimated needs for one day

Note: Comparison to the DRIs is assumed, but other reference intake standards may be used.

Recommended Body Weight/ Body Mass Index/Growth

Definition

Estimated reference ideal body weight (known as desirable body weight), body mass index, and/or growth parameter used to evaluate nutritional status.

Purpose

Identify appropriate reference standard for body weight for clients. Utilized as a basis of comparison to assess client's body weight as compared to recommendations and for development of the nutrition prescription

Indicators (Measures)

- Ideal/reference body weight (IBW)
- Recommended body mass index (BMI)* (kg/m2)—defined as advised weight in kilograms divided by the square height in meters
- Goal body weight (pounds, ounces, kilograms, or grams)—defined as desired weight
- Goal body weight gain in 24 hours (grams/day)—defined as desired weight gain per day
- Goal body weight for length z score (z score)—defined as desired standard deviation score for body weight in proportion to attained growth in length
- Goal mid upper arm circumference z score (z score)—defined as desired standard deviation score for mid-upper arm circumference
- Goal body mass index (BMI for age z score) (z score)—defined as desired standard deviation score for BMI at the child's age
- Percent median body mass index (BMI) (%)—defined as comparison of the child's BMI to the median BMI-for-age expressed as a percent

Note: Please refer to the Academy Evidence Analysis Library, ***www.andeal.org*** for recommendations related to using actual weight versus IBW or actual body weight (ABW) for estimating energy expenditure.

* BMI is a measure of the weight of an individual scaled according to height. It is a common method for assessing body fat in the clinical setting and is compared to a population reference standard (eg, US National Institutes of Health guidelines or World Health Organization guidelines). BMI was designed for use within a physically inactive population.

Intervention Goal Status

Definition

Evaluation of progress toward meeting goals set in the course of nutrition intervention.

Nutrition Assessment and Monitoring and Evaluation

Indicators

- New goal identified—defined as the goal identified in Nutrition Intervention planning and was not identified in the previous Nutrition Intervention planning
- Goal achieved—defined as the goal has been met
- Goal discontinued—defined as the need for the goal no longer exists because the conditions or situation has changed and goal is no longer appropriate
- Goal not achieved—defined as there is no overall progress toward or away from a goal
- Some progress toward goal—defined as any progress toward the goal
- Some digression away from goal—defined as no overall progress toward the goal and progress overall is worsening

Examples of the measurement methods or data sources for these outcome indicators: Client report, survey data

Typically used with the following domains of nutrition interventions: Food and/or nutrient delivery, education, counseling, coordination of nutrition care by nutrition professional, population based nutrition action

Typically used to determine and to monitor and evaluate change in the following nutrition diagnoses: all nutrition diagnoses

> *Note:* Judgment must be used to select indicators and determine the appropriate measurement techniques and reference standards for a given client population and setting. Once identified, these indicators, measurement techniques, and reference standards should be identified in policies and procedures or other documents for use in client records, quality or performance improvement, or in formal research projects.

Client Example(s)

Example of one (or more) of the nutrition care indicators (includes sample initial and reassessment of documentation for one of the indicators)

Indicator(s) Selected

New goal and Some progress toward goal

Criteria for Evaluation

Comparison to reference standard, recommendation, or goal:

1. Reference standard: Varies depending on the target value (eg, intake, behavior change) of the goal.
2. Recommendation: Varies depending on the target value (eg, intake, behavior change) of the goal.
3. Goal: Varies depending on the client preference.

Intervention Goal Status

Sample Nutrition Assessment and Monitoring and Evaluation Documentation	
Initial encounter	Client identified a goal that they will increase estimated vegetable serving intake in 24 hours to 2 vegetable servings with lunch on 5 of 7 days per week by next encounter in 3 weeks. [New goal]
Reassessment after nutrition intervention	Client identified that they have made some progress toward goal of increasing estimated vegetable serving intake in 24 hours by eating 2 vegetable servings with lunch on 3 of 7 days per week. [Some progress toward goal]

Nutrition Diagnosis Status

Definition

Evaluation of the status of a nutrition diagnosis.

Purpose

To ensure clear communication of the progress toward resolution of each nutrition diagnosis

Nutrition Assessment and Monitoring and Evaluation

Indicators

- New nutrition diagnosis—a nutrition diagnosis identified that was not identified in any nutrition diagnoses made in the previous assessment
- Active nutrition diagnosis—the signs and symptoms in the nutrition diagnosis require nutrition intervention and monitoring and evaluation to meet the goal
- Resolved nutrition diagnosis—the signs and symptoms identified in the nutrition diagnosis have met or exceeded the goal
- Discontinued nutrition diagnosis—the nutrition diagnosis no longer exists because the client's condition or situation has changed; the client's current assessment data no longer support this nutrition diagnosis

Examples of the measurement methods or data sources for these outcome indicators: Not applicable

Typically used with the following domains of nutrition interventions: Not applicable

Typically used to determine and to monitor and evaluate change in the following nutrition diagnoses: All

Note: Judgment must be used to select indicators and determine the appropriate measurement techniques and reference standards for a given client population and setting. Once identified, these indicators, measurement techniques, and reference standards should be identified in policies and procedures or other documents for use in client records, quality or performance improvement, or in formal research projects.

Client Example

Example of one (or more) of the nutrition care indicators (includes sample initial and reassessment of documentation for one of the indicators)

Indicator(s) Selected

New nutrition diagnosis, active nutrition diagnosis

Criteria for Evaluation

Comparison to reference standard, recommendation, or goal:

1. Reference standard: Not applicable
2. Recommendation: Not applicable
3. Goal: Not applicable

Nutrition Diagnosis Status

Sample Nutrition Assessment Documentation

Examples

Altered nutrition related laboratory values: decreased serum potassium *related to* severe illness related pediatric malnutrition *as evidenced by* serum potassium 2.9 mEq/L. **[New nutrition diagnosis] (Physiologic metabolic etiology)**

Altered nutrition related laboratory values: decreased serum magnesium *related to* severe illness related pediatric malnutrition *as evidenced by* serum magnesium 1.1 mEq/L. **[New nutrition diagnosis] (Physiologic metabolic etiology)**

Growth rate below expected *related to* insufficient enteral nutrition and oral feeding prior to admission (PTA) *as evidenced by* length for age z score −4.0, weight for age z score −5.1, and weight for length z score −2. **[Active nutrition diagnosis] (Treatment etiology)**

SNAPSHOT
NCP Step 2: Nutrition Diagnosis

Definition: The purpose of a nutrition diagnosis is to identify and label a nutrition problem that can be resolved or improved through treatment/nutrition intervention by a nutrition and dietetics practitioner. A nutrition diagnosis (eg, inconsistent carbohydrate intake) is different from a medical diagnosis (eg, diabetes).

Determining a nutrition diagnosis: Nutrition and dietetics practitioners use nutrition assessment data to identify and label the client's nutrition diagnosis using standard nutrition diagnostic terminology. This section of the *NCPT Reference Manual* provides a reference sheet for each nutrition diagnosis that includes its definition, possible etiology/causes, and common signs or symptoms identified in the Nutrition Assessment step.

Terminology for Nutrition Diagnosis is organized in four domains (categories):

Intake	Too much or too little of a food or nutrient compared to actual or estimated needs
Clinical	Nutrition problems that relate to medical or physical conditions
Behavioral–Environmental	Knowledge, attitudes, beliefs, physical environment, access to food, or food safety
Nutrition Situation	Nutrition related findings providing additional context relevant to a person's nutrition care

Documenting a nutrition diagnosis: Nutrition and dietetics practitioners write a PES (Problem, Etiology, Signs and Symptoms) statement to describe each problem, the root causes, and the assessment data that provide evidence for the nutrition diagnosis(es).

The format for the PES statement is "[Nutrition diagnosis term (**P**roblem)] related to [**E**tiology] as evidenced by [**S**igns/**S**ymptoms]."

(P) Problem or Nutrition Diagnosis Term
Describes alterations in the client's nutritional status or contributing factors to alterations in the client's nutritional status.

(E) Etiology Cause/Contributing Risk Factors
Linked to the nutrition diagnosis term by the words "related to."

(S) Signs/Symptoms
Data or indicators used to determine the client's nutrition diagnosis. Linked to the etiology by the words "as evidenced by."

No nutrition diagnosis at this time (NO) may be documented if the assessment indicates that no nutrition problem exists to justify a nutrition intervention.

Guidelines for writing a clear PES statement: Select the most important and urgent problem to be addressed. When writing the PES statement, nutrition and dietetics practitioners can ask a series of questions that help clarify the nutrition diagnosis.

P: Can the nutrition and dietetics practitioner resolve or improve the client's nutrition diagnosis? When all things are equal and there is a choice between stating a PES statement using two nutrition diagnoses from different domains, consider the intake nutrition diagnosis as the one more specific to the role of the RDN.

E: Evaluate whether the etiology for each problem is the specific "root cause" that can be addressed with a nutrition intervention. If addressing the etiology cannot resolve the problem, can the RDN intervention at least lessen the signs and symptoms?

S: Will measuring the signs and symptoms indicate if the problem is resolved or improved? Are the signs and symptoms specific enough to monitor (measure/evaluate changes) and communicate resolution or improvement of a nutrition diagnosis?

General PES Statement: Do the nutrition assessment data support the nutrition diagnoses, etiologies, and signs and symptoms?

Critical Thinking Skills

- Finding patterns and relationships among the data and possible causes
- Making inferences
- Stating each problem clearly and singularly
- Ruling in or ruling out specific diagnoses
- Identifying an etiology, and the etiology category to which it is assigned, for each problem that may be resolved, lessened, or managed by the intervention(s)
- Identifying signs and symptoms that are measurable, or their change may be tracked
- Prioritizing identified problems

For more detailed information about the Nutrition Diagnosis step, log in as a subscriber to www.nutritioncareprocess.org.

NCP Step 2: Nutrition Diagnosis

The following is a quick reference outline of the Nutrition Diagnosis Step. This outline does not include all the terms in this step.

Key: ◆ = NCP Domain; ▲ = NCP Class; ● = NCP Subclass; □ = NCP Term

Each term is designated with a a five-digit (eg, 99999) Academy unique identifier (ANDUID). This should not be used in nutrition documentation. The ANDUID is for data-tracking purposes in electronic health records.

◆ INTAKE NUTRITION DIAGNOSES

Actual problems related to intake of energy, nutrients, fluids, bioactive constituents through oral diet or nutrition support

	ANDUID
▲ Energy Balance Nutrition Diagnoses	**10632**

Actual or estimated changes in energy (calorie/kcal/kJ) balance

❑ Increased energy expenditure	10633
❑ Inadequate energy intake	10634
❑ Excessive energy intake	10635
❑ Predicted inadequate energy intake	10636
❑ Predicted excessive energy intake	10637
▲ Oral or Nutrition Support Intake Nutrition Diagnoses	**10638**

Actual or estimated food and beverage intake from oral diet or nutrition support compared with client goal

❑ Inadequate oral intake	10639
❑ Excessive oral intake	10640
❑ Inadequate enteral nutrition infusion	10641
❑ Excessive enteral nutrition infusion	10642
❑ Enteral nutrition composition inconsistent with needs	11142
❑ Enteral nutrition administration inconsistent with needs	11143
❑ Inadequate parenteral nutrition infusion	10644
❑ Excessive parenteral nutrition infusion	10645
❑ Parenteral nutrition composition inconsistent with needs	11144
❑ Parenteral nutrition administration inconsistent with needs	11145
❑ Unbalanced diet pattern	10779
▲ Fluid Intake Nutrition Diagnoses	**10648**

Actual or estimated fluid intake compared with client goal

❑ Inadequate fluid intake	10649
❑ Excessive fluid intake	10650
▲ Bioactive Constituent Intake Nutrition Diagnoses	**10651**

Actual or estimated intake of bioactive substances, including single or multiple functional food components, ingredients, dietary supplements, alcohol

	ANDUID
❑ Inadequate bioactive substance intake	10859
❑ Inadequate plant stanol ester intake	11077
❑ Inadequate plant sterol ester intake	11078
❑ Inadequate soy protein intake	11080
❑ Inadequate psyllium intake	11079
❑ Inadequate beta glucan intake	11076
❑ Excessive bioactive substance intake	10653
❑ Excessive plant stanol ester intake	11084
❑ Excessive plant sterol ester intake	11085
❑ Excessive soy protein intake	11087
❑ Excessive psyllium intake	11086
❑ Excessive beta glucan intake	11081
❑ Excessive food additive intake	11083
❑ Excessive caffeine intake	11082
❑ Excessive alcohol intake	10654
▲ Nutrient Intake Nutrition Diagnoses	**10655**

Actual or estimated intake of specific nutrient groups or single nutrients as compared with desired levels

❑ Increased nutrient needs	10656
❑ Inadequate protein energy intake	10658
❑ Decreased nutrient needs	10659
❑ Imbalance of nutrients	10660
● Fat and Cholesterol Intake Nutrition Diagnoses	**10661**
❑ Inadequate fat intake	10662
❑ Excessive fat intake	10663
❑ Intake of types of fats inconsistent with needs	10854
● Protein Intake Nutrition Diagnoses	**10665**
❑ Inadequate protein intake	10666
❑ Excessive protein intake	10667
❑ Intake of types of proteins inconsistent with needs	10855
● Amino Acid Intake Nutrition Diagnoses	**12006**
❑ Intake of types of amino acids inconsistent with needs	12007
● Carbohydrate and Fiber Intake Nutrition Diagnoses	**10669**
❑ Inadequate carbohydrate intake	10670
❑ Excessive carbohydrate intake	10671
❑ Intake of types of carbohydrate inconsistent with needs	10856
❑ Inconsistent carbohydrate intake	10673
❑ Inadequate fiber intake	10675
❑ Excessive fiber intake	10676

Key: ◆ = NCP Domain; ▲ = NCP Class; ● = NCP Subclass; ❑ = NCP Term

	ANDUID
● **Vitamin Intake Nutrition Diagnoses**	**10677**
❑ Inadequate vitamin intake	10678
❑ Inadequate intake of vitamin A	10679
❑ Inadequate intake of vitamin C	10680
❑ Inadequate intake of vitamin D	10681
❑ Inadequate intake of vitamin E	10682
❑ Inadequate intake of vitamin K	10683
❑ Inadequate intake of thiamin	10684
❑ Inadequate intake of riboflavin	10685
❑ Inadequate intake of niacin	10686
❑ Inadequate intake of folate	10687
❑ Inadequate intake of vitamin B6	10688
❑ Inadequate intake of vitamin B12	10689
❑ Inadequate intake of pantothenic acid	10690
❑ Inadequate intake of biotin	10691
❑ Excessive vitamin intake	10693
❑ Excessive intake of vitamin A	10694
❑ Excessive intake of vitamin C	10695
❑ Excessive intake of vitamin D	10696
❑ Excessive intake of vitamin E	10697
❑ Excessive intake of vitamin K	10698
❑ Excessive intake of thiamin	10699
❑ Excessive intake of riboflavin	10700
❑ Excessive intake of niacin	10701
❑ Excessive intake of folate	10702
❑ Excessive intake of vitamin B6	10703
❑ Excessive intake of vitamin B12	10704
❑ Excessive intake of pantothenic acid	10705
❑ Excessive intake of biotin	10706
● **Mineral Intake Nutrition Diagnoses**	**10708**
❑ Inadequate mineral intake	10709
❑ Inadequate intake of calcium	10710
❑ Inadequate intake of chloride	10711
❑ Inadequate intake of iron	10712
❑ Inadequate intake of magnesium	10713
❑ Inadequate intake of potassium	10714
❑ Inadequate intake of phosphorus	10715
❑ Inadequate intake of sodium	10716
❑ Inadequate intake of zinc	10717
❑ Inadequate intake of sulfate	10718
❑ Inadequate intake of fluoride	10719
❑ Inadequate intake of copper	10720
❑ Inadequate intake of iodine	10721
❑ Inadequate intake of selenium	10722
❑ Inadequate intake of manganese	10723
❑ Inadequate intake of chromium	10724
❑ Inadequate intake of molybdenum	10725
❑ Inadequate intake of boron	10726
❑ Inadequate intake of cobalt	10727
❑ Excessive mineral intake	10729
❑ Excessive intake of calcium	10730

	ANDUID
❑ Excessive intake of chloride	10731
❑ Excessive intake of iron	10732
❑ Excessive intake of magnesium	10733
❑ Excessive intake of potassium	10734
❑ Excessive intake of phosphorus	10735
❑ Excessive intake of sodium	10736
❑ Excessive intake of zinc	10737
❑ Excessive intake of sulfate	10738
❑ Excessive intake of fluoride	10739
❑ Excessive intake of copper	10740
❑ Excessive intake of iodine	10741
❑ Excessive intake of selenium	10742
❑ Excessive intake of manganese	10743
❑ Excessive intake of chromium	10744
❑ Excessive intake of molybdenum	10745
❑ Excessive intake of boron	10746
❑ Excessive intake of cobalt	10747
● **Multinutrient Intake Nutrition Diagnoses**	**10749**
❑ Predicted inadequate nutrient intake	10750
❑ Predicted excessive nutrient intake	10751

◆ CLINICAL NUTRITION DIAGNOSES

Nutritional findings/problems identified that relate to medical or physical conditions

▲ Functional Nutrition Diagnoses **10753**

Change in body's physical and/or mechanical function compared to expected function

❑ Swallowing difficulty	10754
❑ Difficulty chewing	10755
❑ Breastfeeding difficulty	10756
❑ Altered GI function	10757
❑ Predicted breastfeeding difficulty	11146
❑ Sarcopenia	30090

▲ Biochemical Nutrition Diagnoses **10758**

Change in capacity to metabolize nutrients as a result of medications, surgery, or as indicated by altered laboratory values

❑ Impaired nutrient utilization	10759
❑ Altered nutrition related laboratory values	10760
❑ Food medication interaction	10761
❑ Predicted food medication interaction	10762

▲ Weight Nutrition Diagnoses **10763**

Chronic weight or changed weight status when compared with usual or desired body weight

❑ Underweight	10764
❑ Unintended weight loss	10765
❑ Overweight/obesity	10766
❑ Overweight, adult or pediatric	10767
❑ Obesity, adult or pediatric	82233

Key: ◆ = NCP Domain; ▲ = NCP Class; ● = NCP Subclass; ❑ = NCP Term

	ANDUID
❑ Obesity pediatric	10768
❑ Obesity class I	10769
❑ Obesity class II	10818
❑ Obesity class III	10819
❑ Unintended weight gain	10770
❑ Growth rate below expected	10802
❑ Excessive growth rate	10803

▲ Malnutrition Disorders Diagnoses 12008

Health consequences resulting from insufficient or excessive energy and/or nutrient intake compared to physiologic needs and/or utilization

- ❑ Malnutrition (undernutrition) 10657
  - ❑ Starvation related malnutrition 11130
    - ❑ Moderate starvation related malnutrition 13210
    - ❑ Severe starvation related malnutrition 13211
  - ❑ Chronic disease or condition related malnutrition 11131
    - ❑ Moderate chronic disease or condition related malnutrition 13212
    - ❑ Severe chronic disease or condition related malnutrition 13213
  - ❑ Acute disease or injury related malnutrition 11132
    - ❑ Moderate acute disease or injury related malnutrition 13214
    - ❑ Severe acute disease or injury related malnutrition 13215
  - ❑ Non illness related pediatric malnutrition 13017
    - ❑ Mild non illness related pediatric malnutrition 13216
    - ❑ Moderate non illness related pediatric malnutrition 13217
    - ❑ Severe non illness related pediatric malnutrition 13218
  - ❑ Illness related pediatric malnutrition 13018
    - ❑ Mild illness related pediatric malnutrition 13219
    - ❑ Moderate illness related pediatric malnutrition 13220
- ❑ Severe illness related pediatric malnutrition 13221

◆ BEHAVIORAL-ENVIRONMENTAL NUTRITION DIAGNOSES

Nutritional findings/problems identified that relate to knowledge, attitudes/beliefs, physical environment, access to food, or food safety

ANDUID

▲ Knowledge and Beliefs Nutrition Diagnoses 10772

Actual knowledge and beliefs as related, observed, or documented

- ❑ Food and nutrition related knowledge deficit 10773
- ❑ Belief finding that hinders food and/or nutrition behavior change 10857
- ❑ Not ready for nutrition related behavior change 10775
- ❑ Self monitoring deficit 10776
- ❑ Disordered eating pattern 10777
- ❑ Limited adherence to nutrition related recommendations 10778
- ❑ Limited food acceptance 10647
- ❑ Limited food and nutrition related skill 30091
- ❑ Attitude finding that hinders food and/or nutrition behavior change 30093

▲ Physical Activity and Function Nutrition Diagnoses 10781

Actual physical activity, self care, and quality of life problems as reported, observed, or documented

- ❑ Physical inactivity 10782
- ❑ Excessive physical activity 10783
- ❑ Inability to manage self care 10780
- ❑ Limited ability to prepare food for eating 10785
- ❑ Poor food and/or nutrition quality of life 10786
- ❑ Self feeding difficulty 10787

▲ Food Safety and Access Nutrition Diagnoses 10788

Actual problems with food safety or access to food, water, or nutrition related supplies

- ❑ Intake of unsafe food 10789
- ❑ Food insecurity 12009
- ❑ Limited access to nutrition related supplies 10791
- ❑ Limited access to potable water 12010

◆ NUTRITION SITUATION 30092

Nutrition related findings providing additional context relevant to a person's nutrition care.

- ❑ No nutrition diagnosis at this time 10795

Key: ◆ = NCP Domain; ▲ = NCP Class; ● = NCP Subclass; ☐ = NCP Term

Increased Energy Expenditure

Definition

Resting metabolic rate (RMR) more than predicted requirements due to body composition; medications; or endocrine, neurologic, or genetic changes.

Note: RMR is the sum of metabolic processes of active cell mass related to the maintenance of normal body functions and regulatory balance during rest.

Etiology (Cause/Contributing Risk Factors)

Factors gathered during the nutrition assessment process that contribute to the existence or the maintenance of pathophysiological, psychosocial, situational, developmental, cultural, and/or environmental problems:

- Physiological causes increasing nutrient needs due to anabolism, growth, maintenance of body temperature
- Voluntary or involuntary physical activity/movement

Etiology Category

Etiologies are grouped by the type of cause or contributing risk factor. Communicate the etiology category by selecting the appropriate Nutrition Assessment, Monitoring, and Evaluation term.

NCP Term	ANDUID
Beliefs attitudes etiology	14567
Cultural etiology	14568
Knowledge etiology	14569
Physical function etiology	14570
Physiologic metabolic etiology	14571
Psychological etiology	14572
Social personal etiology	14573
Treatment etiology	14574
Access etiology	14575
Behavior etiology	14576

Visit the Nutrition Diagnosis Etiology Category Identification reference sheet on page 185 for more details on etiology categories. An additional useful resource to determine the etiology category is the Nutrition Diagnosis Matrix on page 528.

Signs/Symptoms (Defining Characteristics)

A typical cluster of subjective and objective signs and symptoms gathered during the nutrition assessment process that provide evidence that a problem exists; quantify the problem and describe its severity.

Increased Energy Expenditure

Nutrition Assessment Category	Potential Indicators of This Nutrition Diagnosis (one or more must be present)
Biochemical Data, Medical Tests and Procedures	
Anthropometric Measurements	• Unintentional weight loss of ≥ 10% in 6 months, ≥ 5% in 1 month (adults and pediatrics), and > 2% in 1 week (pediatrics) • Evidence of need for accelerated or catch-up growth or weight gain in children; absence of normal growth • Increased proportion of lean body mass
Physical Exam Findings	• Fever • Measured RMR > estimated or expected RMR
Food/Nutrition-Related History	• Increased physical activity, eg, endurance athlete • Medications that increase energy expenditure
Client History*	Conditions associated with a diagnosis or treatment, eg, Parkinson's disease, cerebral palsy, Alzheimer's disease, cystic fibrosis, chronic obstructive pulmonary disease (COPD)
Assessment, Monitoring, and Evaluation Tools	
Comparative Standards	

** Client History terms are used for Nutrition Assessment but not for Nutrition Monitoring and Evaluation.*

Progress Evaluation

Communicate the progress toward the resolution of a nutrition diagnosis by selecting the appropriate nutrition diagnosis status value from the Nutrition Assessment, Monitoring, and Evaluation terms.

NCP Term	ANDUID
New nutrition diagnosis	14586
Active nutrition diagnosis	14587
Resolved nutrition diagnosis	14588
Discontinued nutrition diagnosis	14589

For details on these terms, visit the Nutrition Diagnosis Status reference sheet on page 200.

Inadequate Energy Intake

Definition

Energy intake that is less than energy expenditure, established reference standards, or recommendations based on physiological needs.

Note: May not be an appropriate nutrition diagnosis when the goal is weight loss, during end-of-life care, upon initiation of EN/PN, or acute stressed state (eg, surgery, organ failure).

Whenever possible, nutrient intake data should be considered in combination with clinical, biochemical, anthropometric information, medical diagnosis, clinical status, and/or other factors to provide a valid assessment of nutritional status based on a totality of the evidence. (Institute of Medicine. *Dietary Reference Intakes: Applications in Dietary Assessment.* National Academies Press; 2000.)

Etiology Cause/Contributing Risk Factors

Factors gathered during the nutrition assessment process that contribute to the existence or the maintenance of pathophysiological, psychosocial, situational, developmental, cultural, and/or environmental problems:

- Pathological or physiological causes that result in increased energy requirements, eg, increased nutrient needs due to prolonged catabolic illness
- Decreased ability to consume sufficient energy
- Food insecurity
- Limited access to nutrition-related supplies (eg, artificial nutrition)
- Cultural practices that affect ability to access food
- Food and nutrition related knowledge deficit concerning energy intake
- Psychological causes such as depression and disordered eating

Etiology Category

Etiologies are grouped by the type of cause or contributing risk factor. Communicate the etiology category by selecting the appropriate Nutrition Assessment, Monitoring, and Evaluation term.

NCP Term	ANDUID
Beliefs attitudes etiology	14567
Cultural etiology	14568
Knowledge etiology	14569
Physical function etiology	14570
Physiologic metabolic etiology	14571
Psychological etiology	14572
Social personal etiology	14573
Treatment etiology	14574
Access etiology	14575
Behavior etiology	14576

Visit the Nutrition Diagnosis Etiology Category Identification reference sheet on page 185 for more details on etiology categories. An additional useful resource to determine the etiology category is the Nutrition Diagnosis Matrix on page 528.

Inadequate Energy Intake

Signs/Symptoms (Defining Characteristics)

A typical cluster of subjective and objective signs and symptoms gathered during the nutrition assessment process that provide evidence that a problem exists; quantify the problem and describe its severity.

Nutrition Assessment Category	Potential Indicators of This Nutrition Diagnosis (one or more must be present)
Biochemical Data, Medical Tests and Procedures	
Anthropometric Measurements	Failure to gain or maintain appropriate body weight
Physical Exam Findings	Poor dentition
Food/Nutrition-Related History	Reports or observations of: • Estimated energy intake from diet less than needs based on estimated or measured RMR • Restriction or omission of energy-dense foods from diet • Food avoidance and/or lack of interest in food • Limited ability to independently consume foods/fluids (diminished joint mobility of wrist, hand, or digits) • Estimated parenteral or enteral nutrition intake insufficient to meet needs based on estimated or measured RMR • Excessive consumption of alcohol or other drugs that reduce hunger • Medications that affect appetite
Client History*	Conditions associated with diagnosis or treatment, eg, mental illness, eating disorders, dementia, alcoholism, substance abuse, and acute or chronic pain management
Assessment, Monitoring, and Evaluation Tools	
Comparative Standards	• Total energy estimated needs in 24 hours • Method for estimating total 24 hour energy needs • Energy estimated needs per kg of body weight in 24 hours

** Client History terms are used for Nutrition Assessment but not for Nutrition Monitoring and Evaluation.*

Progress Evaluation

Communicate the progress toward the resolution of a nutrition diagnosis by selecting the appropriate nutrition diagnosis status value from the Nutrition Assessment, Monitoring, and Evaluation terms.

NCP Term	ANDUID
New nutrition diagnosis	14586
Active nutrition diagnosis	14587
Resolved nutrition diagnosis	14588
Discontinued nutrition diagnosis	14589

For details on these terms, visit the Nutrition Diagnosis Status reference sheet on page 200.

Excessive Energy Intake

Definition

Energy intake that exceeds energy expenditure, established reference standards, or recommendations based on physiological needs.

Note: May not be appropriate nutrition diagnosis when weight gain is desired.

Etiology (Cause/Contributing Risk Factors)

Factors gathered during the nutrition assessment process that contribute to the existence or the maintenance of pathophysiological, psychosocial, situational, developmental, cultural, and/or environmental problems:

- Belief finding that hinders food and/or nutrition behavior change
- Attitude finding that hinders food and/or nutrition behavior change
- Food and nutrition related knowledge deficit concerning energy intake
- Food insecurity
- Limited value for behavior change, competing values
- Medications that increase appetite, eg, steroids, antidepressants
- Overfeeding of parenteral/enteral nutrition (PN/EN)
- Calories/kcal/kJ unaccounted for from IV infusion and/or medications
- Limited interest in reducing energy intake
- Limited adjustment for lifestyle changes and decreased metabolism (eg, aging)
- Limited adjustment for restricted mobility due to recovery from injury, surgical procedure, or other
- Resolution of prior hypermetabolism without reduction in intake
- Limited food- and nutrition-related skill

Etiology Category

Etiologies are grouped by the type of cause or contributing risk factor. Communicate the etiology category by selecting the appropriate Nutrition Assessment, Monitoring, and Evaluation term.

NCP Term	ANDUID
Beliefs attitudes etiology	14567
Cultural etiology	14568
Knowledge etiology	14569
Physical function etiology	14570
Physiologic metabolic etiology	14571
Psychological etiology	14572
Social personal etiology	14573
Treatment etiology	14574
Access etiology	14575
Behavior etiology	14576

Visit the Nutrition Diagnosis Etiology Category Identification reference sheet on page 185 for more details on etiology categories. An additional useful resource to determine the etiology category is the Nutrition Diagnosis Matrix on page 528.

Excessive Energy Intake

Signs/Symptoms (Defining Characteristics)

A typical cluster of subjective and objective signs and symptoms gathered during the nutrition assessment process that provide evidence that a problem exists; quantify the problem and describe its severity.

Nutrition Assessment Category	Potential Indicators of This Nutrition Diagnosis (one or more must be present)
Biochemical Data, Medical Tests and Procedures	• Abnormal LFTs after prolonged exposure (3 to 6 weeks) to PN • ↑ Respiratory quotient >1.0
Anthropometric Measurements	• Body fat percentage > 25% for men and > 32% for women • BMI > 25 (adults); BMI > 95th percentile (pediatrics) • Body weight gain
Physical Exam Findings	• Increased body adiposity • Increased respiratory rate
Food/Nutrition-Related History	Reports or observations of: • Intake of energy in excess of estimated or measured energy needs • Intake of high caloric density or large portions of foods/beverages • EN/PN more than estimated or measured (eg, indirect calorimetry) energy expenditure
Client History*	
Assessment, Monitoring, and Evaluation Tools	
Comparative Standards	• Total energy estimated needs in 24 hours • Method for estimating total 24 hour energy needs • Energy estimated needs per kg of body weight in 24 hours

Arrows used with laboratory values: ↑ represents above reference standard and ↓ represents below reference standard.
** Client History terms are used for Nutrition Assessment but not for Nutrition Monitoring and Evaluation.*

Progress Evaluation

Communicate the progress toward the resolution of a nutrition diagnosis by selecting the appropriate nutrition diagnosis status value from the Nutrition Assessment, Monitoring, and Evaluation terms.

NCP Term	ANDUID
New nutrition diagnosis	14586
Active nutrition diagnosis	14587
Resolved nutrition diagnosis	14588
Discontinued nutrition diagnosis	14589

For details on these terms, visit the Nutrition Diagnosis Status reference sheet on page 200.

Predicted Inadequate Energy Intake

Definition

Future energy intake that is anticipated, based on observation, experience, or scientific reason, to be less than estimated energy expenditure, established reference standards, or recommendations based on physiological needs.

Note: May not be an appropriate nutrition diagnosis during weight loss. Use Inadequate Energy Intake when current energy intake is less than energy expenditure.

Etiology (Cause/Contributing Risk Factors)

Factors gathered during the nutrition assessment process that contribute to the existence or the maintenance of pathophysiological, psychosocial, situational, developmental, cultural, and/or environmental problems:

- Scheduled or planned procedure or medical therapy that is predicted to increase energy requirements
- Scheduled or planned medical therapy or medication that is predicted to decrease ability to consume sufficient energy
- Anticipated change in physical demands of work or leisure activities (eg, job change, training for competitive sports)
- Stressful life event or living situation (eg, death in family, divorce, loss of home) that, in the past, resulted in inadequate energy intake

Etiology Category

Etiologies are grouped by the type of cause or contributing risk factor. Communicate the etiology category by selecting the appropriate Nutrition Assessment, Monitoring, and Evaluation term.

NCP Term	ANDUID
Beliefs attitudes etiology	14567
Cultural etiology	14568
Knowledge etiology	14569
Physical function etiology	14570
Physiologic metabolic etiology	14571
Psychological etiology	14572
Social personal etiology	14573
Treatment etiology	14574
Access etiology	14575
Behavior etiology	14576

Visit the Nutrition Diagnosis Etiology Category Identification reference sheet on page 185 for more details on etiology categories. An additional useful resource to determine the etiology category is the Nutrition Diagnosis Matrix on page 528.

Signs/Symptoms (Defining Characteristics)

A typical cluster of subjective and objective signs and symptoms gathered during the nutrition assessment process that provide evidence that a problem exists; quantify the problem and describe its severity.

Predicted Inadequate Energy Intake

Nutrition Assessment Category	Potential Indicators of This Nutrition Diagnosis (one or more must be present)
Biochemical Data, Medical Tests and Procedures	
Anthropometric Measurements	Population-based anthropometric data indicating inadequate energy intake
Physical Exam Findings	
Food/Nutrition-Related History	Reports or observations of: • Estimated energy intake from all sources less than projected needs • History of marginal or inadequate energy intake • Projected change in ability to shop, prepare, and/or consume sufficient energy • Medications that are anticipated to decrease appetite or affect ability to consume sufficient energy • No prior knowledge of need for food- and nutrition-related recommendations • Projected increase in level of physical activity
Client History*	• Scheduled procedure or therapy known to increase energy need or change ability to consume sufficient energy • History or presence of a condition for which research shows an increased incidence of increased energy expenditure • History or presence of a condition for which research shows an increased incidence of inadequate energy intake • Client report of recent or anticipated life stress or change
Assessment, Monitoring, and Evaluation Tools	
Comparative Standards	

** Client History terms are used for Nutrition Assessment but not for Nutrition Monitoring and Evaluation.*

Progress Evaluation

Communicate the progress toward the resolution of a nutrition diagnosis by selecting the appropriate nutrition diagnosis status value from the Nutrition Assessment, Monitoring, and Evaluation terms.

NCP Term	ANDUID
New nutrition diagnosis	14586
Active nutrition diagnosis	14587
Resolved nutrition diagnosis	14588
Discontinued nutrition diagnosis	14589

For details on these terms, visit the Nutrition Diagnosis Status reference sheet on page 200.

Predicted Excessive Energy Intake

Definition

Future energy intake that is anticipated, based on observation, experience, or scientific reason, to exceed estimated energy expenditure, established reference standards, or recommendations based on physiological needs.

Note: May not be appropriate nutrition diagnosis when weight gain is desired. Use Excessive Energy Intake when current energy intake is more than energy expenditure.

Etiology (Cause/Contributing Risk Factors)

Factors gathered during the nutrition assessment process that contribute to the existence or the maintenance of pathophysiological, psychosocial, situational, developmental, cultural, and/or environmental problems:

- Anticipated change in physical demands with periods of immobility or reduced physical activity
- Family or social history or culture of overeating
- Genetic predisposition to overweight/obesity
- Physiological condition associated with altered metabolism
- Scheduled or planned medical therapy or medication that is predicted to reduce metabolic rate/metabolism
- Stressful life event or living situation (eg, death in family, divorce, loss of home) that, in the past, resulted in excessive energy intake

Etiology Category

Etiologies are grouped by the type of cause or contributing risk factor. Communicate the etiology category by selecting the appropriate Nutrition Assessment, Monitoring, and Evaluation term.

NCP Term	ANDUID
Beliefs attitudes etiology	14567
Cultural etiology	14568
Knowledge etiology	14569
Physical function etiology	14570
Physiologic metabolic etiology	14571
Psychological etiology	14572
Social personal etiology	14573
Treatment etiology	14574
Access etiology	14575
Behavior etiology	14576

Visit the Nutrition Diagnosis Etiology Category Identification reference sheet on page 185 for more details on etiology categories. An additional useful resource to determine the etiology category is the Nutrition Diagnosis Matrix on page 528.

Signs/Symptoms (Defining Characteristics)

A typical cluster of subjective and objective signs and symptoms gathered during the nutrition assessment process that provide evidence that a problem exists; quantify the problem and describe its severity.

Predicted Excessive Energy Intake

Nutrition Assessment Category	Potential Indicators of This Nutrition Diagnosis (one or more must be present)
Biochemical Data, Medical Tests and Procedures	
Anthropometric Measurements	Population-based anthropometric data indicating excessive energy intake
Physical Exam Findings	
Food/Nutrition-Related History	Reports or observations of: • Estimated energy intake from all sources more than projected needs at new lower metabolic level • Estimated energy intake from all sources more than projected needs at new lower physical activity level • History of excessive energy intake at previous metabolic level • History of excessive energy intake at previous physical activity level • Recent or planned change in mobility and/or ability to engage in physical activity • Projected change in ability to shop and/or prepare food • Medications that increase appetite • Recent or planned change in physical activity • No prior knowledge of need for food- and nutrition-related recommendations
Client History*	• Scheduled surgical procedure or medical therapy known to decrease energy need • History or presence of a condition for which research shows an increased incidence of decreased energy expenditure • History or presence of a condition for which research shows an increased incidence of excessive energy intake
Assessment, Monitoring, and Evaluation Tools	
Comparative Standards	

** Client History terms are used for Nutrition Assessment but not for Nutrition Monitoring and Evaluation.*

Progress Evaluation

Communicate the progress toward the resolution of a nutrition diagnosis by selecting the appropriate nutrition diagnosis status value from the Nutrition Assessment, Monitoring, and Evaluation terms.

NCP Term	ANDUID
New nutrition diagnosis	14586
Active nutrition diagnosis	14587
Resolved nutrition diagnosis	14588
Discontinued nutrition diagnosis	14589

For details on these terms, visit the Nutrition Diagnosis Status reference sheet on page 200.

Inadequate Oral Intake

Definition

Oral food/beverage intake that is less than established reference standards or recommendations based on physiological needs.

Note: This nutrition diagnosis does not include intake via oroenteric tube.

May not be an appropriate nutrition diagnosis when the goal is weight loss, during end-of-life care, upon initiation of feeding, or during combined oral/EN/PN therapy.

Whenever possible, nutrient intake data should be considered in combination with clinical, biochemical, anthropometric information, medical diagnosis, clinical status, and/or other factors to provide a valid assessment of nutritional status based on a totality of the evidence. (Institute of Medicine. *Dietary Reference Intakes: Applications in Dietary Assessment.* National Academies Press; 2000.)

Etiology (Cause/Contributing Risk Factors)

Factors gathered during the nutrition assessment process that contribute to the existence or the maintenance of pathophysiological, psychosocial, situational, developmental, cultural, and/or environmental problems:

- Physiological causes increasing nutrient needs, eg, due to prolonged catabolic illness
- Decreased ability to consume sufficient energy, eg, increased nutrient needs due to prolonged catabolic illness
- Food insecurity
- Limited food acceptance
- Belief finding that hinders food and/or nutrition behavior change
- Attitude finding that hinders food and/or nutrition behavior change
- Cultural practices that affect ability to access food
- Food and nutrition related knowledge deficit concerning appropriate oral food/beverage intake
- Psychological causes such as depression and disordered eating

Etiology Category

Etiologies are grouped by the type of cause or contributing risk factor. Communicate the etiology category by selecting the appropriate Nutrition Assessment, Monitoring, and Evaluation term.

NCP Term	ANDUID
Beliefs attitudes etiology	14567
Cultural etiology	14568
Knowledge etiology	14569
Physical function etiology	14570
Physiologic metabolic etiology	14571
Psychological etiology	14572
Social personal etiology	14573
Treatment etiology	14574

Continued on next page

Inadequate Oral Intake

Continued from previous page

NCP Term	ANDUID
Access etiology	14575
Behavior etiology	14576

Visit the Nutrition Diagnosis Etiology Category Identification reference sheet on page 185 for more details on etiology categories. An additional useful resource to determine the etiology category is the Nutrition Diagnosis Matrix on page 528.

Signs/Symptoms (Defining Characteristics)

A typical cluster of subjective and objective signs and symptoms gathered during the nutrition assessment process that provide evidence that a problem exists; quantify the problem and describe its severity.

Nutrition Assessment Category	Potential Indicators of This Nutrition Diagnosis (one or more must be present)
Biochemical Data, Medical Tests and Procedures	
Anthropometric Measurements	Body weight loss, insufficient growth velocity
Physical Exam Findings	• Dry skin, mucous membranes, poor skin turgor • Anorexia, nausea, or vomiting • Change in appetite or taste • Clinical evidence of vitamin/mineral deficiency
Food/Nutrition-Related History	Reports or observations of: • Estimates of insufficient intake of energy or high-quality protein from diet when compared to requirements • Economic constraints that limit food availability • Excessive consumption of alcohol or other drugs that reduce hunger • Medications that cause anorexia • Limited food/beverage intake inconsistent with nutrition reference standards for type, variety, diet quality • Less than optimal reliance on foods, food groups, supplements or nutrition support
Client History*	• Conditions associated with a diagnosis or treatment of catabolic illness such as AIDS, tuberculosis, anorexia nervosa, sepsis or infection from recent surgery, depression, acute or chronic pain • Protein and/or nutrient malabsorption
Assessment, Monitoring, and Evaluation Tools	
Comparative Standards	

** Client History terms are used for Nutrition Assessment but not for Nutrition Monitoring and Evaluation.*

Inadequate Oral Intake

Progress Evaluation

Communicate the progress toward the resolution of a nutrition diagnosis by selecting the appropriate nutrition diagnosis status value from the Nutrition Assessment, Monitoring, and Evaluation terms.

NCP Term	ANDUID
New nutrition diagnosis	14586
Active nutrition diagnosis	14587
Resolved nutrition diagnosis	14588
Discontinued nutrition diagnosis	14589

For details on these terms, visit the Nutrition Diagnosis Status reference sheet on page 200.

Excessive Oral Intake

Definition

Oral food/beverage intake that exceeds estimated energy needs, established reference standards, or recommendations based on physiological needs.

Note: This nutrition diagnosis does not include intake via oroenteric tube.

May not be an appropriate nutrition diagnosis when weight gain is desired.

Etiology (Cause/Contributing Risk Factors)

Factors gathered during the nutrition assessment process that contribute to the existence or the maintenance of pathophysiological, psychosocial, situational, developmental, cultural, and/or environmental problems:

- Belief finding that hinders food and/or nutrition behavior change
- Attitude finding that hinders food and/or nutrition behavior change
- Food and nutrition related knowledge deficit concerning appropriate oral food/beverage intake
- Limited access to healthful food choices, eg, healthful food choices not provided as an option by caregiver or parent, client experiencing homelessness
- Limited value for behavior change, competing values
- Inability to limit or refuse offered foods
- Limited food planning, purchasing, and preparation skills
- Loss of appetite awareness
- Medications that increase appetite, eg, steroids, antidepressants
- Psychological causes such as depression and disordered eating
- Unwilling or disinterested in reducing intake

Etiology Category

Etiologies are grouped by the type of cause or contributing risk factor. Communicate the etiology category by selecting the appropriate Nutrition Assessment, Monitoring, and Evaluation term.

NCP Term	ANDUID
Beliefs attitudes etiology	14567
Cultural etiology	14568
Knowledge etiology	14569
Physical function etiology	14570
Physiologic metabolic etiology	14571
Psychological etiology	14572
Social personal etiology	14573
Treatment etiology	14574
Access etiology	14575
Behavior etiology	14576

Visit the Nutrition Diagnosis Etiology Category Identification reference sheet on page 185 for more details on etiology categories. An additional useful resource to determine the etiology category is the Nutrition Diagnosis Matrix on page 528.

Excessive Oral Intake

Signs/Symptoms (Defining Characteristics)

A typical cluster of subjective and objective signs and symptoms gathered during the nutrition assessment process that provide evidence that a problem exists; quantify the problem and describe its severity.

Nutrition Assessment Category	Potential Indicators of This Nutrition Diagnosis (one or more must be present)
Biochemical Data, Medical Tests and Procedures	
Anthropometric Measurements	Weight gain not attributed to fluid retention or normal growth
Physical Exam Findings	
Food/Nutrition-Related History	Reports or observations of: • Intake of energy-dense foods/beverages (juice, soda, or alcohol) at meals and/or snacks • Intake of large portions of foods/beverages, food groups, or specific food items • Estimated intake that exceeds estimated or measured energy needs • Highly variable estimated daily energy intake • Binge eating patterns • Frequent, excessive fast food or restaurant intake
Client History*	Conditions associated with a diagnosis or treatment, eg, obesity, overweight, or metabolic syndrome, depression, anxiety disorder
Assessment, Monitoring, and Evaluation Tools	
Comparative Standards	

** Client History terms are used for Nutrition Assessment but not for Nutrition Monitoring and Evaluation.*

Progress Evaluation

Communicate the progress toward the resolution of a nutrition diagnosis by selecting the appropriate nutrition diagnosis status value from the Nutrition Assessment, Monitoring, and Evaluation terms.

NCP Term	ANDUID
New nutrition diagnosis	14586
Active nutrition diagnosis	14587
Resolved nutrition diagnosis	14588
Discontinued nutrition diagnosis	14589

For details on these terms, visit the Nutrition Diagnosis Status reference sheet on page 200.

Inadequate Enteral Nutrition Infusion

Definition

Enteral infusion that provides fewer calories/kcal/kJ or nutrients compared to established reference standards or recommendations based on physiological needs.

Note: May not be an appropriate nutrition diagnosis when recommendation is for weight loss, during end-of-life care, upon initiation of feeding, or during acute stressed states (eg, surgery, organ failure).

Whenever possible, nutrient intake data should be considered in combination with clinical, biochemical, anthropometric information, medical diagnosis, clinical status, and/or other factors to provide a valid assessment of nutritional status based on a totality of the evidence. (Institute of Medicine. *Dietary Reference Intakes: Applications in Dietary Assessment*. National Academies Press; 2000.)

Etiology (Cause/Contributing Risk Factors)

Factors gathered during the nutrition assessment process that contribute to the existence or the maintenance of pathophysiological, psychosocial, situational, developmental, cultural, and/or environmental problems:

- Altered absorption or metabolism of nutrients, eg, medications
- Food and nutrition related knowledge deficit concerning appropriate formula/formulation given for EN
- Lack of, compromised, or incorrect access for delivering EN
- Physiological causes increasing nutrient needs, eg, due to accelerated growth, wound healing, chronic infection, multiple fractures
- Intolerance of EN
- Infusion volume not reached or schedule for infusion interrupted
- Limited food- and nutrition-related skill

Etiology Category

Etiologies are grouped by the type of cause or contributing risk factor. Communicate the etiology category by selecting the appropriate Nutrition Assessment, Monitoring, and Evaluation term.

NCP Term	ANDUID
Beliefs attitudes etiology	14567
Cultural etiology	14568
Knowledge etiology	14569
Physical function etiology	14570
Physiologic metabolic etiology	14571
Psychological etiology	14572
Social personal etiology	14573
Treatment etiology	14574
Access etiology	14575
Behavior etiology	14576

Visit the Nutrition Diagnosis Etiology Category Identification reference sheet on page 185 for more details on etiology categories. An additional useful resource to determine the etiology category is the Nutrition Diagnosis Matrix on page 528.

Inadequate Enteral Nutrition Infusion

Signs/Symptoms (Defining Characteristics)

A typical cluster of subjective and objective signs and symptoms gathered during the nutrition assessment process that provide evidence that a problem exists; quantify the problem and describe its severity.

Nutrition Assessment Category	Potential Indicators of This Nutrition Diagnosis (one or more must be present)
Biochemical Data, Medical Tests and Procedures	• ↓ Metabolic cart/indirect calorimetry measurement, eg, respiratory quotient < 0.7 • Vitamin/mineral abnormalities: ○ ↓ Calcium < 9.2 mg/dL (2.3 mmol/L) ○ Vitamin K: abnormal INR ○ ↓ Copper < 70 μg/dL (11 μmol/L) ○ ↓ Zinc < 78 μg/dL (12 μmol/L) ○ ↓ Iron < 50 μg/dL (8.9 nmol/L); iron-binding capacity < 250 μg/dL (44.8 μmol/L)
Anthropometric Measurements	• Growth failure, based on reference growth standards, eg National Center for Health Statistics (NCHS) and fetal growth failure • Insufficient maternal weight gain • Limited planned weight gain • Unintentional weight loss of ≥ 5% in 1 month or ≥ 10% in 6 months (not attributed to fluid) in adults • Any weight loss in infants or children • Underweight (BMI < 18.5)
Physical Exam Findings	• Clinical evidence of vitamin/mineral deficiency (eg, hair loss, bleeding gums, pale nail beds, neurologic changes) • Evidence of dehydration, eg, dry mucous membranes, poor skin turgor • Loss of skin integrity, delayed wound healing, or pressure ulcers • Loss of muscle mass and/or subcutaneous fat • Nausea, vomiting, diarrhea
Food/Nutrition-Related History	Reports or observations of: • Inadequate EN volume compared to estimated or measured (indirect calorimetry) requirements • Feeding tube in wrong position or removed • Altered capacity for desired levels of physical activity or exercise, easy fatigue with increased activity • Suboptimal feeding position
Client History*	Conditions associated with a diagnosis or treatment, eg, intestinal resection, Crohn's disease, HIV/AIDS, burns, preterm birth, malnutrition
Assessment, Monitoring, and Evaluation Tools	
Comparative Standards	

Arrows used with laboratory values: ↑ represents above reference standard and ↓ represents below reference standard.
** Client History terms are used for Nutrition Assessment but not for Nutrition Monitoring and Evaluation.*

Inadequate Enteral Nutrition Infusion

Progress Evaluation

Communicate the progress toward the resolution of a nutrition diagnosis by selecting the appropriate nutrition diagnosis status value from the Nutrition Assessment, Monitoring, and Evaluation terms.

NCP Term	ANDUID
New nutrition diagnosis	14586
Active nutrition diagnosis	14587
Resolved nutrition diagnosis	14588
Discontinued nutrition diagnosis	14589

For details on these terms, visit the Nutrition Diagnosis Status reference sheet on page 200.

Excessive Enteral Nutrition Infusion

Definition

Enteral infusion that provides more calories/kcal/kJ or nutrients compared to established reference standards or recommendations based on physiological needs.

Etiology (Cause/Contributing Risk Factors)

Factors gathered during the nutrition assessment process that contribute to the existence or the maintenance of pathophysiological, psychosocial, situational, developmental, cultural, and/or environmental problems:

- Physiological causes, eg, decreased needs related to low activity levels with critical illness or organ failure
- Food and nutrition related knowledge deficit concerning appropriate amount of enteral nutrition
- Limited food- and nutrition-related skill

Etiology Category

Etiologies are grouped by the type of cause or contributing risk factor. Communicate the etiology category by selecting the appropriate Nutrition Assessment, Monitoring, and Evaluation term.

NCP Term	ANDUID
Beliefs attitudes etiology	14567
Cultural etiology	14568
Knowledge etiology	14569
Physical function etiology	14570
Physiologic metabolic etiology	14571
Psychological etiology	14572
Social personal etiology	14573
Treatment etiology	14574
Access etiology	14575
Behavior etiology	14576

Visit the Nutrition Diagnosis Etiology Category Identification reference sheet on page 185 for more details on etiology categories. An additional useful resource to determine the etiology category is the Nutrition Diagnosis Matrix on page 528.

Signs/Symptoms (Defining Characteristics)

A typical cluster of subjective and objective signs and symptoms gathered during the nutrition assessment process that provide evidence that a problem exists; quantify the problem and describe its severity.

Excessive Enteral Nutrition Infusion

Nutrition Assessment Category	Potential Indicators of This Nutrition Diagnosis (one or more must be present)
Biochemical Data, Medical Tests and Procedures	• ↑ BUN:creatinine ratio (protein) • Hyperglycemia (carbohydrate) • Hypercapnia
Anthropometric Measurements	Weight gain in excess of lean tissue accretion
Physical Exam Findings	Edema with excess fluid administration
Food/Nutrition-Related History	Reports or observations of: • Estimated intake from enteral nutrients that is consistently more than recommended intake for carbohydrate, protein, and fat • Use of drugs that reduce requirements or impair metabolism of energy, protein, fat, or fluid. • Unrealistic expectations of weight gain or ideal weight
Client History*	
Assessment, Monitoring, and Evaluation Tools	
Comparative Standards	

Arrows used with laboratory values: ↑ represents above reference standard and ↓ represents below reference standard.
** Client History terms are used for Nutrition Assessment but not for Nutrition Monitoring and Evaluation.*

Progress Evaluation

Communicate the progress toward the resolution of a nutrition diagnosis by selecting the appropriate nutrition diagnosis status value from the Nutrition Assessment, Monitoring, and Evaluation terms.

NCP Term	ANDUID
New nutrition diagnosis	14586
Active nutrition diagnosis	14587
Resolved nutrition diagnosis	14588
Discontinued nutrition diagnosis	14589

For details on these terms, visit the Nutrition Diagnosis Status reference sheet on page 200.

Enteral Nutrition Composition Inconsistent With Needs

Definition

Enteral nutrition (EN) formula that varies from established reference standards or recommendations based on physiological needs.

Etiology (Cause/Contributing Risk Factors)

Factors gathered during the nutrition assessment process that contribute to the existence or the maintenance of pathophysiological, psychosocial, situational, developmental, cultural, and/or environmental problems:

- Physiological causes, eg, improvement in client status, allowing return to total or partial oral diet; changes in the course of disease resulting in changes in feeding and/or nutrient requirements
- Food and nutrition related knowledge deficit concerning EN product
- End-of-life care if client or family does not desire nutrition support

Etiology Category

Etiologies are grouped by the type of cause or contributing risk factor. Communicate the etiology category by selecting the appropriate Nutrition Assessment, Monitoring, and Evaluation term.

NCP Term	ANDUID
Beliefs attitudes etiology	14567
Cultural etiology	14568
Knowledge etiology	14569
Physical function etiology	14570
Physiologic metabolic etiology	14571
Psychological etiology	14572
Social personal etiology	14573
Treatment etiology	14574
Access etiology	14575
Behavior etiology	14576

Visit the Nutrition Diagnosis Etiology Category Identification reference sheet on page 185 for more details on etiology categories. An additional useful resource to determine the etiology category is the Nutrition Diagnosis Matrix on page 528.

Signs/Symptoms (Defining Characteristics)

A typical cluster of subjective and objective signs and symptoms gathered during the nutrition assessment process that provide evidence that a problem exists; quantify the problem and describe its severity.

Nutrition Assessment Category	Potential Indicators of This Nutrition Diagnosis (one or more must be present)
Biochemical Data, Medical Tests and Procedures	Abnormal levels of markers specific for various nutrients, eg, hyperphosphatemia in patient/client receiving feedings with a high phosphorus content, hypokalemia in patient/client receiving feedings with low potassium content

Continued on next page

Enteral Nutrition Composition Inconsistent With Needs

Continued from previous page

Nutrition Assessment Category	Potential Indicators of This Nutrition Diagnosis (one or more must be present)
Anthropometric Measurements	• Weight gain in excess of lean tissue accretion • Weight loss
Physical Exam Findings	• Edema with excess fluid administration • Loss of subcutaneous fat and muscle stores • Diarrhea, constipation
Food/Nutrition-Related History	Reports or observations of: • Estimated intake from enteral nutrients that is consistently more or less than recommended intake for carbohydrate, proteins or amino acids, fat or fatty acids, and/or micronutrients • Formula composition that is inconsistent with ability to digest and absorb nutrients • Formula composition or concentration that is inconsistent with evidence-based practice • Verbalizations or written responses that are inaccurate or incomplete for EN formula prescribed
Client History*	• Improved or diminished gastrointestinal function • Conditions associated with a diagnosis or treatment, eg, major elective surgery, trauma, burns, or head and neck cancer, and critically ill patients, acute lung injury, acute respiratory distress syndrome, treatments/therapy requiring interruption of infusion, transfer of nutrition care to a new setting or level of care, or end-of-life care
Assessment, Monitoring, and Evaluation Tools	
Comparative Standards	

** Client History terms are used for Nutrition Assessment but not for Nutrition Monitoring and Evaluation.*

Progress Evaluation

Communicate the progress toward the resolution of a nutrition diagnosis by selecting the appropriate nutrition diagnosis status value from the Nutrition Assessment, Monitoring, and Evaluation terms.

NCP Term	ANDUID
New nutrition diagnosis	14586
Active nutrition diagnosis	14587
Resolved nutrition diagnosis	14588
Discontinued nutrition diagnosis	14589

For details on these terms, visit the Nutrition Diagnosis Status reference sheet on page 200.

Enteral Nutrition Administration Inconsistent With Needs

Definition

Enteral nutrition (EN) provision that varies from established reference standards or recommendations based on physiological needs.

Etiology (Cause/Contributing Risk Factors)

Factors gathered during the nutrition assessment process that contribute to the existence or the maintenance of pathophysiological, psychosocial, situational, developmental, cultural, and/or environmental problems:

- Physiological causes, eg, improvement in client status, allowing return to total or partial oral diet; changes in the course of disease resulting in changes in feeding
- Food and nutrition related knowledge deficit concerning EN product provision
- End-of-life care if client or family does not desire nutrition support
- Limited food- and nutrition-related skill

Etiology Category

Etiologies are grouped by the type of cause or contributing risk factor. Communicate the etiology category by selecting the appropriate Nutrition Assessment, Monitoring, and Evaluation term.

NCP Term	ANDUID
Beliefs attitudes etiology	14567
Cultural etiology	14568
Knowledge etiology	14569
Physical function etiology	14570
Physiologic metabolic etiology	14571
Psychological etiology	14572
Social personal etiology	14573
Treatment etiology	14574
Access etiology	14575
Behavior etiology	14576

Visit the Nutrition Diagnosis Etiology Category Identification reference sheet on page 185 for more details on etiology categories. An additional useful resource to determine the etiology category is the Nutrition Diagnosis Matrix on page 528.

Signs/Symptoms (Defining Characteristics)

A typical cluster of subjective and objective signs and symptoms gathered during the nutrition assessment process that provide evidence that a problem exists; quantify the problem and describe its severity.

Enteral Nutrition Administration Inconsistent With Needs

Nutrition Assessment Category	Potential Indicators of This Nutrition Diagnosis (one or more must be present)
Biochemical Data, Medical Tests and Procedures	↑ or ↓ serum glucose
Anthropometric Measurements	
Physical Exam Findings	• Nausea, vomiting, diarrhea, high gastric residual volume • Satiety
Food/Nutrition-Related History	Reports or observations of: • Access route that may warrant modification • Access type that may warrant modification • Administration that may conflict with oral intake • Administration that may conflict with therapies (including medications) or procedures • EN that may contribute to poor food and/or nutrition quality of life • Intolerance of feeding method • Intolerance of rate of delivery • Verbalizations or written responses that are inaccurate or incomplete regarding EN administration • History of EN intolerance
Client History*	• Improved/diminished gastrointestinal function • Conditions associated with a diagnosis or treatment, eg, major elective surgery, trauma, burns, or head and neck cancer, and critical illness, acute lung injury, acute respiratory distress syndrome, treatments/therapy requiring interruption of infusion, transfer of nutrition care to a new setting or level of care, or end-of-life care
Assessment, Monitoring, and Evaluation Tools	
Comparative Standards	

Arrows used with laboratory values: ↑ represents above reference standard and ↓ represents below reference standard.
** Client History terms are used for Nutrition Assessment but not for Nutrition Monitoring and Evaluation.*

Progress Evaluation

Communicate the progress toward the resolution of a nutrition diagnosis by selecting the appropriate nutrition diagnosis status value from the Nutrition Assessment, Monitoring, and Evaluation terms.

NCP Term	ANDUID
New nutrition diagnosis	14586
Active nutrition diagnosis	14587
Resolved nutrition diagnosis	14588
Discontinued nutrition diagnosis	14589

For details on these terms, visit the Nutrition Diagnosis Status reference sheet on page 200.

Inadequate Parenteral Nutrition Infusion

Definition

Parenteral infusion that provides fewer calories/kcal/kJ or nutrients compared to established reference standards or recommendations based on physiological needs.

Note: May not be an appropriate nutrition diagnosis when recommendation is for weight loss, during end-of-life care, upon initiation of feeding, or during acute stressed states (eg, surgery, organ failure).

Whenever possible, nutrient intake data should be considered in combination with clinical, biochemical, anthropometric information, medical diagnosis, clinical status, and/or other factors to provide a valid assessment of nutritional status based on a totality of the evidence. (Institute of Medicine. *Dietary Reference Intakes: Applications in Dietary Assessment*. National Academies Press; 2000.)

Etiology (Cause/Contributing Risk Factors)

Factors gathered during the nutrition assessment process that contribute to the existence or the maintenance of pathophysiological, psychosocial, situational, developmental, cultural, and/or environmental problems:

- Altered absorption or metabolism of nutrients, eg, medications
- Food and nutrition related knowledge deficit concerning appropriate formula/formulation given for PN
- Lack of, compromised, or incorrect access for delivering PN
- Physiological causes increasing nutrient needs, eg, due to accelerated growth, wound healing, chronic infection, multiple fractures
- Intolerance of PN
- Infusion volume not reached or schedule for infusion interrupted
- Limited food- and nutrition-related skill

Etiology Category

Etiologies are grouped by the type of cause or contributing risk factor. Communicate the etiology category by selecting the appropriate Nutrition Assessment, Monitoring, and Evaluation term.

NCP Term	ANDUID
Beliefs attitudes etiology	14567
Cultural etiology	14568
Knowledge etiology	14569
Physical function etiology	14570
Physiologic metabolic etiology	14571
Psychological etiology	14572
Social personal etiology	14573
Treatment etiology	14574
Access etiology	14575
Behavior etiology	14576

Visit the Nutrition Diagnosis Etiology Category Identification reference sheet on page 185 for more details on etiology categories. An additional useful resource to determine the etiology category is the Nutrition Diagnosis Matrix on page 528.

Inadequate Parenteral Nutrition Infusion

Signs/Symptoms (Defining Characteristics)

A typical cluster of subjective and objective signs and symptoms gathered during the nutrition assessment process that provide evidence that a problem exists; quantify the problem and describe its severity.

Nutrition Assessment Category	Potential Indicators of This Nutrition Diagnosis (one or more must be present)
Biochemical Data, Medical Tests and Procedures	• ↓ Metabolic cart/indirect calorimetry measurement, eg, respiratory quotient < 0.7 • Vitamin/mineral abnormalities: ○ ↓ Calcium < 9.2 mg/dL (2.3 mmol/L) ○ Vitamin K: abnormal INR ○ ↓ Copper < 70 µg/dL (11 µmol/L) ○ ↓ Zinc < 78 µg/dL (12 µmol/L) ○ ↓ Iron < 50 µg/dL(nmol/L); iron-binding capacity < 250 µg/dL (44.8 µmol/L)
Anthropometric Measurements	• Growth failure, based on reference growth standards, eg National Center for Health Statistics (NCHS) and fetal growth failure • Insufficient maternal weight gain • Lack of planned weight gain • Unintentional weight loss of 5% in 1 month or 10% in 6 months (not attributed to fluid) in adults • Any weight loss in infants or children • Underweight (BMI < 18.5)
Physical Exam Findings	• Clinical evidence of vitamin/mineral deficiency (eg, hair loss, bleeding gums, pale nail beds, neurologic changes) • Evidence of dehydration, eg, dry mucous membranes, poor skin turgor • Loss of skin integrity, delayed wound healing, or pressure ulcers • Loss of muscle mass and/or subcutaneous fat • Nausea, vomiting, diarrhea
Food/Nutrition-Related History	Reports or observations of: • Inadequate PN volume compared to estimated or measured (indirect calorimetry) requirements • Feeding tube or venous access in wrong position or removed • Altered capacity for desired levels of physical activity or exercise, easy fatigue with increased activity
Client History*	Conditions associated with a diagnosis or treatment, eg, intestinal resection, Crohn's disease, HIV/AIDS, burns, preterm birth, malnutrition
Assessment, Monitoring, and Evaluation Tools	
Comparative Standards	

Arrows used with laboratory values: ↑ represents above reference standard and ↓ represents below reference standard.
** Client History terms are used for Nutrition Assessment but not for Nutrition Monitoring and Evaluation.*

Inadequate Parenteral Nutrition Infusion

Progress Evaluation

Communicate the progress toward the resolution of a nutrition diagnosis by selecting the appropriate nutrition diagnosis status value from the Nutrition Assessment, Monitoring, and Evaluation terms.

NCP Term	ANDUID
New nutrition diagnosis	14586
Active nutrition diagnosis	14587
Resolved nutrition diagnosis	14588
Discontinued nutrition diagnosis	14589

For details on these terms, visit the Nutrition Diagnosis Status reference sheet on page 200.

Excessive Parenteral Nutrition Infusion

Definition

Parenteral infusion that provides more calories/kcal/kJ or nutrients compared to established reference standards or recommendations based on physiological needs.

Etiology (Cause/Contributing Risk Factors)

Factors gathered during the nutrition assessment process that contribute to the existence or the maintenance of pathophysiological, psychosocial, situational, developmental, cultural, and/or environmental problems:

- Physiological causes, eg, decreased needs related to low activity levels with critical illness or organ failure
- Food and nutrition related knowledge deficit concerning appropriate amount of parenteral nutrition
- Limited food- and nutrition-related skill

Etiology Category

Etiologies are grouped by the type of cause or contributing risk factor. Communicate the etiology category by selecting the appropriate Nutrition Assessment, Monitoring, and Evaluation term.

NCP Term	ANDUID
Beliefs attitudes etiology	14567
Cultural etiology	14568
Knowledge etiology	14569
Physical function etiology	14570
Physiologic metabolic etiology	14571
Psychological etiology	14572
Social personal etiology	14573
Treatment etiology	14574
Access etiology	14575
Behavior etiology	14576

Visit the Nutrition Diagnosis Etiology Category Identification reference sheet on page 185 for more details on etiology categories. An additional useful resource to determine the etiology category is the Nutrition Diagnosis Matrix on page 528.

Signs/Symptoms (Defining Characteristics)

A typical cluster of subjective and objective signs and symptoms gathered during the nutrition assessment process that provide evidence that a problem exists; quantify the problem and describe its severity.

Excessive Parenteral Nutrition Infusion

Nutrition Assessment Category	Potential Indicators of This Nutrition Diagnosis (one or more must be present)
Biochemical Data, Medical Tests and Procedures	• ↑ BUN:creatinine ratio (protein) • Hyperglycemia (carbohydrate) • Hypercapnia • ↑ Liver enzymes
Anthropometric Measurements	Weight gain in excess of lean tissue accretion
Physical Exam Findings	Edema with excess fluid administration
Food/Nutrition-Related History	Reports or observations of: • Estimated intake from parenteral nutrients that is consistently more than recommended intake for carbohydrate, protein, and fat • Use of drugs that reduce requirements or impair metabolism of energy, protein, fat, or fluid • Unrealistic expectations of weight gain or ideal weight
Client History*	
Assessment, Monitoring, and Evaluation Tools	
Comparative Standards	

Arrows used with laboratory values: ↑ represents above reference standard and ↓ represents below reference standard.
** Client History terms are used for Nutrition Assessment but not for Nutrition Monitoring and Evaluation.*

Progress Evaluation

Communicate the progress toward the resolution of a nutrition diagnosis by selecting the appropriate nutrition diagnosis status value from the Nutrition Assessment, Monitoring, and Evaluation terms.

NCP Term	ANDUID
New nutrition diagnosis	14586
Active nutrition diagnosis	14587
Resolved nutrition diagnosis	14588
Discontinued nutrition diagnosis	14589

For details on these terms, visit the Nutrition Diagnosis Status reference sheet on page 200.

Parenteral Nutrition Composition Inconsistent With Needs

Definition

Parenteral nutrition solution that varies from established reference standards or recommendations based on physiological needs.

Etiology (Cause/Contributing Risk Factors)

Factors gathered during the nutrition assessment process that contribute to the existence or the maintenance of pathophysiological, psychosocial, situational, developmental, cultural, and/or environmental problems:

- Physiological causes, eg, improvement in client status, allowing return to total or partial oral diet or enteral nutrition; changes in the course of disease resulting in changes in feeding and/or nutrient requirements
- Food and nutrition related knowledge deficit concerning parenteral nutrition (PN) composition
- End-of-life care if client or family does not desire nutrition support

Etiology Category

Etiologies are grouped by the type of cause or contributing risk factor. Communicate the etiology category by selecting the appropriate Nutrition Assessment, Monitoring, and Evaluation term.

NCP Term	ANDUID
Beliefs attitudes etiology	14567
Cultural etiology	14568
Knowledge etiology	14569
Physical function etiology	14570
Physiologic metabolic etiology	14571
Psychological etiology	14572
Social personal etiology	14573
Treatment etiology	14574
Access etiology	14575
Behavior etiology	14576

Visit the Nutrition Diagnosis Etiology Category Identification reference sheet on page 185 for more details on etiology categories. An additional useful resource to determine the etiology category is the Nutrition Diagnosis Matrix on page 528.

Signs/Symptoms (Defining Characteristics)

A typical cluster of subjective and objective signs and symptoms gathered during the nutrition assessment process that provide evidence that a problem exists; quantify the problem and describe its severity. (See the next page for the nutrition assessment category and potential indicators.)

Parenteral Nutrition Composition Inconsistent With Needs

Nutrition Assessment Category	Potential Indicators of This Nutrition Diagnosis (one or more must be present)
Biochemical Data, Medical Tests and Procedures	• ↑ LFTs in client on long-term (more than 3 to 6 weeks) nutrition support • Abnormal levels of markers specific for various nutrients, eg, hyperphosphatemia in patient/client receiving feedings with a high phosphorus content, hypokalemia in patient/client receiving feedings with low potassium content
Anthropometric Measurements	• Weight gain in excess of lean tissue accretion • Weight loss
Physical Exam Findings	• Edema with excess fluid administration • Loss of subcutaneous fat and muscle stores • Nausea
Food/Nutrition-Related History	Reports or observations of: • Estimated intake from parenteral nutrients that is consistently more or less than recommended intake for carbohydrate, protein or amino acids, fat or fatty acids, vitamins, and/or minerals • Estimated intake of other nutrients that is consistently more or less than recommended • Formula composition or type that is inconsistent with evidence-based practice • Verbalizations or written responses that are inaccurate or incomplete regarding PN solution • History of PN intolerance
Client History*	• Complications such as fatty liver in the absence of other causes • Resolving or improved GI function • Conditions associated with a diagnosis or treatment, eg, major elective surgery, trauma, burns, or head and neck cancer, and critically ill clients, acute lung injury, acute respiratory distress syndrome, treatments/therapy requiring interruption of infusion, transfer of nutrition care to a new setting or level of care, or end-of-life care
Assessment, Monitoring, and Evaluation Tools	
Comparative Standards	

Arrows used with laboratory values: ↑ represents above reference standard and ↓ represents below reference standard.
** Client History terms are used for Nutrition Assessment but not for Nutrition Monitoring and Evaluation.*

Parenteral Nutrition Composition Inconsistent With Needs

Progress Evaluation

Communicate the progress toward the resolution of a nutrition diagnosis by selecting the appropriate nutrition diagnosis status value from the Nutrition Assessment, Monitoring, and Evaluation terms.

NCP Term	ANDUID
New nutrition diagnosis	14586
Active nutrition diagnosis	14587
Resolved nutrition diagnosis	14588
Discontinued nutrition diagnosis	14589

For details on these terms, visit the Nutrition Diagnosis Status reference sheet on page 200.

Parenteral Nutrition Administration Inconsistent With Needs

Definition

Parenteral nutrition provision that varies from established reference standards or recommendations based on physiological needs

Etiology (Cause/Contributing Risk Factors)

Factors gathered during the nutrition assessment process that contribute to the existence or the maintenance of pathophysiological, psychosocial, situational, developmental, cultural, and/or environmental problems:

- Physiological causes, eg, improvement in client status, allowing return to total or partial oral diet or enteral nutrition; changes in the course of disease resulting in changes in feeding provision
- Food and nutrition related knowledge deficit concerning PN provision
- End-of-life care, client or family does not desire nutrition support

Etiology Category

Etiologies are grouped by the type of cause or contributing risk factor. Communicate the etiology category by selecting the appropriate Nutrition Assessment, Monitoring, and Evaluation term.

NCP Term	ANDUID
Beliefs attitudes etiology	14567
Cultural etiology	14568
Knowledge etiology	14569
Physical function etiology	14570
Physiologic metabolic etiology	14571
Psychological etiology	14572
Social personal etiology	14573
Treatment etiology	14574
Access etiology	14575
Behavior etiology	14576

Visit the Nutrition Diagnosis Etiology Category Identification reference sheet on page 185 for more details on etiology categories. An additional useful resource to determine the etiology category is the Nutrition Diagnosis Matrix on page 528.

Signs/Symptoms (Defining Characteristics)

A typical cluster of subjective and objective signs and symptoms gathered during the nutrition assessment process that provide evidence that a problem exists; quantify the problem and describe its severity.

Parenteral Nutrition Administration Inconsistent With Needs

Nutrition Assessment Category	Potential Indicators of This Nutrition Diagnosis (one or more must be present)
Biochemical Data, Medical Tests and Procedures	↑ LFTs in client on long-term (more than 3 to 6 weeks) nutrition support
Anthropometric Measurements	
Physical Exam Findings	• Infusion site compromise • Nausea
Food/Nutrition-Related History	Reports or observations of: • Access route that may warrant modification • Access type that may warrant modification • PN that may conflict with oral or enteral nutrition intake • PN that may conflict with therapies or procedures • PN that may contribute to poor food and/or nutrition quality of life • Intolerance of rate of delivery • Verbalizations or written responses that are inaccurate or incomplete regarding PN administration • History of PN intolerance
Client History*	• Complications such as fatty liver in the absence of other causes • Resolving or improved GI function • Conditions associated with a diagnosis or treatment, eg, major elective surgery, trauma, burns, head and neck cancer, and critically ill clients, acute lung injury, acute respiratory distress syndrome, treatments/therapy requiring interruption of infusion, transfer of nutrition care to a new setting or level of care, end-of-life care
Assessment, Monitoring, and Evaluation Tools	
Comparative Standards	

Arrows used with laboratory values: ↑ represents above reference standard and ↓ represents below reference standard.
** Client History terms are used for Nutrition Assessment but not for Nutrition Monitoring and Evaluation.*

Progress Evaluation

Communicate the progress toward the resolution of a nutrition diagnosis by selecting the appropriate nutrition diagnosis status value from the Nutrition Assessment, Monitoring, and Evaluation terms.

NCP Term	ANDUID
New nutrition diagnosis	14586
Active nutrition diagnosis	14587
Resolved nutrition diagnosis	14588
Discontinued nutrition diagnosis	14589

For details on these terms, visit the Nutrition Diagnosis Status reference sheet on page 200.

Unbalanced Diet Pattern

Definition

Food (ie, solid, liquid) intake, representative of usual food intake, that is inconsistent with dietary reference intake standards (eg, Dietary Reference Intakes, reference intakes by country), national food guidelines (eg, U.S. Dietary Guidelines, country diet guidelines), diet quality index standards (eg, Healthy Eating Index) or as defined in the nutrition prescription.

Etiology (Cause/Contributing Risk Factors)

Factors gathered during the nutrition assessment process that contribute to the existence or the maintenance of pathophysiological, psychosocial, situational, developmental, cultural, and/or environmental problems:

- Limited exposure to accurate nutrition-related information
- Cultural belief that contributes to unbalanced diet
- Limited cognitive ability, including learning differences
- Fatigue or side effect of treatment
- Food insecurity
- Perception that limited resources (eg, time, financial, or interpersonal) prevent balanced food intake
- Food allergies, food intolerance
- Limited motivation and/or readiness to apply or support systems change
- Limited interest in learning information and/or applying skills
- Psychological causes such as depression
- Limited social support in personal or broader social environment to support food choices
- Limited physical ability to obtain varied food consistently
- Biological differences in food preference
- Physiological causes, eg, pain, discomfort, functional issues in the GI tract, neurological changes
- Behavioral concerns, eg, caregiver issues, eating behavior that serves another purpose
- Belief finding that hinders food and/or nutrition behavior change
- Attitude finding that hinders food and/or nutrition behavior change

Etiology Category

Etiologies are grouped by the type of cause or contributing risk factor. Communicate the etiology category by selecting the appropriate Nutrition Assessment, Monitoring, and Evaluation term.

NCP Term	ANDUID
Beliefs attitudes etiology	14567
Cultural etiology	14568
Knowledge etiology	14569
Physical function etiology	14570
Physiologic metabolic etiology	14571
Psychological etiology	14572
Social personal etiology	14573
Treatment etiology	14574

Continued on next page

Unbalanced Diet Pattern

Continued from previous page

NCP Term	ANDUID
Access etiology	14575
Behavior etiology	14576

Visit the Nutrition Diagnosis Etiology Category Identification reference sheet on page 185 for more details on etiology categories. An additional useful resource to determine the etiology category is the Nutrition Diagnosis Matrix on page 528.

Signs/Symptoms (Defining Characteristics)

A typical cluster of subjective and objective signs and symptoms gathered during the nutrition assessment process that provide evidence that a problem exists; quantify the problem and describe its severity.

Nutrition Assessment Category	Potential Indicators of This Nutrition Diagnosis (one or more must be present)
Biochemical Data, Medical Tests and Procedures	• ↑ Lipid panel • ↓ and/or ↑ micronutrient levels • ↓ Urine pH, 24 hour • ↓ Urine citrate, 24 hour
Anthropometric Measurements	• ↑ Body weight • ↓ Body weight
Physical Exam Findings	Findings consistent with vitamin and/or /mineral deficiency and/or excess
Food/Nutrition-Related History	• Reports or observations of: • Estimated intake inconsistent with dietary reference intake standards (eg, DRIs, reference intakes by country), national food guidelines (eg, US Dietary Guidelines, country diet guidelines), diet quality index standards (eg, Healthy Eating Index), or nutrition prescription • Intake reflecting limited consumption of nutrient rich foods, eg, vegetables and fruits • Low intake of fruit and vegetables and/or high intake of protein foods that may result in ↓ urine pH, 24 hour • Limited access to food consistent with guidelines • Fatigue during eating • None to basic nutrition knowledge • None to basic nutrition skill ability • Limited readiness to change nutrition-related behavior score • Precontemplation stage for readiness to change • Negative emotions about food and nutrition
Client History*	Conditions associated with a diagnosis or treatment that might contribute to unbalanced diet pattern

Continued on next page

Unbalanced Diet Pattern

Continued from previous page

Nutrition Assessment Category	Potential Indicators of This Nutrition Diagnosis (one or more must be present)
Assessment, Monitoring, and Evaluation Tools	Low Minimum Dietary Diversity for Women (MDD-W) indicator score
Comparative Standards	• Ideal/reference body weight (IBW) • Recommended body mass index (BMI) • Goal body weight • Goal body weight for length *z* score • Goal body mass index (BMI) for age *z* score • Percent median body mass index (BMI)

Arrows used with laboratory values: ↑ represents above reference standard and ↓ represents below reference standard.
** Client History terms are used for Nutrition Assessment but not for Nutrition Monitoring and Evaluation.*

Progress Evaluation

Communicate the progress toward the resolution of a nutrition diagnosis by selecting the appropriate nutrition diagnosis status value from the Nutrition Assessment, Monitoring, and Evaluation terms.

NCP Term	ANDUID
New nutrition diagnosis	14586
Active nutrition diagnosis	14587
Resolved nutrition diagnosis	14588
Discontinued nutrition diagnosis	14589

For details on these terms, visit the Nutrition Diagnosis Status reference sheet on page 200.

Inadequate Fluid Intake

Definition

Lower intake of fluid-containing foods or substances compared to established reference standards or recommendations based on physiological needs.

Note: Whenever possible, nutrient intake data should be considered in combination with clinical, biochemical, anthropometric information, medical diagnosis, clinical status, and/or other factors to provide a valid assessment of nutritional status based on a totality of the evidence. (Institute of Medicine. *Dietary Reference Intakes: Applications in Dietary Assessment*. National Academies Press; 2000.)

Etiology (Cause/Contributing Risk Factors)

Factors gathered during the nutrition assessment process that contribute to the existence or the maintenance of pathophysiological, psychosocial, situational, developmental, cultural, and/or environmental problems:

- Physiological causes increasing fluid needs due to climate/temperature change, increased exercise or conditions leading to increased fluid losses, fever causing increased insensible losses, decreased thirst sensation, or use of drugs that reduce thirst
- Limited access to potable water, eg, economic constraints, unable to access fluid independently such as elderly or children
- Cultural practices that affect the ability to access fluid
- Food and nutrition related knowledge deficit concerning appropriate fluid intake
- Psychological causes, eg, depression or disordered eating
- Impaired cognitive ability, including learning disabilities, neurological or sensory impairment, and/or dementia
- Limited food- and nutrition-related skill

Etiology Category

Etiologies are grouped by the type of cause or contributing risk factor. Communicate the etiology category by selecting the appropriate Nutrition Assessment, Monitoring, and Evaluation term.

NCP Term	ANDUID
Beliefs attitudes etiology	14567
Cultural etiology	14568
Knowledge etiology	14569
Physical function etiology	14570
Physiologic metabolic etiology	14571
Psychological etiology	14572
Social personal etiology	14573
Treatment etiology	14574
Access etiology	14575
Behavior etiology	14576

Visit the Nutrition Diagnosis Etiology Category Identification reference sheet on page 185 for more details on etiology categories. An additional useful resource to determine the etiology category is the Nutrition Diagnosis Matrix on page 528.

Inadequate Fluid Intake

Signs/Symptoms (Defining Characteristics)

A typical cluster of subjective and objective signs and symptoms gathered during the nutrition assessment process that provide evidence that a problem exists; quantify the problem and describe its severity.

Nutrition Assessment Category	Potential Indicators of This Nutrition Diagnosis (one or more must be present)
Biochemical Data, Medical Tests and Procedures	• Plasma or serum osmolality greater than 290 mOsm/kg • Abnormal BUN, Na • ↓ Urine volume • ↑ Urine specific gravity • Hyperglycemia in diabetic client
Anthropometric Measurements	Acute body weight loss
Physical Exam Findings	• Dry skin and mucous membranes, poor skin turgor, tachycardia and normal or hypotensive blood pressure, fever, increased respirations, flattened neck veins • Thirst • Difficulty swallowing • Increased insensible loss
Food/Nutrition-Related History	Reports or observations of: • Estimated intake of fluid less than requirements (eg, per body surface area for pediatrics) • Use of drugs that reduce thirst
Client History*	Conditions associated with a diagnosis or treatment, eg, dementia resulting in decreased recognition of thirst, dehydration, diabetes mellitus, alterations in renal function, diarrhea, vomiting, ileostomy, colostomy, infection
Assessment, Monitoring, and Evaluation Tools	
Comparative Standards	• Total fluid estimated needs in 24 hours • Method for estimating 24 hour fluid needs

Arrows used with laboratory values: ↑ represents above reference standard and ↓ represents below reference standard.
** Client History terms are used for Nutrition Assessment but not for Nutrition Monitoring and Evaluation.*

Progress Evaluation

Communicate the progress toward the resolution of a nutrition diagnosis by selecting the appropriate nutrition diagnosis status value from the Nutrition Assessment, Monitoring, and Evaluation terms.

NCP Term	ANDUID
New nutrition diagnosis	14586
Active nutrition diagnosis	14587
Resolved nutrition diagnosis	14588
Discontinued nutrition diagnosis	14589

For details on these terms, visit the Nutrition Diagnosis Status reference sheet on page 200.

Excessive Fluid Intake

Definition

Higher intake of fluid compared to established reference standards or recommendations based on physiological needs.

Etiology (Cause/Contributing Risk Factors)

Factors gathered during the nutrition assessment process that contribute to the existence or the maintenance of pathophysiological, psychosocial, situational, developmental, cultural, and/or environmental problems:

- Physiological causes, eg, kidney, liver, cardiac, endocrine, neurological, and/or pulmonary dysfunction; diminished water and sodium losses due to changes in exercise or climate, syndrome of inappropriate antidiuretic hormone (SIADH)
- Food and nutrition related knowledge deficit concerning appropriate fluid intake
- Psychological causes such as depression and disordered eating
- Limited food- and nutrition-related skill

Etiology Category

Etiologies are grouped by the type of cause or contributing risk factor. Communicate the etiology category by selecting the appropriate Nutrition Assessment, Monitoring, and Evaluation term.

NCP Term	ANDUID
Beliefs attitudes etiology	14567
Cultural etiology	14568
Knowledge etiology	14569
Physical function etiology	14570
Physiologic metabolic etiology	14571
Psychological etiology	14572
Social personal etiology	14573
Treatment etiology	14574
Access etiology	14575
Behavior etiology	14576

Visit the Nutrition Diagnosis Etiology Category Identification reference sheet on page 185 for more details on etiology categories. An additional useful resource to determine the etiology category is the Nutrition Diagnosis Matrix on page 528.

Signs/Symptoms (Defining Characteristics)

A typical cluster of subjective and objective signs and symptoms gathered during the nutrition assessment process that provide evidence that a problem exists; quantify the problem and describe its severity. (See the next page for the nutrition assessment category and potential indicators.)

Excessive Fluid Intake

Nutrition Assessment Category	Potential Indicators of This Nutrition Diagnosis (one or more must be present)
Biochemical Data, Medical Tests and Procedures	• ↓ Plasma osmolality (270-280 mOsm/kg), only if positive fluid balance is in excess of positive sodium balance • ↓ Serum sodium in SIADH • ↓ Urine specific gravity
Anthropometric Measurements	Body weight gain
Physical Exam Findings	• Edema in the skin of the legs, sacral area, or diffusely; weeping of fluids from lower legs • Ascites • Pulmonary edema as evidenced by shortness of breath; orthopnea; crackles or rales • Nausea, vomiting, anorexia, headache, muscle spasms, convulsions • Shortness of breath or dyspnea with exertion or at rest • Providing medications in large amounts of fluid • Use of drugs that impair fluid excretion
Food/Nutrition-Related History	Reports or observations of: • Estimated intake of fluid more than requirements (eg, per body surface area for pediatrics) • Estimated salt intake in excess of recommendations
Client History*	• Conditions associated with a diagnosis or treatment, eg, end-stage renal disease, nephrotic syndrome, heart failure, or liver disease • Coma (SIADH)
Assessment, Monitoring, and Evaluation Tools	
Comparative Standards	• Total fluid estimated needs in 24 hours • Method for estimating 24 hour fluid needs

Arrows used with laboratory values: ↑ represents above reference standard and ↓ represents below reference standard.
** Client History terms are used for Nutrition Assessment but not for Nutrition Monitoring and Evaluation.*

Progress Evaluation

Communicate the progress toward the resolution of a nutrition diagnosis by selecting the appropriate nutrition diagnosis status value from the Nutrition Assessment, Monitoring, and Evaluation terms.

NCP Term	ANDUID
New nutrition diagnosis	14586
Active nutrition diagnosis	14587
Resolved nutrition diagnosis	14588
Discontinued nutrition diagnosis	14589

For details on these terms, visit the Nutrition Diagnosis Status reference sheet on page 200.

Inadequate Bioactive Substance Intake

Definition

Lower intake of bioactive substances compared to established reference standards or recommendations based on physiological needs.

> *Note:* Bioactive substances are not part of the Dietary Reference Intakes, and therefore there are no established minimum requirements or Tolerable Upper Intake Levels. However, nutrition and dietetics practitioners can assess whether estimated intakes are adequate or excessive using the client goal or nutrition prescription for comparison.
>
> Working definition of bioactive substances—physiologically active components of foods that may have an effect on health. There is no scientific consensus about a definition for bioactive substances/components.

Etiology (Cause/Contributing Risk Factors)

Factors gathered during the nutrition assessment process that contribute to the existence or the maintenance of pathophysiological, psychosocial, situational, developmental, cultural, and/or environmental problems:

- Food and nutrition related knowledge deficit concerning recommended bioactive substance intake
- Lack of or limited access to food that contains a bioactive substance
- Alteration in gastrointestinal tract structure and/or function
- Limited food- and nutrition-related skill

Etiology Category

Etiologies are grouped by the type of cause or contributing risk factor. Communicate the etiology category by selecting the appropriate Nutrition Assessment, Monitoring, and Evaluation term.

NCP Term	ANDUID
Beliefs attitudes etiology	14567
Cultural etiology	14568
Knowledge etiology	14569
Physical function etiology	14570
Physiologic metabolic etiology	14571
Psychological etiology	14572
Social personal etiology	14573
Treatment etiology	14574
Access etiology	14575
Behavior etiology	14576

Visit the Nutrition Diagnosis Etiology Category Identification reference sheet on page 185 for more details on etiology categories. An additional useful resource to determine the etiology category is the Nutrition Diagnosis Matrix on page 528.

Inadequate Bioactive Substance Intake

Signs/Symptoms (Defining Characteristics)

A typical cluster of subjective and objective signs and symptoms gathered during the nutrition assessment process that provide evidence that a problem exists; quantify the problem and describe its severity.

Nutrition Assessment Category	Potential Indicators of This Nutrition Diagnosis (one or more must be present)
Biochemical Data, Medical Tests and Procedures	
Anthropometric Measurements	
Physical Exam Findings	
Food/Nutrition-Related History	Reports or observations of: • Estimated intake of foods containing the following lower than recommended: ○ Psyllium (↓ total and LDL cholesterol) ○ Soy protein (↓ total and LDL cholesterol) ○ Beta glucan, eg, whole oat products (↓ total and LDL cholesterol) ○ Plant sterol and stanol esters, eg, fortified margarines (↓ total and LDL cholesterol) ○ Probiotics • Verbalizes inaccurate or incomplete knowledge about bioactive substances
Client History*	Conditions associated with a diagnosis or treatment, eg, cardiovascular disease, elevated cholesterol
Assessment, Monitoring, and Evaluation Tools	
Comparative Standards	

Arrows used with laboratory values: ↑ represents above reference standard and ↓ represents below reference standard.
** Client History terms are used for Nutrition Assessment but not for Nutrition Monitoring and Evaluation.*

Progress Evaluation

Communicate the progress toward the resolution of a nutrition diagnosis by selecting the appropriate nutrition diagnosis status value from the Nutrition Assessment, Monitoring, and Evaluation terms.

NCP Term	ANDUID
New nutrition diagnosis	14586
Active nutrition diagnosis	14587
Resolved nutrition diagnosis	14588
Discontinued nutrition diagnosis	14589

For details on these terms, visit the Nutrition Diagnosis Status reference sheet on page 200.

Excessive Bioactive Substance Intake

Definition

Higher intake of bioactive substances compared to established reference standards or recommendations based on physiological needs.

Note: Bioactive substances are not part of the Dietary Reference Intakes, and therefore there are no established minimum requirements or Tolerable Upper Intake Levels. However, nutrition and dietetics practitioners can assess whether estimated intakes are adequate or excessive using the client goal or nutrition prescription for comparison.

Working definition of bioactive substances—physiologically active components of foods that may have an effect on health. There is no scientific consensus about a definition for bioactive substances/components.

Etiology (Cause/Contributing Risk Factors)

Factors gathered during the nutrition assessment process that contribute to the existence or the maintenance of pathophysiological, psychosocial, situational, developmental, cultural, and/or environmental problems:

- Food and nutrition related knowledge deficit concerning recommended bioactive substance intake including food additives
- Contamination, misname, mislabel or lack of labeling, misuse, recent brand change, recent dose increase, recent formulation change of substance consumed
- Frequent intake of foods containing bioactive substances
- Alteration in gastrointestinal tract structure and/or function
- Lack of or limited access to appropriate foods, eg, inadequate markets with labeled food
- Limited food- and nutrition-related skill

Etiology Category

Etiologies are grouped by the type of cause or contributing risk factor. Communicate the etiology category by selecting the appropriate Nutrition Assessment, Monitoring, and Evaluation term.

NCP Term	ANDUID
Beliefs attitudes etiology	14567
Cultural etiology	14568
Knowledge etiology	14569
Physical function etiology	14570
Physiologic metabolic etiology	14571
Psychological etiology	14572
Social personal etiology	14573
Treatment etiology	14574
Access etiology	14575
Behavior etiology	14576

Visit the Nutrition Diagnosis Etiology Category Identification reference sheet on page 185 for more details on etiology categories. An additional useful resource to determine the etiology category is the Nutrition Diagnosis Matrix on page 528.

Excessive Bioactive Substance Intake

Signs/Symptoms (Defining Characteristics)

A typical cluster of subjective and objective signs and symptoms gathered during the nutrition assessment process that provide evidence that a problem exists; quantify the problem and describe its severity.

Nutrition Assessment Category	Potential Indicators of This Nutrition Diagnosis (one or more must be present)
Biochemical Data, Medical Tests and Procedures	• Lab values indicating excessive intake of the specific substance, such as rapid ↓ in cholesterol from intake of stanol or sterol esters and a statin drug and related dietary changes or medications • ↑ Hepatic enzyme reflecting hepatocellular damage
Anthropometric Measurements	Body weight loss as a result of malabsorption or maldigestion
Physical Exam Findings	Constipation, diarrhea, nausea, stomach pain, gas, cramps or bloating, vomiting, heartburn Neurologic changes, eg, anxiety, mental status changes Cardiovascular changes, eg, heart rate, blood pressure Discomfort or pain associated with intake of foods rich in bioactive substances, eg, soluble fiber, beta glucan, soy protein Headache/migraine Hives, flushing Irritability or nervousness
Food/Nutrition-Related History	Reports or observations of: • High intake of plant foods containing: ○ Soy protein (↓ total and LDL cholesterol) ○ Beta glucan, eg, whole oat products (↓ total and LDL cholesterol) ○ Plant sterol and stanol esters, eg, fortified margarines (↓ total and LDL cholesterol) or other foods based on dietary substance, concentrate, metabolite, constituent, extract, or combination ○ Substances that interfere with digestion or absorption of foodstuffs ○ Ready access to available foods/products with bioactive substance, eg, as from dietary supplement vendors ○ Attempts to use supplements or bioactive substances for weight loss, to treat constipation, or to prevent or cure chronic or acute disease ○ Other substances (for which scientific evidence exists and a recommended intake level has been established) ○ Intake of food additives for which client is intolerant, eg, yellow 5, yellow 6, safrole, FD&C Red #4, carmine, monosodium glutamate, sulfites ○ Verbalizes inaccurate or incomplete knowledge about bioactive substances

Continued on next page

Excessive Bioactive Substance Intake

Continued from previous page

Nutrition Assessment Category	Potential Indicators of This Nutrition Diagnosis (one or more must be present)
Client History*	• Conditions associated with a diagnosis or treatment, eg, cardiovascular disease, elevated cholesterol, hypertension, asthma • Cardiovascular changes, eg, electrocardiogram changes
Assessment, Monitoring, and Evaluation Tools	
Comparative Standards	

Arrows used with laboratory values: ↑ represents above reference standard and ↓ represents below reference standard.
** Client History terms are used for Nutrition Assessment but not for Nutrition Monitoring and Evaluation.*

Progress Evaluation

Communicate the progress toward the resolution of a nutrition diagnosis by selecting the appropriate nutrition diagnosis status value from the Nutrition Assessment, Monitoring, and Evaluation terms:

NCP Term	ANDUID
New nutrition diagnosis	14586
Active nutrition diagnosis	14587
Resolved nutrition diagnosis	14588
Discontinued nutrition diagnosis	14589

For details on these terms, visit the Nutrition Diagnosis Status reference sheet on page 200.

Excessive Alcohol Intake

Definition

Intake more than the suggested limits for alcohol.

Etiology (Cause/Contributing Risk Factors)

Factors gathered during the nutrition assessment process that contribute to the existence or the maintenance of pathophysiological, psychosocial, situational, developmental, cultural, and/or environmental problems:

- Belief finding that hinders food and/or nutrition behavior change
- Attitude finding that hinders food and/or nutrition behavior change
- Food and nutrition related knowledge deficit concerning appropriate alcohol intake
- Limited value for behavior change, competing values
- Alcohol addiction
- Limited food and nutrition related skill

Etiology Category

Etiologies are grouped by the type of cause or contributing risk factor. Communicate the etiology category by selecting the appropriate Nutrition Assessment, Monitoring and Evaluation term.

NCP Term	ANDUID
Beliefs attitudes etiology	14567
Cultural etiology	14568
Knowledge etiology	14569
Physical function etiology	14570
Physiologic metabolic etiology	14571
Psychological etiology	14572
Social personal etiology	14573
Treatment etiology	14574
Access etiology	14575
Behavior etiology	14576

Visit the Nutrition Diagnosis Etiology Category Identification reference sheet on page 185 for more details on etiology categories. An additional useful resource to determine the etiology category is the Nutrition Diagnosis Matrix on page 528.

Signs/Symptoms (Defining Characteristics)

A typical cluster of subjective and objective signs and symptoms gathered during the nutrition assessment process that provide evidence that a problem exists; quantify the problem and describe its severity.

Excessive Alcohol Intake

Nutrition Assessment Category	Potential Indicators of This Nutrition Diagnosis (one or more must be present)
Biochemical Data, Medical Tests and Procedures	↑ AST, gamma-glutamyl transferase (GGT), carbohydrate-deficient transferrin, MCV, blood alcohol levels
Anthropometric Measurements	
Physical Exam Findings	
Food/Nutrition-Related History	Reports or observations of: • Intake of > 2 drinks*/day (men) • Intake of > 1 drink*/day (women) • Binge drinking • Consumption of any alcohol when contraindicated, eg, during pregnancy
Client History[+]	• Conditions associated with a diagnosis or treatment, eg, severe hypertriglyceridemia, elevated blood pressure, depression, liver disease, pancreatitis • New medical diagnosis or change in existing diagnosis or condition • History of estimated alcohol intake in excess of recommendation • Giving birth to an infant with fetal alcohol syndrome
Assessment, Monitoring, and Evaluation Tools	
Comparative Standards	

Arrows used with laboratory values: ↑ represents above reference standard and ↓ represents below reference standard.
**1 drink = 5 oz (150 mL) wine, 12 oz (350 mL) beer, 1.5 oz (45 mL) distilled alcohol*
[+] Client History terms are used for Nutrition Assessment but not for Nutrition Monitoring and Evaluation.

Progress Evaluation

Communicate the progress toward the resolution of a nutrition diagnosis by selecting the appropriate nutrition diagnosis status value from the Nutrition Assessment, Monitoring, and Evaluation terms.

NCP Term	ANDUID
New nutrition diagnosis	14586
Active nutrition diagnosis	14587
Resolved nutrition diagnosis	14588
Discontinued nutrition diagnosis	14589

For details on these terms, visit the Nutrition Diagnosis Status reference sheet on page 200.

Increased Nutrient Needs

Definition

Increased need for a specific nutrient compared to established reference standards or recommendations based on physiological needs.

Etiology (Cause/Contributing Risk Factors)

Factors gathered during the nutrition assessment process that contribute to the existence or the maintenance of pathophysiological, psychosocial, situational, developmental, cultural, and/or environmental problems:

- Altered absorption or metabolism of nutrient, eg, from medications
- Compromise of organs related to GI function, eg, pancreas, liver
- Decreased functional length of intestine, eg, short bowel syndrome
- Decreased or compromised function of intestine, eg, celiac disease, Crohn's disease
- Increased demand for nutrient, eg, accelerated growth, wound healing, chronic infection

Etiology Category

Etiologies are grouped by the type of cause or contributing risk factor. Communicate the etiology category by selecting the appropriate Nutrition Assessment, Monitoring and Evaluation term:

NCP Term	ANDUID
Beliefs attitudes etiology	14567
Cultural etiology	14568
Knowledge etiology	14569
Physical function etiology	14570
Physiologic metabolic etiology	14571
Psychological etiology	14572
Social personal etiology	14573
Treatment etiology	14574
Access etiology	14575
Behavior etiology	14576

Visit the Nutrition Diagnosis Etiology Category Identification reference sheet on page 185 for more details on etiology categories. An additional useful resource to determine the etiology category is the Nutrition Diagnosis Matrix on page 528.

Signs/Symptoms (Defining Characteristics)

A typical cluster of subjective and objective signs and symptoms gathered during the nutrition assessment process that provide evidence that a problem exists; quantify the problem and describe its severity.

Increased Nutrient Needs

Nutrition Assessment Category	Potential Indicators of This Nutrition Diagnosis (one or more must be present)
Biochemical Data, Medical Tests and Procedures	• ↓ total cholesterol < 160 mg/dL, albumin, prealbumin, C-reactive protein, indicating increased stress and increased metabolic needs • Electrolyte/mineral (eg, potassium, magnesium, phosphorus) abnormalities • Urinary or fecal losses of specific or related nutrient (eg, fecal fat, d-xylose test) • Vitamin and/or mineral deficiency
Anthropometric Measurements	• Growth failure, based on reference growth standards, eg National Center for Health Statistics (NCHS) and fetal growth failure • Unintentional weight loss of ≥ 5% in 1 month or ≥ 10% in 6 months • Underweight (BMI < 18.5) • Low percent body fat and muscle mass
Physical Exam Findings	• Clinical evidence of vitamin/mineral deficiency (eg, hair loss, bleeding gums, pale nail beds) • Loss of skin integrity, delayed wound healing, or pressure ulcers • Loss of muscle mass, subcutaneous fat
Food/Nutrition-Related History	Reports or observations of: • Estimated intake of foods/supplements containing needed nutrient less than estimated requirements • Intake of foods that do not contain sufficient quantities of available nutrient (eg, overprocessed, overcooked, or stored improperly) • Food and nutrition related knowledge deficit (eg, lack of information, incorrect information or nonadherence with intake of needed nutrient) • Medications affecting absorption or metabolism of needed nutrient • Athletes or active individuals engaged in intense physical activity
Client History*	Conditions associated with a diagnosis or treatment, eg, intestinal resection, Crohn's disease, HIV/AIDS, burns, pre-term birth, malnutrition
Assessment, Monitoring, and Evaluation Tools	
Comparative Standards	

Arrows used with laboratory values: ↑ represents above reference standard and ↓ represents below reference standard.
** Client History terms are used for Nutrition Assessment but not for Nutrition Monitoring and Evaluation.*

Increased Nutrient Needs

Progress Evaluation

Communicate the progress toward the resolution of a nutrition diagnosis by selecting the appropriate nutrition diagnosis status value from the Nutrition Assessment, Monitoring, and Evaluation terms.

NCP Term	ANDUID
New nutrition diagnosis	14586
Active nutrition diagnosis	14587
Resolved nutrition diagnosis	14588
Discontinued nutrition diagnosis	14589

For details on these terms, visit the Nutrition Diagnosis Status reference sheet on page 200.

Inadequate Protein Energy Intake

Definition

Inadequate intake of protein and energy compared to established reference standards or recommendations based on physiological needs of short or recent duration.

> *Note:* Whenever possible, nutrient intake data should be considered in combination with clinical, biochemical, anthropometric information, medical diagnosis, clinical status, and/or other factors to provide a valid assessment of nutritional status based on a totality of the evidence. (Institute of Medicine. *Dietary Reference Intakes: Applications in Dietary Assessment*. National Academies Press; 2000.)

Etiology (Cause/Contributing Risk Factors)

Factors gathered during the nutrition assessment process that contribute to the existence or the maintenance of pathophysiological, psychosocial, situational, developmental, cultural, and/or environmental problems:

- Physiological causes increasing nutrient needs due to catabolic illness, malabsorption
- Decreased ability to consume sufficient protein and/or energy
- Food insecurity
- Cultural or religious practices that affect ability to access food
- Food and nutrition related knowledge deficit concerning appropriate amount and type of dietary fat and/or protein
- Psychological causes such as depression and disordered eating
- Limited food and nutrition related skill

Etiology Category

Etiologies are grouped by the type of cause or contributing risk factor. Communicate the etiology category by selecting the appropriate Nutrition Assessment, Monitoring, and Evaluation term.

NCP Term	ANDUID
Beliefs attitudes etiology	14567
Cultural etiology	14568
Knowledge etiology	14569
Physical function etiology	14570
Physiologic metabolic etiology	14571
Psychological etiology	14572
Social personal etiology	14573
Treatment etiology	14574
Access etiology	14575
Behavior etiology	14576

Visit the Nutrition Diagnosis Etiology Category Identification reference sheet on page 185 for more details on etiology categories. An additional useful resource to determine the etiology category is the Nutrition Diagnosis Matrix on page 528.

Inadequate Protein Energy Intake

Signs/Symptoms (Defining Characteristics)

A typical cluster of subjective and objective signs and symptoms gathered during the nutrition assessment process that provide evidence that a problem exists; quantify the problem and describe its severity.

Nutrition Assessment Category	Potential Indicators of This Nutrition Diagnosis (one or more must be present)
Biochemical Data, Medical Tests and Procedures	Normal albumin (in the setting of normal liver function despite decreased protein-energy intake)
Anthropometric Measurements	• Inadequate maternal weight gain (mild but not severe) • Weight loss of 7% in 3 months, >5% in 1 month, or 1% to 2% in 1 week in adults; any weight loss or failure to gain weight in children • Growth failure in children
Physical Exam Findings	Slow wound healing in pressure ulcer or surgical site
Food/Nutrition-Related History	Reports or observations of: • Estimated energy intake from diet less than estimated or measured RMR or recommended levels • Restriction or omission of food groups • Recent food avoidance and/or lack of interest in food • Lack of ability to prepare meals • Excessive consumption of alcohol or other drugs that reduce hunger • Hunger in the face of inadequate access to food supply
Client History*	• Conditions associated with a diagnosis or treatment of mild protein-energy malnutrition, recent illness (eg, pulmonary or cardiac failure, flu, infection, surgery) • Nutrient malabsorption (eg, bariatric surgery, diarrhea, steatorrhea) • Lack of funds to purchase appropriate foods
Assessment, Monitoring, and Evaluation Tools	
Comparative Standards	

** Client History terms are used for Nutrition Assessment but not for Nutrition Monitoring and Evaluation.*

Progress Evaluation

Communicate the progress toward the resolution of a nutrition diagnosis by selecting the appropriate nutrition diagnosis status value from the Nutrition Assessment, Monitoring, and Evaluation terms.

NCP Term	ANDUID
New nutrition diagnosis	14586
Active nutrition diagnosis	14587
Resolved nutrition diagnosis	14588
Discontinued nutrition diagnosis	14589

For details on these terms, visit the Nutrition Diagnosis Status reference sheet on page 200.

Decreased Nutrient Needs

Definition

Decreased need for a specific nutrient compared to established reference standards or recommendations based on physiological needs.

Etiology (Cause/Contributing Risk Factors)

Factors gathered during the nutrition assessment process that contribute to the existence or the maintenance of pathophysiological, psychosocial, situational, developmental, cultural, and/or environmental problems:

- Renal dysfunction
- Liver dysfunction
- Altered cholesterol metabolism/regulation
- Heart failure
- Food intolerances, eg, irritable bowel syndrome

Etiology Category

Etiologies are grouped by the type of cause or contributing risk factor. Communicate the etiology category by selecting the appropriate Nutrition Assessment, Monitoring, and Evaluation term.

NCP Term	ANDUID
Beliefs attitudes etiology	14567
Cultural etiology	14568
Knowledge etiology	14569
Physical function etiology	14570
Physiologic metabolic etiology	14571
Psychological etiology	14572
Social personal etiology	14573
Treatment etiology	14574
Access etiology	14575
Behavior etiology	14576

Visit the Nutrition Diagnosis Etiology Category Identification reference sheet on page 185 for more details on etiology categories. An additional useful resource to determine the etiology category is the Nutrition Diagnosis Matrix on page 528.

Signs/Symptoms (Defining Characteristics)

A typical cluster of subjective and objective signs and symptoms gathered during the nutrition assessment process that provide evidence that a problem exists; quantify the problem and describe its severity. (See the next page for the nutrition assessment category and potential indicators.)

Decreased Nutrient Needs

Nutrition Assessment Category	Potential Indicators of This Nutrition Diagnosis (one or more must be present)
Biochemical Data, Medical Tests and Procedures	• ↑ Total cholesterol > 200 mg/dL (5.2 mmol/L), ↑ LDL cholesterol > 100 mg/dL (2.59 mmol/L), ↓ HDL cholesterol < 40 mg/dL (1.036 mmol/L), ↑ triglycerides > 150 mg/dL (1.695 mmol/L) • ↑ Phosphorus > 5.5 mg/dL (1.78 mmol/L) • ↓ GFR < 90 mL/min/1.73 m^2 • ↑ BUN, creatinine, potassium • ↑ LFTs indicating severe liver disease
Anthropometric Measurements	Interdialytic weight gain greater than expected
Physical Exam Findings	Edema/fluid retention
Food/Nutrition-Related History	Reports or observations of estimated intake higher than recommended for fat, phosphorus, sodium, protein, fiber
Client History*	• Conditions associated with a diagnosis or treatment that require a specific type and/or amount of nutrient, eg, cardiovascular disease (fat), early renal disease (protein, phosphorus), end-stage renal disease (ESRD) (phosphorus, sodium, potassium, fluid), advanced liver disease (protein), heart failure (sodium, fluid), irritable bowel disease/Crohn's flare up (fiber) • Diagnosis of hypertension, confusion related to liver disease
Assessment, Monitoring, and Evaluation Tools	
Comparative Standards	

Arrows used with laboratory values: ↑ represents above reference standard and ↓ represents below reference standard.
** Client History terms are used for Nutrition Assessment but not for Nutrition Monitoring and Evaluation.*

Progress Evaluation

Communicate the progress toward the resolution of a nutrition diagnosis by selecting the appropriate nutrition diagnosis status value from the Nutrition Assessment, Monitoring, and Evaluation terms.

NCP Term	ANDUID
New nutrition diagnosis	14586
Active nutrition diagnosis	14587
Resolved nutrition diagnosis	14588
Discontinued nutrition diagnosis	14589

For details on these terms, visit the Nutrition Diagnosis Status reference sheet on page 200.

Imbalance of Nutrients

Definition

An undesirable combination of nutrients, such that the amount of one nutrient interferes with or alters absorption and/or utilization of another nutrient.

Etiology (Cause/Contributing Risk Factors)

Factors gathered during the nutrition assessment process that contribute to the existence or the maintenance of pathophysiological, psychosocial, situational, developmental, cultural, and/or environmental problems:

- Consumption of high-dose nutrient supplements
- Food and nutrition related knowledge deficit concerning nutrient interactions
- Belief finding that hinders food and/or nutrition behavior change
- Attitude finding that hinders food and/or nutrition behavior change
- Food faddism
- Insufficient electrolyte replacement when initiating feeding (PN/EN, including oral)
- Limited food and nutrition related skill

Etiology Category

Etiologies are grouped by the type of cause or contributing risk factor. Communicate the etiology category by selecting the appropriate Nutrition Assessment, Monitoring, and Evaluation term.

NCP Term	ANDUID
Beliefs attitudes etiology	14567
Cultural etiology	14568
Knowledge etiology	14569
Physical function etiology	14570
Physiologic metabolic etiology	14571
Psychological etiology	14572
Social personal etiology	14573
Treatment etiology	14574
Access etiology	14575
Behavior etiology	14576

Visit the Nutrition Diagnosis Etiology Category Identification reference sheet on page 185 for more details on etiology categories. An additional useful resource to determine the etiology category is the Nutrition Diagnosis Matrix on page 528.

Signs/Symptoms (Defining Characteristics)

A typical cluster of subjective and objective signs and symptoms gathered during the nutrition assessment process that provide evidence that a problem exists; quantify the problem and describe its severity. (See the next page for the nutrition assessment category and potential indicators.)

Imbalance of Nutrients

Nutrition Assessment Category	Potential Indicators of This Nutrition Diagnosis (one or more must be present)
Biochemical Data, Medical Tests and Procedures	• Severe hypophosphatemia (in the presence of increased carbohydrate) • Severe hypokalemia (in the presence of increased protein) • Severe hypomagnesemia (in the presence of increased carbohydrate)
Anthropometric Measurements	
Physical Exam Findings	• Diarrhea or constipation (iron supplements) • Epigastric pain, nausea, vomiting, diarrhea (zinc supplements)
Food/Nutrition-Related History	Reports or observations of: • Estimated intake of iron supplements (decreased zinc absorption) higher than recommended • Estimated intake of zinc supplements (decreased copper status) higher than recommended • Estimated intake of manganese (decreased iron status) higher than recommended
Client History*	Refeeding syndrome
Assessment, Monitoring, and Evaluation Tools	
Comparative Standards	

** Client History terms are used for Nutrition Assessment but not for Nutrition Monitoring and Evaluation.*

Progress Evaluation

Communicate the progress toward the resolution of a nutrition diagnosis by selecting the appropriate nutrition diagnosis status value from the Nutrition Assessment, Monitoring, and Evaluation terms.

NCP Term	ANDUID
New nutrition diagnosis	14586
Active nutrition diagnosis	14587
Resolved nutrition diagnosis	14588
Discontinued nutrition diagnosis	14589

For details on these terms, visit the Nutrition Diagnosis Status reference sheet on page 200.

Inadequate Fat Intake

Definition

Lower fat intake compared to established reference standards or recommendations based on physiological needs.

> *Note:* May not be an appropriate nutrition diagnosis when the goal is weight loss or during end-of-life care.
>
> Whenever possible, nutrient intake data should be considered in combination with clinical, biochemical, anthropometric information, medical diagnosis, clinical status, and/or other factors to provide a valid assessment of nutritional status based on a totality of the evidence. (Institute of Medicine. *Dietary Reference Intakes: Applications in Dietary Assessment*. National Academies Press; 2000.)

Etiology (Cause/Contributing Risk Factors)

Factors gathered during the nutrition assessment process that contribute to the existence or the maintenance of pathophysiological, psychosocial, situational, developmental, cultural, and/or environmental problems:

- Alteration in gastrointestinal tract structure and/or function
- Less than optimal food choices, eg, economic constraints, restricting food given to elderly and/or children, specific food choices
- Cultural practices that affect ability to make appropriate food choices
- Food and nutrition related knowledge deficit concerning appropriate amount of dietary fat
- Psychological causes such as depression and disordered eating
- Limited food and nutrition related skill

Etiology Category

Etiologies are grouped by the type of cause or contributing risk factor. Communicate the etiology category by selecting the appropriate Nutrition Assessment, Monitoring, and Evaluation term.

NCP Term	ANDUID
Beliefs attitudes etiology	14567
Cultural etiology	14568
Knowledge etiology	14569
Physical function etiology	14570
Physiologic metabolic etiology	14571
Psychological etiology	14572
Social personal etiology	14573
Treatment etiology	14574
Access etiology	14575
Behavior etiology	14576

Visit the Nutrition Diagnosis Etiology Category Identification reference sheet on page 185 for more details on etiology categories. An additional useful resource to determine the etiology category is the Nutrition Diagnosis Matrix on page 528.

Inadequate Fat Intake

Signs/Symptoms (Defining Characteristics)

A typical cluster of subjective and objective signs and symptoms gathered during the nutrition assessment process that provide evidence that a problem exists; quantify the problem and describe its severity.

Nutrition Assessment Category	Potential Indicators of This Nutrition Diagnosis (one or more must be present)
Biochemical Data, Medical Tests and Procedures	↑ Triene:tetraene ratio > 0.2
Anthropometric Measurements	• Impaired growth • Body weight loss if insufficient calories/kcal/kJ consumed
Physical Exam Findings	Scaly skin and dermatitis consistent with essential fatty acid deficiency
Food/Nutrition-Related History	Reports or observations of: • Estimated intake of essential fatty acids less than 10% of energy (primarily associated with parenteral nutrition) • Verbalizes inaccurate or incomplete knowledge • Cultural or religious practices that affect intake
Client History*	• Conditions associated with a diagnosis or treatment, eg, prolonged catabolic illness (eg, AIDS, tuberculosis, anorexia nervosa, sepsis or severe infection from recent surgery) • Severe fat malabsorption with bowel resection, pancreatic insufficiency, or hepatic disease accompanied by steatorrhea
Assessment, Monitoring, and Evaluation Tools	
Comparative Standards	• Total fat estimated needs in 24 hours • Fat estimated needs per kg of body weight in 24 hours • Method for estimating total 24 hour fat needs • Proportion of energy needs from fat in 24 hours

Arrows used with laboratory values: ↑ represents above reference standard and ↓ represents below reference standard.
** Client History terms are used for Nutrition Assessment but not for Nutrition Monitoring and Evaluation.*

Progress Evaluation

Communicate the progress toward the resolution of a nutrition diagnosis by selecting the appropriate nutrition diagnosis status value from the Nutrition Assessment, Monitoring, and Evaluation terms.

NCP Term	ANDUID
New nutrition diagnosis	14586
Active nutrition diagnosis	14587
Resolved nutrition diagnosis	14588
Discontinued nutrition diagnosis	14589

For details on these terms, visit the Nutrition Diagnosis Status reference sheet on page 200.

Excessive Fat Intake

Definition

Higher fat intake compared to established reference standards or recommendations based on physiological needs.

Etiology (Cause/Contributing Risk Factors)

Factors gathered during the nutrition assessment process that contribute to the existence or the maintenance of pathophysiological, psychosocial, situational, developmental, cultural, and/or environmental problems:

- Food and nutrition related knowledge deficit concerning appropriate amount of dietary fat
- Belief finding that hinders food and/or nutrition behavior change
- Attitude finding that hinders food and/or nutrition behavior change
- Food insecurity
- Changes in taste and appetite or preference
- Limited value for behavior change, competing values
- Physiological causes decreasing total fat needs or recommendations
- Limited food- and nutrition-related skill

Etiology Category

Etiologies are grouped by the type of cause or contributing risk factor. Communicate the etiology category by selecting the appropriate Nutrition Assessment, Monitoring and Evaluation term.

NCP Term	ANDUID
Beliefs attitudes etiology	14567
Cultural etiology	14568
Knowledge etiology	14569
Physical function etiology	14570
Physiologic metabolic etiology	14571
Psychological etiology	14572
Social personal etiology	14573
Treatment etiology	14574
Access etiology	14575
Behavior etiology	14576

Visit the Nutrition Diagnosis Etiology Category Identification reference sheet on page 185 for more details on etiology categories. An additional useful resource to determine the etiology category is the Nutrition Diagnosis Matrix on page 528.

Signs/Symptoms (Defining Characteristics)

A typical cluster of subjective and objective signs and symptoms gathered during the nutrition assessment process that provide evidence that a problem exists; quantify the problem and describe its severity. (See the next page for the nutrition assessment category and potential indicators.)

Excessive Fat Intake

Nutrition Assessment Category	Potential Indicators of This Nutrition Diagnosis (one or more must be present)
Biochemical Data, Medical Tests and Procedures	• ↑ Cholesterol > 200 mg/dL (5.2 mmol/L), ↑ LDL cholesterol > 100 mg/dL (2.59 mmol/L), ↓ HDL cholesterol < 40 mg/dL (1.036 mmol/L), ↑ triglycerides > 150 mg/dL (1.695 mmol/L) • ↑ Serum amylase and/or lipase • ↑ LFTs, total bilirubin • ↑ Fecal fat > 7g/24 hours
Anthropometric Measurements	
Physical Exam Findings	• Evidence of xanthomas • Diarrhea, cramping, steatorrhea, epigastric pain
Food/Nutrition-Related History	Reports or observations of: • Frequent or large portions of high-fat foods • Frequent food preparation with added fat • Frequent consumption of high-risk lipids (ie, saturated fat, *trans* fat, cholesterol) • Report of foods containing fat more than diet prescription • Medication, eg, pancreatic enzymes, cholesterol- or other lipid-lowering medications • Verbalizes inaccurate or incomplete knowledge • Verbalizes unsupported beliefs and attitudes
Client History*	• Conditions associated with a diagnosis or treatment, eg, hyperlipidemia; cystic fibrosis; angina; atherosclerosis; pancreatic; liver; and biliary diseases; post-transplantation, chyle fluid leak • Family history of hyperlipidemia, atherosclerosis, or pancreatitis
Assessment, Monitoring, and Evaluation Tools	
Comparative Standards	• Total fat estimated needs in 24 hours • Fat estimated needs per kg of body weight in 24 hours • Method for estimating total 24 hour fat needs • Proportion of energy needs from fat in 24 hours

Arrows used with laboratory values: ↑ represents above reference standard and ↓ represents below reference standard.
** Client History terms are used for Nutrition Assessment but not for Nutrition Monitoring and Evaluation.*

Progress Evaluation

Communicate the progress toward the resolution of a nutrition diagnosis by selecting the appropriate nutrition diagnosis status value from the Nutrition Assessment, Monitoring, and Evaluation terms.

NCP Term	ANDUID
New nutrition diagnosis	14586
Active nutrition diagnosis	14587
Resolved nutrition diagnosis	14588
Discontinued nutrition diagnosis	14589

For details on these terms, visit the Nutrition Diagnosis Status reference sheet on page 200.

Intake of Types of Fats Inconsistent With Needs

Definition

Intake of wrong type or quality of fats compared to established reference standards or recommendations based on physiological needs.

Etiology (Cause/Contributing Risk Factors)

Factors gathered during the nutrition assessment process that contribute to the existence or the maintenance of pathophysiological, psychosocial, situational, developmental, cultural, and/or environmental problems:

- Food and nutrition related knowledge deficit concerning type of fat (eg, fats added to food, formula/breastmilk)
- Belief finding that hinders food and/or nutrition behavior change
- Attitude finding that hinders food and/or nutrition behavior change
- Food insecurity
- Changes in taste and appetite or preference
- Limited value for behavior change, competing values
- Physiological causes altering fatty acid needs or recommendations
- Limited food- and nutrition-related skill

Etiology Category

Etiologies are grouped by the type of cause or contributing risk factor. Communicate the etiology category by selecting the appropriate Nutrition Assessment, Monitoring, and Evaluation term.

NCP Term	ANDUID
Beliefs attitudes etiology	14567
Cultural etiology	14568
Knowledge etiology	14569
Physical function etiology	14570
Physiologic metabolic etiology	14571
Psychological etiology	14572
Social personal etiology	14573
Treatment etiology	14574
Access etiology	14575
Behavior etiology	14576

Visit the Nutrition Diagnosis Etiology Category Identification reference sheet on page 185 for more details on etiology categories. An additional useful resource to determine the etiology category is the Nutrition Diagnosis Matrix on page 528.

Intake of Types of Fats Inconsistent With Needs

Signs/Symptoms (Defining Characteristics)

A typical cluster of subjective and objective signs and symptoms gathered during the nutrition assessment process that provide evidence that a problem exists; quantify the problem and describe its severity.

Nutrition Assessment Category	Potential Indicators of This Nutrition Diagnosis (one or more must be present)
Biochemical Data, Medical Tests and Procedures	• ↑ Cholesterol > 200 mg/dL (5.2 mmol/L), ↑ LDL cholesterol > 100 mg/dL (2.59 mmol/L), ↓ HDL cholesterol < 40 mg/dL (1.036 mmol/L) men, ↓ HDL cholesterol < 50 mg/dL (1.3 mmol/L) women, ↑ triglycerides > 150 mg/dL (1.695 mmol/L) • ↑ Serum amylase and/or lipase • ↑ LFTs, total bilirubin, C-reactive protein • Altered acylcarnitine, carnitine, and other measures of fatty acid metabolism • Elevated triene:tetraene ratio (> 0.2) • Altered fatty acid panel mitochondrial C8-C18, serum or plasma (μmol/L) • Altered fatty acid panel mitochondrial C2-C22, serum or plasma (μmol/L) • Altered fatty acid panel mitochondrial C22-C26, serum or plasma (μmol/L)
Anthropometric Measurements	
Physical Exam Findings	• Evidence of dermatitis • Diarrhea, cramping, steatorrhea, epigastric pain
Food/Nutrition-Related History	Reports or observations of: • Frequent food preparation with added fat that is not of desired type for condition • Frequent consumption of fats that are undesirable for condition (eg, saturated fat, *trans* fat, cholesterol, n-6 fatty acids, fatty acid chain length) • Estimated intake of monounsaturated, polyunsaturated, n-3 fatty acids, or DHA/ARA, fatty acid chain length less than recommended or in suboptimal ratio • Verbalizes inaccurate or incomplete knowledge • Verbalizes beliefs and attitudes that may not support food and/or nutrition behavior change
Client History*	• Conditions associated with a diagnosis or treatment, eg, diabetes mellitus, cardiac diseases, obesity, liver or biliary disorders, chyle fluid leak, inborn errors of metabolism • Family history of diabetes-related heart disease, hyperlipidemia, atherosclerosis, or pancreatitis

Continued on next page

Intake of Types of Fats Inconsistent With Needs

Continued from previous page

Nutrition Assessment Category	Potential Indicators of This Nutrition Diagnosis (one or more must be present)
Assessment, Monitoring, and Evaluation Tools	
Comparative Standards	

Arrows used with laboratory values: ↑ represents above reference standard and ↓ represents below reference standard.
** Client History terms are used for Nutrition Assessment but not for Nutrition Monitoring and Evaluation.*

Progress Evaluation

Communicate the progress toward the resolution of a nutrition diagnosis by selecting the appropriate nutrition diagnosis status value from the Nutrition Assessment, Monitoring, and Evaluation terms.

NCP Term	ANDUID
New nutrition diagnosis	14586
Active nutrition diagnosis	14587
Resolved nutrition diagnosis	14588
Discontinued nutrition diagnosis	14589

For details on these terms, visit the Nutrition Diagnosis Status reference sheet on page 200.

Inadequate Protein Intake

Definition

Lower intake of protein compared to established reference standards or recommendations based on physiological needs.

> *Note:* Whenever possible, nutrient intake data should be considered in combination with clinical, biochemical, anthropometric information, medical diagnosis, clinical status, and/or other factors to provide a valid assessment of nutritional status based on a totality of the evidence. (Institute of Medicine. *Dietary Reference Intakes: Applications in Dietary Assessment.* National Academies Press; 2000.)

Etiology (Cause/Contributing Risk Factors)

Factors gathered during the nutrition assessment process that contribute to the existence or the maintenance of pathophysiological, psychosocial, situational, developmental, cultural, and/or environmental problems:

- Physiological causes increasing nutrient needs due to prolonged catabolic illness, malabsorption, age, or condition
- Decreased ability to consume sufficient protein
- Food insecurity
- Cultural practices that affect the ability to access food
- Food and nutrition related knowledge deficit concerning amount of protein
- Psychological causes such as depression and disordered eating
- Limited food- and nutrition-related skill

Etiology Category

Etiologies are grouped by the type of cause or contributing risk factor. Communicate the etiology category by selecting the appropriate Nutrition Assessment, Monitoring, and Evaluation term.

NCP Term	ANDUID
Beliefs attitudes etiology	14567
Cultural etiology	14568
Knowledge etiology	14569
Physical function etiology	14570
Physiologic metabolic etiology	14571
Psychological etiology	14572
Social personal etiology	14573
Treatment etiology	14574
Access etiology	14575
Behavior etiology	14576

Visit the Nutrition Diagnosis Etiology Category Identification reference sheet on page 185 for more details on etiology categories. An additional useful resource to determine the etiology category is the Nutrition Diagnosis Matrix on page 528.

Inadequate Protein Intake

Signs/Symptoms (Defining Characteristics)

A typical cluster of subjective and objective signs and symptoms gathered during the nutrition assessment process that provide evidence that a problem exists; quantify the problem and describe its severity.

Nutrition Assessment Category	Potential Indicators of This Nutrition Diagnosis (one or more must be present)
Biochemical Data, Medical Tests and Procedures	
Anthropometric Measurements	
Physical Exam Findings	Edema, failure to thrive (infants/children), poor musculature, dull skin, thin and fragile hair
Food/Nutrition-Related History	Reports or observation of: • Estimated intake of protein insufficient to meet requirements • Cultural or religious practices that limit protein intake • Economic constraints that limit food availability • Prolonged adherence to a very-low-protein weight loss diet • Verbalizes inaccurate or incomplete knowledge
Client History*	Conditions associated with a diagnosis or treatment, eg, severe protein malabsorption such as bowel resection
Assessment, Monitoring, and Evaluation Tools	
Comparative Standards	• Total protein estimated needs in 24 hours • Protein estimated needs per kg of body weight in 24 hours • Method for estimating total 24 hour protein needs • Proportion of energy needs from protein in 24 hours

** Client History terms are used for Nutrition Assessment but not for Nutrition Monitoring and Evaluation.*

Progress Evaluation

Communicate the progress toward the resolution of a nutrition diagnosis by selecting the appropriate nutrition diagnosis status value from the Nutrition Assessment, Monitoring, and Evaluation terms.

NCP Term	ANDUID
New nutrition diagnosis	14586
Active nutrition diagnosis	14587
Resolved nutrition diagnosis	14588
Discontinued nutrition diagnosis	14589

For details on these terms, visit the Nutrition Diagnosis Status reference sheet on page 200.

Excessive Protein Intake

Definition

Intake more than the recommended level of protein compared to established reference standards or recommendations based on physiological needs.

Etiology (Cause/Contributing Risk Factors)

Factors gathered during the nutrition assessment process that contribute to the existence or the maintenance of pathophysiological, psychosocial, situational, developmental, cultural, and/or environmental problems:

- Liver dysfunction
- Renal dysfunction
- Belief finding that hinders food and/or nutrition behavior change
- Attitude finding that hinders food and/or nutrition behavior change
- Food and nutrition related knowledge deficit
- Lack of or limited access to specialized protein products
- Metabolic abnormality
- Food faddism
- Limited food- and nutrition-related skill

Etiology Category

Etiologies are grouped by the type of cause or contributing risk factor. Communicate the etiology category by selecting the appropriate Nutrition Assessment, Monitoring, and Evaluation term.

NCP Term	ANDUID
Beliefs attitudes etiology	14567
Cultural etiology	14568
Knowledge etiology	14569
Physical function etiology	14570
Physiologic metabolic etiology	14571
Psychological etiology	14572
Social personal etiology	14573
Treatment etiology	14574
Access etiology	14575
Behavior etiology	14576

Visit the Nutrition Diagnosis Etiology Category Identification reference sheet on page 185 for more details on etiology categories. An additional useful resource to determine the etiology category is the Nutrition Diagnosis Matrix on page 528.

Signs/Symptoms (Defining Characteristics)

A typical cluster of subjective and objective signs and symptoms gathered during the nutrition assessment process that provide evidence that a problem exists; quantify the problem and describe its severity.

Excessive Protein Intake

Nutrition Assessment Category	Potential Indicators of This Nutrition Diagnosis (one or more must be present)
Biochemical Data, Medical Tests and Procedures	Altered laboratory values, eg, ↑ BUN, ↓ GFR (altered renal status)
Anthropometric Measurements	Growth stunting or failure based on National Center for Health Statistics growth charts (metabolic disorders)
Physical Exam Findings	
Food/Nutrition-Related History	Reports or observations of: • Estimated total protein intake higher than recommended, eg, early renal disease, advanced liver disease with confusion • Excess protein supplementation • Verbalizes inaccurate or incomplete knowledge • Verbalizes unsupported beliefs and attitudes
Client History*	Conditions associated with a diagnosis or treatment, eg, early renal disease or advanced liver disease with confusion
Assessment, Monitoring, and Evaluation Tools	
Comparative Standards	• Total protein estimated needs in 24 hours • Protein estimated needs per kg of body weight in 24 hours • Method for estimating total 24 hour protein needs • Proportion of energy needs from protein in 24 hours

Arrows used with laboratory values: ↑ represents above reference standard and ↓ represents below reference standard.
** Client History terms are used for Nutrition Assessment but not for Nutrition Monitoring and Evaluation.*

Progress Evaluation

Communicate the progress toward the resolution of a nutrition diagnosis by selecting the appropriate nutrition diagnosis status value from the Nutrition Assessment, Monitoring, and Evaluation terms.

NCP Term	ANDUID
New nutrition diagnosis	14586
Active nutrition diagnosis	14587
Resolved nutrition diagnosis	14588
Discontinued nutrition diagnosis	14589

For details on these terms, visit the Nutrition Diagnosis Status reference sheet on page 200.

Intake of Types of Proteins Inconsistent With Needs

Definition

Intake of an amount of a specific type of protein compared to established reference standards or recommendations based on physiological needs.

Etiology (Cause/Contributing Risk Factors)

Factors gathered during the nutrition assessment process that contribute to the existence or the maintenance of pathophysiological, psychosocial, situational, developmental, cultural, and/or environmental problems:

- Liver dysfunction
- Renal dysfunction
- Belief finding that hinders food and/or nutrition behavior change
- Attitude finding that hinders food and/or nutrition behavior change
- Misused specialized protein products
- Metabolic abnormality
- Food faddism
- Inborn errors of metabolism
- Celiac disease, dermatitis herpetiformis, or other GI disease
- Cultural or religious practices that affect the ability to regulate types of protein or amino acids consumed
- Food and nutrition related knowledge deficit concerning an appropriate amount of a specific types of proteins or amino acids
- Food and nutrition adherence limitations
- Insufficient access to appropriate protein sources
- Limited food- and nutrition-related skill

Etiology Category

Etiologies are grouped by the type of cause or contributing risk factor. Communicate the etiology category by selecting the appropriate Nutrition Assessment, Monitoring, and Evaluation term.

NCP Term	ANDUID
Beliefs attitudes etiology	14567
Cultural etiology	14568
Knowledge etiology	14569
Physical function etiology	14570
Physiologic metabolic etiology	14571
Psychological etiology	14572
Social personal etiology	14573
Treatment etiology	14574
Access etiology	14575
Behavior etiology	14576

Visit the Nutrition Diagnosis Etiology Category Identification reference sheet on page 185 for more details on etiology categories. An additional useful resource to determine the etiology category is the Nutrition Diagnosis Matrix on page 528.

Intake of Types of Proteins Inconsistent With Needs

Signs/Symptoms (Defining Characteristics)

A typical cluster of subjective and objective signs and symptoms gathered during the nutrition assessment process that provide evidence that a problem exists; quantify the problem and describe its severity.

Nutrition Assessment Category	Potential Indicators of This Nutrition Diagnosis (one or more must be present)
Biochemical Data, Medical Tests and Procedures	• Altered laboratory values, eg, ↑ BUN, ↓ GFR (altered renal status) • ↑ Specific amino acids (inborn errors of metabolism) • ↑ Homocysteine or ammonia • Positive autoantibody levels (Anti-tTG antibodies, EmA IgA tissue transglutaminase [tTG] and IgA endomysial antibodies [EMA]) • Positive small bowel biopsy for celiac or other GI disease
Anthropometric Measurements	Weight loss, inability to gain weight, delayed growth
Physical Exam Findings	• Physical or neurological changes (inborn errors of metabolism) • Diarrhea in response to certain types of protein in specific carbohydrate-rich foods, supplements, and medications • Abdominal pain, distention, constipation, reflux, gastroesophageal reflux disease, vomiting
Food/Nutrition-Related History	Reports or observation of: • Estimated protein intake from all sources higher or lower than recommended • Estimated energy intake from all sources lower than recommended • Less than optimal supplementation of specific types of protein • Limited knowledge of protein composition or of protein metabolism • Chronic use of medications containing proteins not recommended
Client History*	• Conditions associated with a diagnosis or treatment of illness that requires EN/PN therapy, celiac disease, dermatitis herpetiformis, allergies, inborn errors of metabolism • Uremia, azotemia (clients with renal conditions)
Assessment, Monitoring, and Evaluation Tools	
Comparative Standards	

Arrows used with laboratory values: ↑ represents above reference standard and ↓ represents below reference standard.
** Client History terms are used for Nutrition Assessment but not for Nutrition Monitoring and Evaluation.*

Intake of Types of Proteins Inconsistent With Needs

Progress Evaluation

Communicate the progress toward the resolution of a nutrition diagnosis by selecting the appropriate nutrition diagnosis status value from the Nutrition Assessment, Monitoring, and Evaluation terms.

NCP Term	ANDUID
New nutrition diagnosis	14586
Active nutrition diagnosis	14587
Resolved nutrition diagnosis	14588
Discontinued nutrition diagnosis	14589

For details on these terms, visit the Nutrition Diagnosis Status reference sheet on page 200.

Intake of Types of Amino Acids Inconsistent With Needs

Definition

Intake of an amount of a specific type of amino acid compared to established reference standards or recommendations based on physiological needs.

Etiology (Cause/Contributing Risk Factors)

Factors gathered during the nutrition assessment process that contribute to the existence or the maintenance of pathophysiological, psychosocial, situational, developmental, cultural, and/or environmental problems:

- Liver dysfunction
- Renal dysfunction
- Belief finding that hinders food and/or nutrition behavior change
- Attitude finding that hinders food and/or nutrition behavior change
- Misused specialized amino acid products
- Metabolic demand or abnormality
- Medication with an amino acid interaction
- Inborn errors of metabolism
- Food and nutrition related knowledge deficit concerning an appropriate amount of specific amino acids
- Limited adherence to recommendation to modify amino acid intake
- Insufficient access to appropriate amino acid sources
- Limited food and nutrition related skill

Etiology Category

Etiologies are grouped by the type of cause or contributing risk factor. Communicate the etiology category by selecting the appropriate Nutrition Assessment, Monitoring and Evaluation term.

NCP Term	ANDUID
Beliefs attitudes etiology	14567
Cultural etiology	14568
Knowledge etiology	14569
Physical function etiology	14570
Physiologic metabolic etiology	14571
Psychological etiology	14572
Social personal etiology	14573
Treatment etiology	14574
Access etiology	14575
Behavior etiology	14576

Visit the Nutrition Diagnosis Etiology Category Identification reference sheet on page 185 for more details on etiology categories. An additional useful resource to determine the etiology category is the Nutrition Diagnosis Matrix on page 528.

Intake of Types of Amino Acids Inconsistent With Needs

Signs/Symptoms (Defining Characteristics)

A typical cluster of subjective and objective signs and symptoms gathered during the nutrition assessment process that provide evidence that a problem exists; quantify the problem and describe its severity.

Nutrition Assessment Category	Potential Indicators of This Nutrition Diagnosis (one or more must be present)
Biochemical Data, Medical Tests and Procedures	• ↑ or ↓ specific amino acids, serum, plasma or urine • ↑ ammonia, serum
Anthropometric Measurements	Weight loss, inability to gain weight, delayed growth
Physical Exam Findings	• Physical or neurological changes • Vomiting • Diarrhea • Fever
Food/Nutrition-Related History	Reports or observation of: • Estimated amino acid intake higher or lower than recommended via all routes • Less than optimal amino acid supplementation • Incomplete knowledge of amino acid composition or of amino acid metabolism • Estimated energy intake from all sources lower than recommended
Client History*	Conditions associated with a diagnosis or treatment of illness that requires EN/PN therapy, food allergy or intolerance, inborn errors of metabolism, liver disease, kidney disease
Assessment, Monitoring, and Evaluation Tools	
Comparative Standards	

Arrows used with laboratory values: ↑ represents above reference standard and ↓ represents below reference standard.
** Client History terms are used for Nutrition Assessment but not for Nutrition Monitoring and Evaluation.*

Progress Evaluation

Communicate the progress toward the resolution of a nutrition diagnosis by selecting the appropriate nutrition diagnosis status value from the Nutrition Assessment, Monitoring, and Evaluation terms.

NCP Term	ANDUID
New nutrition diagnosis	14586
Active nutrition diagnosis	14587
Resolved nutrition diagnosis	14588
Discontinued nutrition diagnosis	14589

For details on these terms, visit the Nutrition Diagnosis Status reference sheet on page 200.

Inadequate Carbohydrate Intake

Definition

Lower intake of carbohydrate compared to established reference standards or recommendations based on physiological needs.

> *Note:* Whenever possible, nutrient intake data should be considered in combination with clinical, biochemical, anthropometric information, medical diagnosis, clinical status, and/or other factors to provide a valid assessment of nutritional status based on a totality of the evidence. (Institute of Medicine. *Dietary Reference Intakes: Applications in Dietary Assessment*. National Academies Press; 2000.)

Etiology (Cause/Contributing Risk Factors)

Factors gathered during the nutrition assessment process that contribute to the existence or the maintenance of pathophysiological, psychosocial, situational, developmental, cultural, and/or environmental problems:

- Physiological causes, eg, increased energy needs due to increased activity level or metabolic change, malabsorption
- Food insecurity
- Cultural practices that affect the ability to access food
- Food and nutrition related knowledge deficit concerning appropriate amount of dietary carbohydrate
- Psychological causes such as depression and disordered eating
- Limited food- and nutrition-related skill

Etiology Category

Etiologies are grouped by the type of cause or contributing risk factor. Communicate the etiology category by selecting the appropriate Nutrition Assessment, Monitoring, and Evaluation term.

NCP Term	ANDUID
Beliefs attitudes etiology	14567
Cultural etiology	14568
Knowledge etiology	14569
Physical function etiology	14570
Physiologic metabolic etiology	14571
Psychological etiology	14572
Social personal etiology	14573
Treatment etiology	14574
Access etiology	14575
Behavior etiology	14576

Visit the Nutrition Diagnosis Etiology Category Identification reference sheet on page 185 for more details on etiology categories. An additional useful resource to determine the etiology category is the Nutrition Diagnosis Matrix on page 528.

Inadequate Carbohydrate Intake

Signs/Symptoms (Defining Characteristics)

A typical cluster of subjective and objective signs and symptoms gathered during the nutrition assessment process that provide evidence that a problem exists; quantify the problem and describe its severity.

Nutrition Assessment Category	Potential Indicators of This Nutrition Diagnosis (one or more must be present)
Biochemical Data, Medical Tests and Procedures	
Anthropometric Measurements	
Physical Exam Findings	Ketone smell on breath
Food/Nutrition-Related History	Reports or observation of: • Estimated carbohydrate intake less than recommended amounts • Limited ability to independently consume foods/fluids, eg, diminished mobility in hand, wrist, or digits • Verbalizes inaccurate or incomplete knowledge
Client History*	Conditions associated with a diagnosis or treatment, eg, pancreatic insufficiency, hepatic disease, celiac disease, seizure disorder, or carbohydrate malabsorption
Assessment, Monitoring, and Evaluation Tools	
Comparative Standards	• Total carbohydrate estimated needs in 24 hours • Carbohydrate estimated needs per kg of body weight in 24 hours • Method for estimating total 24 hour carbohydrate needs • Proportion of energy needs from carbohydrate in 24 hours

** Client History terms are used for Nutrition Assessment but not for Nutrition Monitoring and Evaluation.*

Progress Evaluation

Communicate the progress toward the resolution of a nutrition diagnosis by selecting the appropriate nutrition diagnosis status value from the Nutrition Assessment, Monitoring, and Evaluation terms.

NCP Term	ANDUID
New nutrition diagnosis	14586
Active nutrition diagnosis	14587
Resolved nutrition diagnosis	14588
Discontinued nutrition diagnosis	14589

For details on these terms, visit the Nutrition Diagnosis Status reference sheet on page 200.

Excessive Carbohydrate Intake

Definition

Intake more than the recommended level and type of carbohydrate compared to established reference standards or recommendations based on physiological needs.

Etiology (Cause/Contributing Risk Factors)

Factors gathered during the nutrition assessment process that contribute to the existence or the maintenance of pathophysiological, psychosocial, situational, developmental, cultural, and/or environmental problems:

- Physiological causes requiring modified carbohydrate intake, eg, diabetes mellitus, lactase deficiency, sucrase-isomaltase deficiency, aldolase-B deficiency
- Cultural practices that affect the ability to reduce carbohydrate intake
- Food and nutrition related knowledge deficit concerning appropriate amount of carbohydrate intake
- Limited adherence with recommendations to modify carbohydrate intake
- Psychological causes such as depression and disordered eating
- Limited food- and nutrition-related skill

Etiology Category

Etiologies are grouped by the type of cause or contributing risk factor. Communicate the etiology category by selecting the appropriate Nutrition Assessment, Monitoring, and Evaluation term.

NCP Term	ANDUID
Beliefs attitudes etiology	14567
Cultural etiology	14568
Knowledge etiology	14569
Physical function etiology	14570
Physiologic metabolic etiology	14571
Psychological etiology	14572
Social personal etiology	14573
Treatment etiology	14574
Access etiology	14575
Behavior etiology	14576

Visit the Nutrition Diagnosis Etiology Category Identification reference sheet on page 185 for more details on etiology categories. An additional useful resource to determine the etiology category is the Nutrition Diagnosis Matrix on page 528.

Signs/Symptoms (Defining Characteristics)

A typical cluster of subjective and objective signs and symptoms gathered during the nutrition assessment process that provide evidence that a problem exists; quantify the problem and describe its severity. (See the next page for the nutrition assessment category and potential indicators.)

Excessive Carbohydrate Intake

Nutrition Assessment Category	Potential Indicators of This Nutrition Diagnosis (one or more must be present)
Biochemical Data, Medical Tests and Procedures	• Hyperglycemia (↑ fasting blood glucose > 126 mg/dL) • ↑ Hemoglobin A1C > 6% • ↑ Oral glucose tolerance test (2-hour post load glucose > 200 mg/dL)
Anthropometric Measurements	
Physical Exam Findings	• Dental caries • Diarrhea
Food/Nutrition-Related History	Reports or observation of: • Cultural or religious practices that do not support modification of dietary carbohydrate intake • Estimated carbohydrate intake that is consistently more than recommended amounts • Chronic use of medications that cause hyperglycemia, eg, steroids • Verbalizes inaccurate or incomplete knowledge
Client History*	• Conditions associated with a diagnosis or treatment, eg, diabetes mellitus, inborn errors of carbohydrate metabolism, lactase deficiency, severe infection, sepsis, or obesity • Pancreatic insufficiency resulting in reduced insulin production • Economic constraints that limit availability of appropriate foods
Assessment, Monitoring, and Evaluation Tools	
Comparative Standards	• Total carbohydrate estimated needs in 24 hours • Carbohydrate estimated needs per kg of body weight in 24 hours • Method for estimating total 24 hour carbohydrate needs • Proportion of energy needs from carbohydrate in 24 hours

Arrows used with laboratory values: ↑ represents above reference standard and ↓ represents below reference standard.
** Client History terms are used for Nutrition Assessment but not for Nutrition Monitoring and Evaluation.*

Progress Evaluation

Communicate the progress toward the resolution of a nutrition diagnosis by selecting the appropriate nutrition diagnosis status value from the Nutrition Assessment, Monitoring, and Evaluation terms.

NCP Term	ANDUID
New nutrition diagnosis	14586
Active nutrition diagnosis	14587
Resolved nutrition diagnosis	14588
Discontinued nutrition diagnosis	14589

For details on these terms, visit the Nutrition Diagnosis Status reference sheet on page 200.

Intake of Types of Carbohydrate Inconsistent With Needs

Definition

Intake of an amount of a specific type of carbohydrate compared to the established reference standards or recommendations based on physiological needs.

Note: Intolerance to the protein component of grains (eg, gluten) should be documented using the Intake of Types of Proteins Inconsistent With Needs reference sheet on page 276.

Etiology (Cause/Contributing Risk Factors)

Factors gathered during the nutrition assessment process that contribute to the existence or the maintenance of pathophysiological, psychosocial, situational, developmental, cultural, and/or environmental problems:

- Physiological causes altering carbohydrate digestion or metabolism, eg, intolerance, inborn errors of carbohydrate metabolism.

Note: Although research does not support restriction of individual types of carbohydrate for glycemic control, nutrition and dietetics practitioners may determine that restriction is warranted in unique client situations for glycemic control and/or for other reasons, such as promotion of healthful eating.

- Cultural or religious practices that affect the ability to regulate types of carbohydrate consumed
- Food and nutrition related knowledge deficit concerning an appropriate amount of a specific type of carbohydrate
- Limited adherence to recommendation to modify type of carbohydrate intake
- Psychological causes such as depression and disordered eating
- Limited food and nutrition related skill

Etiology Category

Etiologies are grouped by the type of cause or contributing risk factor. Communicate the etiology category by selecting the appropriate Nutrition Assessment, Monitoring and Evaluation term.

NCP Term	ANDUID
Beliefs attitudes etiology	14567
Cultural etiology	14568
Knowledge etiology	14569
Physical function etiology	14570
Physiologic metabolic etiology	14571
Psychological etiology	14572
Social personal etiology	14573
Treatment etiology	14574
Access etiology	14575
Behavior etiology	14576

Visit the Nutrition Diagnosis Etiology Category Identification reference sheet on page 185 for more details on etiology categories. An additional useful resource to determine the etiology category is the Nutrition Diagnosis Matrix on page 528.

Intake of Types of Carbohydrate Inconsistent With Needs

Signs/Symptoms (Defining Characteristics)

A typical cluster of subjective and objective signs and symptoms gathered during the nutrition assessment process that provide evidence that a problem exists; quantify the problem and describe its severity.

Nutrition Assessment Category	Potential Indicators of This Nutrition Diagnosis (one or more must be present)
Biochemical Data, Medical Tests and Procedures	• Hypoglycemia or hyperglycemia • ↓ galactose-1-phosphate in red blood cells, ↓ galactose-1-phosphate uridyl transferase, ↓ fructose
Anthropometric Measurements	• Weight loss, inability to gain weight, delayed growth • Weight gain
Physical Exam Findings	• Diarrhea in response to certain types of carbohydrates • Abdominal pain, distention, constipation, reflux, gastroesophageal reflux disease (GERD)
Food/Nutrition-Related History	Reports or observations of: • Carbohydrate intake that is a different type or exceeds amount recommended for that specific type of carbohydrate • Limited knowledge of carbohydrate composition of foods or of carbohydrate metabolism • Chronic use of medications that cause altered glucose levels, eg, steroids, diabetes medication, antidepressants, antipsychotics, or contains a type of carbohydrate not recommended • Cultural or religious practices that affect intake
Client History*	• Conditions associated with a diagnosis or treatment, eg, intolerance, inborn errors of metabolism • Allergic reactions or intolerance to certain carbohydrate foods or food groups • Economic constraints that limit availability of appropriate foods
Assessment, Monitoring, and Evaluation Tools	
Comparative Standards	

Arrows used with laboratory values: ↑ represents above reference standard and ↓ represents below reference standard.
** Client History terms are used for Nutrition Assessment but not for Nutrition Monitoring and Evaluation.*

Progress Evaluation

Communicate the progress toward the resolution of a nutrition diagnosis by selecting the appropriate nutrition diagnosis status value from the Nutrition Assessment, Monitoring, and Evaluation terms.

Intake of Types of Carbohydrate Inconsistent With Needs

NCP Term	ANDUID
New nutrition diagnosis	14586
Active nutrition diagnosis	14587
Resolved nutrition diagnosis	14588
Discontinued nutrition diagnosis	14589

For details on these terms, visit the Nutrition Diagnosis Status reference sheet on page 200.

Inconsistent Carbohydrate Intake

Definition

Inconsistent timing of carbohydrate intake throughout the day, day to day, or a pattern of carbohydrate intake that is not consistent with recommended pattern based on physiological or medication needs.

Etiology (Cause/Contributing Risk Factors)

Factors gathered during the nutrition assessment process that contribute to the existence or the maintenance of pathophysiological, psychosocial, situational, developmental, cultural, and/or environmental problems:

- Physiological causes requiring careful timing and consistency in the amount of carbohydrate, eg, diabetes mellitus, hypoglycemia, PN/EN delivery
- Cultural practices that affect the ability to regulate timing of carbohydrate consumption
- Food and nutrition related knowledge deficit concerning appropriate timing of carbohydrate intake
- Limited adherence to recommendations to modify carbohydrate timing
- Psychological causes such as depression and disordered eating
- Limited food- and nutrition-related skill

Etiology Category

Etiologies are grouped by the type of cause or contributing risk factor. Communicate the etiology category by selecting the appropriate Nutrition Assessment, Monitoring, and Evaluation term.

NCP Term	ANDUID
Beliefs attitudes etiology	14567
Cultural etiology	14568
Knowledge etiology	14569
Physical function etiology	14570
Physiologic metabolic etiology	14571
Psychological etiology	14572
Social personal etiology	14573
Treatment etiology	14574
Access etiology	14575
Behavior etiology	14576

Visit the Nutrition Diagnosis Etiology Category Identification reference sheet on page 185 for more details on etiology categories. An additional useful resource to determine the etiology category is the Nutrition Diagnosis Matrix on page 528.

Signs/Symptoms (Defining Characteristics)

A typical cluster of subjective and objective signs and symptoms gathered during the nutrition assessment process that provide evidence that a problem exists; quantify the problem and describe its severity.

Inconsistent Carbohydrate Intake

Nutrition Assessment Category	Potential Indicators of This Nutrition Diagnosis (one or more must be present)
Biochemical Data, Medical Tests and Procedures	• Hypoglycemia or hyperglycemia documented on regular basis associated with inconsistent carbohydrate intake • Wide variations in blood glucose levels
Anthropometric Measurements	
Physical Exam Findings	
Food/Nutrition-Related History	Reports or observations of: • Estimated carbohydrate intake that is different from recommended types or ingested on an irregular basis • Use of insulin or insulin secretagogues • Chronic use of medications that cause altered glucose levels, eg, steroids, antidepressants, antipsychotics • Verbalizes inaccurate or incomplete knowledge • Cultural or religious practices that affect intake
Client History*	• Conditions associated with a diagnosis or treatment, eg, diabetes mellitus, obesity, metabolic syndrome, hypoglycemia • Economic constraints that limit availability of appropriate foods
Assessment, Monitoring, and Evaluation Tools	
Comparative Standards	

** Client History terms are used for Nutrition Assessment but not for Nutrition Monitoring and Evaluation.*

Progress Evaluation

Communicate the progress toward the resolution of a nutrition diagnosis by selecting the appropriate nutrition diagnosis status value from the Nutrition Assessment, Monitoring, and Evaluation terms.

NCP Term	ANDUID
New nutrition diagnosis	14586
Active nutrition diagnosis	14587
Resolved nutrition diagnosis	14588
Discontinued nutrition diagnosis	14589

For details on these terms, visit the Nutrition Diagnosis Status reference sheet on page 200.

Inadequate Fiber Intake

Definition

Lower intake of fiber compared to established reference standards or recommendations based on physiological needs.

Note: Whenever possible, nutrient intake data should be considered in combination with clinical, biochemical, anthropometric information, medical diagnosis, clinical status, and/or other factors to provide a valid assessment of nutritional status based on a totality of the evidence. (Institute of Medicine. *Dietary Reference Intakes: Applications in Dietary Assessment.* National Academies Press; 2000.)

Etiology (Cause/Contributing Risk Factors)

Factors gathered during the nutrition assessment process that contribute to the existence or the maintenance of pathophysiological, psychosocial, situational, developmental, cultural, and/or environmental problems:

- Lack of or limited access to fiber-containing foods/fluids
- Food- and nutrition -related knowledge deficit concerning desirable quantities of fiber
- Psychological causes such as depression and disordered eating
- Prolonged adherence to a low-fiber or low-residue diet
- Difficulty chewing or swallowing high-fiber foods
- Economic constraints that limit availability of higher fiber foods
- Limited ability or limited motivation to purchase or consume fiber-containing foods
- Less than optimal food preparation practices, eg, reliance on overprocessed, overcooked foods
- Limited food- and nutrition -related skill

Etiology Category

Etiologies are grouped by the type of cause or contributing risk factor. Communicate the etiology category by selecting the appropriate Nutrition Assessment, Monitoring, and Evaluation term.

NCP Term	ANDUID
Beliefs attitudes etiology	14567
Cultural etiology	14568
Knowledge etiology	14569
Physical function etiology	14570
Physiologic metabolic etiology	14571
Psychological etiology	14572
Social personal etiology	14573
Treatment etiology	14574
Access etiology	14575
Behavior etiology	14576

Visit the Nutrition Diagnosis Etiology Category Identification reference sheet on page 185 for more details on etiology categories. An additional useful resource to determine the etiology category is the Nutrition Diagnosis Matrix on page 528.

Inadequate Fiber Intake

Signs/Symptoms (Defining Characteristics)

A typical cluster of subjective and objective signs and symptoms gathered during the nutrition assessment process that provide evidence that a problem exists; quantify the problem and describe its severity.

Nutrition Assessment Category	Potential Indicators of This Nutrition Diagnosis (one or more must be present)
Biochemical Data, Medical Tests and Procedures	
Anthropometric Measurements	
Physical Exam Findings	Inadequate fecal bulk
Food/Nutrition-Related History	Reports or observations of: • Estimated intake of fiber that is insufficient when compared to recommended amounts (38 g/day for men and 25 g/day for women) • Verbalizes inaccurate or incomplete knowledge
Client History*	Conditions associated with a diagnosis or treatment, eg, ulcer disease, inflammatory bowel disease, or short-bowel syndrome treated with a low-fiber diet
Assessment, Monitoring, and Evaluation Tools	
Comparative Standards	• Total fiber estimated needs in 24 hours • Method for estimating total 24 hour fiber needs

** Client History terms are used for Nutrition Assessment but not for Nutrition Monitoring and Evaluation.*

Progress Evaluation

Communicate the progress toward the resolution of a nutrition diagnosis by selecting the appropriate nutrition diagnosis status value from the Nutrition Assessment, Monitoring, and Evaluation terms.

NCP Term	ANDUID
New nutrition diagnosis	14586
Active nutrition diagnosis	14587
Resolved nutrition diagnosis	14588
Discontinued nutrition diagnosis	14589

For details on these terms, visit the Nutrition Diagnosis Status reference sheet on page 200.

Excessive Fiber Intake

Definition

Higher intake of fiber compared to recommendations based on client condition.

Etiology (Cause/Contributing Risk Factors)

Factors gathered during the nutrition assessment process that contribute to the existence or the maintenance of pathophysiological, psychosocial, situational, developmental, cultural, and/or environmental problems:

- Food and nutrition related knowledge deficit concerning desirable quantities of fiber
- Belief finding that hinders food and/or nutrition behavior change
- Attitude finding that hinders food and/or nutrition behavior change
- Lack of knowledge about appropriate fiber intake for condition
- Food preparation or eating patterns that involve only high-fiber foods to the exclusion of other nutrient-dense foods
- Limited food- and nutrition-related skill

Etiology Category

Etiologies are grouped by the type of cause or contributing risk factor. Communicate the etiology category by selecting the appropriate Nutrition Assessment, Monitoring and Evaluation term.

NCP Term	ANDUID
Beliefs attitudes etiology	14567
Cultural etiology	14568
Knowledge etiology	14569
Physical function etiology	14570
Physiologic metabolic etiology	14571
Psychological etiology	14572
Social personal etiology	14573
Treatment etiology	14574
Access etiology	14575
Behavior etiology	14576

Visit the Nutrition Diagnosis Etiology Category Identification reference sheet on page 185 for more details on etiology categories. An additional useful resource to determine the etiology category is the Nutrition Diagnosis Matrix on page 528.

Signs/Symptoms (Defining Characteristics)

A typical cluster of subjective and objective signs and symptoms gathered during the nutrition assessment process that provide evidence that a problem exists; quantify the problem and describe its severity.

Excessive Fiber Intake

Nutrition Assessment Category	Potential Indicators of This Nutrition Diagnosis (one or more must be present)
Biochemical Data, Medical Tests and Procedures	
Anthropometric Measurements	
Physical Exam Findings	Nausea, vomiting, excessive flatulence, diarrhea, abdominal cramping, high stool volume or frequency that causes discomfort to the individual
Food/Nutrition-Related History	Reports or observations of: • Estimated fiber intake higher than tolerated or generally recommended for current medical condition • Verbalizes inaccurate or incomplete knowledge • Verbalizes unsupported beliefs and attitudes
Client History*	• Conditions associated with a diagnosis or treatment, eg, ulcer disease, irritable bowel syndrome, inflammatory bowel disease, short-bowel syndrome, diverticulitis, obstructive constipation, prolapsing hemorrhoids, gastrointestinal stricture, eating disorders, or mental illness with obsessive-compulsive tendencies • Obstruction, phytobezoar
Assessment, Monitoring, and Evaluation Tools	
Comparative Standards	• Total fiber estimated needs in 24 hours • Method for estimating total 24 hour fiber needs

** Client History terms are used for Nutrition Assessment but not for Nutrition Monitoring and Evaluation.*

Progress Evaluation

Communicate the progress toward the resolution of a nutrition diagnosis by selecting the appropriate nutrition diagnosis status value from the Nutrition Assessment, Monitoring, and Evaluation terms.

NCP Term	ANDUID
New nutrition diagnosis	14586
Active nutrition diagnosis	14587
Resolved nutrition diagnosis	14588
Discontinued nutrition diagnosis	14589

For details on these terms, visit the Nutrition Diagnosis Status reference sheet on page 200.

Inadequate Vitamin Intake

Definition

Lower intake of one or more vitamins compared to established reference standards or recommendations based on physiological needs.

Note: Whenever possible, nutrient intake data should be considered in combination with clinical, biochemical, anthropometric information, medical diagnosis, clinical status, and/or other factors to provide a valid assessment of nutritional status based on a totality of the evidence. (Institute of Medicine. *Dietary Reference Intakes: Applications in Dietary Assessment.* National Academies Press; 2000.)

Etiology (Cause/Contributing Risk Factors)

Factors gathered during the nutrition assessment process that contribute to the existence or the maintenance of pathophysiological, psychosocial, situational, developmental, cultural, and/or environmental problems:

- Physiological causes increasing nutrient needs, eg, due to prolonged catabolic illness, disease state, malabsorption, or medications
- Decreased ability to consume sufficient amount of a vitamin(s)
- Food insecurity
- Cultural practices that affect ability to access food
- Food and nutrition related knowledge deficit concerning food and supplemental sources of vitamins
- Psychological causes, eg, depression or eating disorders
- Access causes including season, geography, limited access to sunlight
- Limited food- and nutrition-related skill

Etiology Category

Etiologies are grouped by the type of cause or contributing risk factor. Communicate the etiology category by selecting the appropriate Nutrition Assessment, Monitoring, and Evaluation term.

NCP Term	ANDUID
Beliefs attitudes etiology	14567
Cultural etiology	14568
Knowledge etiology	14569
Physical function etiology	14570
Physiologic metabolic etiology	14571
Psychological etiology	14572
Social personal etiology	14573
Treatment etiology	14574
Access etiology	14575
Behavior etiology	14576

Visit the Nutrition Diagnosis Etiology Category Identification reference sheet on page 185 for more details on etiology categories. An additional useful resource to determine the etiology category is the Nutrition Diagnosis Matrix on page 528.

Inadequate Vitamin Intake

Signs/Symptoms (Defining Characteristics)

A typical cluster of subjective and objective signs and symptoms gathered during the nutrition assessment process that provide evidence that a problem exists; quantify the problem and describe its severity.

Nutrition Assessment Category	Potential Indicators of This Nutrition Diagnosis (one or more must be present)
Biochemical Data, Medical Tests and Procedures	• Vitamin A: ↓ serum retinol < 10 μg/dL (0.35 μmol/L) • Vitamin C: ↓ plasma concentrations < 0.2 mg/dL (11.4 μmol/L) • Vitamin D: ↓ 25(OH)D < 50 nmol/L, ↓ ionized calcium < 3.9 mg/dL (0.98 mmol/L) with ↑ parathyroid hormone, normal serum calcium, and ↓ serum phosphorus < 2.6 mg/dL (0.84 mmol/L) • Vitamin E: ↓ plasma alpha-tocopherol < 18 μmol/g (41.8 μmol/L) • Vitamin K: ↑ prothrombin time; altered INR (without anticoagulation therapy) • Thiamin: ↑ erythrocyte transketolase activity > 1.20 μg/mL/h • Riboflavin: ↑ erythrocyte glutathione reductase > 1.2 IU/g hemoglobin • Niacin: ↓ N'methyl-nicotinamide excretion < 5.8 μmol/day • Vitamin B6: ↓ plasma pyridoxal 5'phosphate <5 ng/mL (20 nmol/L) • Vitamin B12: ↓ serum concentration < 24.4 ng/dL (180 pmol/L); ↑ homocysteine • Folic acid: ↓ serum concentration < 0.3 μg/dL (7 nmol/L); ↓ red cell folate < 315 nmol/L • Pantothenic acid: ↓ plasma • Biotin: ↓ serum
Anthropometric Measurements	
Physical Exam Findings	• Vitamin A: night blindness, Bitot spots, xerophthalmia, follicular hyperkeratosis • Vitamin C: follicular hyperkeratosis, petechiae, ecchymosis, coiled hairs, inflamed and bleeding gums, perifollicular hemorrhages, joint effusions, arthralgia, and impaired wound healing • Vitamin D: widening at ends of long bones • Riboflavin: sore throat, hyperemia, edema of pharyngeal and oral mucous membranes, cheilosis, angular stomatitis, glossitis, magenta tongue, seborrheic dermatitis, and normochromic, normocytic anemia with pure erythrocyte cytoplasia of the bone marrow • Niacin: symmetrical, pigmented rash on areas exposed to sunlight; bright red tongue • Vitamin B6: seborrheic dermatitis, stomatitis, cheilosis, glossitis, confusion, depression

Continued on next page

Inadequate Vitamin Intake

Continued from previous page

Nutrition Assessment Category	Potential Indicators of This Nutrition Diagnosis (one or more must be present)
Physical Exam Findings (continued)	• Vitamin B12: tingling and numbness in extremities, diminished vibratory and position sense, motor disturbances including gait disturbances • Pantothenic acid: irritability and restlessness, fatigue, apathy, malaise, sleep disturbances, nausea, vomiting, abdominal cramps, numbness, muscle cramps, hypoglycemia, sensitivity to insulin • Biotin: dermatitis, conjunctivitis, alopecia, depression, lethargy, hallucinations and paresthesia, hypotonia, developmental delays
Food/Nutrition-Related History	Reports or observations of: • Estimated intake of foods containing specific vitamins less than requirements or recommended level • Intake of foods that do not contain available vitamins, eg, overprocessed, overcooked, or improperly stored foods • Prolonged use of substances known to increase vitamin requirements or reduce vitamin absorption • Lack of interest in foods
Client History*	• Conditions associated with a diagnosis or treatment, eg, malabsorption as a result of celiac disease, short bowel syndrome, or inflammatory bowel • Certain environmental conditions, eg, infants exclusively fed breastmilk with limited exposure to sunlight (Vitamin D) • History of chronic kidney disease (decreased conversion of 25[OH]D) • Premature infant, extremely low birth weight infant (vitamin D) • Rachitic rosary in children, rickets, osteomalacia • Pellagra • Vitamin/mineral deficiency
Assessment, Monitoring, and Evaluation Tools	
Comparative Standards	• Estimated vitamin A needs in 24 hours • Estimated vitamin C needs in 24 hours • Estimated vitamin D needs in 24 hours • Estimated vitamin E needs in 24 hours • Estimated vitamin K needs in 24 hours • Estimated thiamin needs in 24 hours • Estimated riboflavin needs in 24 hours • Estimated niacin needs in 24 hours • Estimated folate needs in 24 hours • Estimated vitamin B6 needs in 24 hours

Continued on next page

Inadequate Vitamin Intake

Continued from previous page

Nutrition Assessment Category	Potential Indicators of This Nutrition Diagnosis (one or more must be present)
Comparative Standards (continued)	• Estimated vitamin B12 needs in 24 hours • Estimated pantothenic acid needs in 24 hours • Estimated biotin needs in 24 hours • Method for estimating 24 hour vitamin needs

Arrows used with laboratory values: ↑ represents above reference standard and ↓ represents below reference standard.
** Client History terms are used for Nutrition Assessment but not for Nutrition Monitoring and Evaluation.*

Progress Evaluation

Communicate the progress toward the resolution of a nutrition diagnosis by selecting the appropriate nutrition diagnosis status value from the Nutrition Assessment, Monitoring, and Evaluation terms.

NCP Term	ANDUID
New nutrition diagnosis	14586
Active nutrition diagnosis	14587
Resolved nutrition diagnosis	14588
Discontinued nutrition diagnosis	14589

For details on these terms, visit the Nutrition Diagnosis Status reference sheet on page 200.

Excessive Vitamin Intake

Definition

Higher intake of one or more vitamins compared to established reference standards or recommendations based on physiological needs.

Etiology (Cause/Contributing Risk Factors)

Factors gathered during the nutrition assessment process that contribute to the existence or the maintenance of pathophysiological, psychosocial, situational, developmental, cultural, and/or environmental problems:

- Physiological causes decreasing nutrient needs due to prolonged immobility or chronic renal disease
- Access to foods and supplements in excess of needs, eg, cultural or religious practices; less-than-optimal food and supplements given to pregnant women, elderly, or children
- Food and nutrition related knowledge deficit concerning food and supplemental sources of vitamins
- Psychological causes, eg, depression or eating disorders
- Accidental overdose from oral and supplemental forms, enteral or parenteral sources
- Limited food- and nutrition-related skill

Etiology Category

Etiologies are grouped by the type of cause or contributing risk factor. Communicate the etiology category by selecting the appropriate Nutrition Assessment, Monitoring, and Evaluation term.

NCP Term	ANDUID
Beliefs attitudes etiology	14567
Cultural etiology	14568
Knowledge etiology	14569
Physical function etiology	14570
Physiologic metabolic etiology	14571
Psychological etiology	14572
Social personal etiology	14573
Treatment etiology	14574
Access etiology	14575
Behavior etiology	14576

Visit the Nutrition Diagnosis Etiology Category Identification reference sheet on page 185 for more details on etiology categories. An additional useful resource to determine the etiology category is the Nutrition Diagnosis Matrix on page 528.

Signs/Symptoms (Defining Characteristics)

A typical cluster of subjective and objective signs and symptoms gathered during the nutrition assessment process that provide evidence that a problem exists; quantify the problem and describe its severity.

Excessive Vitamin Intake

Nutrition Assessment Category	Potential Indicators of This Nutrition Diagnosis (one or more must be present)
Biochemical Data, Medical Tests and Procedures	• Vitamin D: ↑ 25(OH) D, ↑ ionized calcium > 5.4 mg/dL (1.35 mol/L) with ↑ parathyroid hormone, normal or ↑ serum calcium, and ↑ serum phosphorus > 2.6 mg/dL (0.84 mmol/L) • Vitamin K: ↓ prothrombin time or altered INR • Niacin: ↑ N'methyl-nicotinamide excretion > 7.3 μmol/day • Vitamin B6: ↑ plasma pyridoxal 5'phosphate > 15.7 ng/mL (94 nmol/L) • Vitamin A: ↑ serum retinol concentration > 60 μg/dL (2.09 μmol/L) • Pantothenic acid: ↑ plasma • Biotin: ↑ serum
Anthropometric Measurements	Vitamin D: growth retardation
Physical Exam Findings	• Vitamin A: changes in the skin and mucous membranes; dry lips (cheilitis); early: dryness of the nasal mucosa and eyes; later: dryness, erythema, scaling and peeling of the skin, hair loss, and nail fragility; headache, nausea, and vomiting. Infants may have bulging fontanelle; children may develop bone alterations. • Vitamin D: calcification of soft tissues (calcinosis), including the kidney, lungs, heart, and even the tympanic membrane of the ear, which can result in deafness. Headache and nausea. Infants given excessive amounts of vitamin D may have gastrointestinal upset and/or bone fragility. • Vitamin K: hemolytic anemia in adults or severe jaundice in infants have been noted on rare occasions • Niacin: histamine release, which causes flushing, aggravation of asthma, or liver disease
Food/Nutrition-Related History	Reports or observations of: • Estimated intake reflects excessive intake of foods and supplements containing vitamins as compared to estimated requirements, including fortified cereals, meal replacements, vitamin-mineral supplements, other dietary supplements (eg, fish liver oils or capsules), tube feeding, and/or parenteral solutions • Estimated intake more than UL for vitamin A based upon reference intake standard • Estimated intake more than UL for vitamin D based upon reference intake standard • Estimated intake more than UL for niacin based upon reference intake standard
Client History*	Conditions associated with a diagnosis or treatment, eg, chronic liver or kidney diseases, heart failure, cancer

Continued on next page

Excessive Vitamin Intake

Continued from previous page

Nutrition Assessment Category	Potential Indicators of This Nutrition Diagnosis (one or more must be present)
Assessment, Monitoring, and Evaluation Tools	
Comparative Standards	• Estimated vitamin A needs in 24 hours • Estimated vitamin C needs in 24 hours • Estimated vitamin D needs in 24 hours • Estimated vitamin E needs in 24 hours • Estimated vitamin K needs in 24 hours • Estimated thiamin needs in 24 hours • Estimated riboflavin needs in 24 hours • Estimated niacin needs in 24 hours • Estimated folate needs in 24 hours • Estimated vitamin B6 needs in 24 hours • Estimated vitamin B12 needs in 24 hours • Estimated pantothenic acid needs in 24 hours • Estimated biotin needs in 24 hours • Method for estimating 24 hour vitamin needs

Arrows used with laboratory values: ↑ represents above reference standard and ↓ represents below reference standard.
** Client History terms are used for Nutrition Assessment but not for Nutrition Monitoring and Evaluation.*

Progress Evaluation

Communicate the progress toward the resolution of a nutrition diagnosis by selecting the appropriate nutrition diagnosis status value from the Nutrition Assessment, Monitoring, and Evaluation terms.

NCP Term	ANDUID
New nutrition diagnosis	14586
Active nutrition diagnosis	14587
Resolved nutrition diagnosis	14588
Discontinued nutrition diagnosis	14589

For details on these terms, visit the Nutrition Diagnosis Status reference sheet on page 200.

Inadequate Mineral Intake

Definition

Lower intake of one or more minerals compared to established reference standards or recommendations based on physiological needs.

Note: Whenever possible, nutrient intake data should be considered in combination with clinical, biochemical, anthropometric information, medical diagnosis, clinical status, and/or other factors to provide a valid assessment of nutritional status based on a totality of the evidence. (Institute of Medicine. *Dietary Reference Intakes: Applications in Dietary Assessment.* National Academies Press; 2000.)

Etiology (Cause/Contributing Risk Factors)

Factors gathered during the nutrition assessment process that contribute to the existence or the maintenance of pathophysiological, psychosocial, situational, developmental, cultural, and/or environmental problems:

- Physiological causes increasing nutrient needs due to prolonged catabolic illness, malabsorption, hyperexcretion, nutrient/drug and nutrient/nutrient interaction, growth and maturation
- Decreased ability to consume sufficient amount of a mineral(s)
- Food insecurity
- Cultural practices that affect ability to access food
- Food and nutrition related knowledge deficit concerning food and supplemental sources of minerals
- Misdiagnosis of lactose intolerance/lactase deficiency; perception of conflicting nutrition messages; less than optimal reliance on supplements
- Psychological causes, eg, depression or eating disorders
- Environmental causes, eg, inadequately tested nutrient bioavailability of fortified foods, beverages, and supplements; less than optimal marketing of fortified foods/beverages/supplements as a substitute for natural food source of nutrient(s)
- Limited food- and nutrition-related skill

Etiology Category

Etiologies are grouped by the type of cause or contributing risk factor. Communicate the etiology category by selecting the appropriate Nutrition Assessment, Monitoring, and Evaluation term.

NCP Term	ANDUID
Beliefs attitudes etiology	14567
Cultural etiology	14568
Knowledge etiology	14569
Physical function etiology	14570
Physiologic metabolic etiology	14571
Psychological etiology	14572
Social personal etiology	14573
Treatment etiology	14574
Access etiology	14575
Behavior etiology	14576

Visit the Nutrition Diagnosis Etiology Category Identification reference sheet on page 185 for more details on etiology categories. An additional useful resource to determine the etiology category is the Nutrition Diagnosis Matrix on page 528.

Inadequate Mineral Intake

Signs/Symptoms (Defining Characteristics)

A typical cluster of subjective and objective signs and symptoms gathered during the nutrition assessment process that provide evidence that a problem exists; quantify the problem and describe its severity.

Nutrition Assessment Category	Potential Indicators of This Nutrition Diagnosis (one or more must be present)
Biochemical Data, Medical Tests and Procedures	• Calcium: bone mineral content (BMC) ↓ the young adult mean; hypocalciuria, serum 25(OH)D < 32 ng/mL • ↓ Phosphorus, < 2.6 mg/dL (0.84 mmol/L) • ↓ Ferritin in client with a ↓ MCV • ↓ Zinc, plasma • ↓ Magnesium, < 1.8 mg/dL (0.7 mmol/L) • Iron: ↓ hemoglobin < 13 g/L (2 mmol/L) (males); < 12 g/L (1.86 mol/L) (females) • Iodine: ↓ urinary excretion < 100 µg/L (788 nmol/L) • Copper: ↓ serum copper < 64 µg/dL (10 µmol/L) • ↓ Selenium, plasma • ↓ Fluoride, plasma • ↓ Manganese, serum • ↓ Molybdenum, serum • ↓ Boron, serum or plasma • Changes in urine labs associated with kidney stones
Anthropometric Measurements	• Calcium: body height loss • Iodine: growth abnormalities • Chromium: unintentional body weight loss
Physical Exam Findings	• Calcium: hypertension, hyperactive reflexes, tetany, muscle spasm, irregular heart rhythm • Iron: pallor of face, mucosa, pale gums, tachycardia, fatigue • Potassium: weakness, constipation, hypoactive reflexes • Phosphorous: fatigue, myalgia, ataxia, confusion, parasthesias • Zinc: dysgeusia, poor wound healing, skin lesions (buttocks, peri-anal area, mouth, nose, eyes), alopecia • Copper: depigmentation of hair and skin, osteoporosis • Selenium: depigmentation of hair and skin • Iodine: enlarged thyroid • Fluoride: dental caries • Manganese: dermatitis
Food/Nutrition-Related History	Reports or observations of: • Estimated mineral intake from diet less than recommended intake • Food avoidance and/or elimination of whole food group(s) from diet

Continued on next page

Inadequate Mineral Intake

Continued from previous page

Nutrition Assessment Category	Potential Indicators of This Nutrition Diagnosis (one or more must be present)
Food/Nutrition-Related History (continued)	• Lack of interest in food • Less than optimal food choices and/or chronic dieting behavior • Verbalizes inaccurate or incomplete knowledge • Cultural or religious practices that affect intake
Client History*	• Conditions associated with a diagnosis or treatment, eg, malabsorption as a result of celiac disease, short bowel syndrome, inflammatory bowel disease, or post-menopausal women without estrogen supplementation and increased calcium need, bariatric surgery, parenteral nutrition • Polycystic ovary syndrome, premenstrual syndrome, kidney stones, colon polyps • Other significant medical diagnoses and therapies • Geographic latitude and history of ultraviolet B exposure/use of sunscreen • Change in living environment/independence • Calcium: obesity • Vitamin/mineral deficiency
Assessment, Monitoring, and Evaluation Tools	
Comparative Standards	• Estimated calcium needs in 24 hours • Estimated chloride needs in 24 hours • Estimated iron needs in 24 hours • Estimated magnesium needs in 24 hours • Estimated potassium needs in 24 hours • Estimated phosphorus needs in 24 hours • Estimated sodium needs in 24 hours • Estimated zinc needs in 24 hours • Estimated sulfate needs in 24 hours • Estimated fluoride needs in 24 hours • Estimated copper needs in 24 hours • Estimated iodine needs in 24 hours • Estimated selenium needs in 24 hours • Estimated manganese needs in 24 hours • Estimated chromium needs in 24 hours • Estimated molybdenum needs in 24 hours • Estimated boron needs in 24 hours • Estimated cobalt needs in 24 hours • Method for estimating 24 hour mineral needs

Arrows used with laboratory values: ↑ represents above reference standard and ↓ represents below reference standard.
** Client History terms are used for Nutrition Assessment but not for Nutrition Monitoring and Evaluation.*

Inadequate Mineral Intake

Progress Evaluation

Communicate the progress toward the resolution of a nutrition diagnosis by selecting the appropriate nutrition diagnosis status value from the Nutrition Assessment, Monitoring, and Evaluation terms.

NCP Term	ANDUID
New nutrition diagnosis	14586
Active nutrition diagnosis	14587
Resolved nutrition diagnosis	14588
Discontinued nutrition diagnosis	14589

For details on these terms, visit the Nutrition Diagnosis Status reference sheet on page 200.

Excessive Mineral Intake

Definition

Higher intake of one or more minerals compared to established reference standards or recommendations based on physiological needs.

Etiology (Cause/Contributing Risk Factors)

Factors gathered during the nutrition assessment process that contribute to the existence or the maintenance of pathophysiological, psychosocial, situational, developmental, cultural, and/or environmental problems:

- Food and nutrition related knowledge deficit concerning food and supplemental sources of minerals
- Belief finding that hinders food and/or nutrition behavior change
- Attitude finding that hinders food and/or nutrition behavior change
- Food faddism
- Accidental over supplementation
- Overconsumption of a limited variety of foods
- Limited knowledge about management of a disorder altering mineral homeostasis
- Limited knowledge about management of a disease state requiring mineral restriction
- Limited food- and nutrition-related skill

Etiology Category

Etiologies are grouped by the type of cause or contributing risk factor. Communicate the etiology category by selecting the appropriate Nutrition Assessment, Monitoring, and Evaluation term.

NCP Term	ANDUID
Beliefs attitudes etiology	14567
Cultural etiology	14568
Knowledge etiology	14569
Physical function etiology	14570
Physiologic metabolic etiology	14571
Psychological etiology	14572
Social personal etiology	14573
Treatment etiology	14574
Access etiology	14575
Behavior etiology	14576

Visit the Nutrition Diagnosis Etiology Category Identification reference sheet on page 185 for more details on etiology categories. An additional useful resource to determine the etiology category is the Nutrition Diagnosis Matrix on page 528.

Signs/Symptoms (Defining Characteristics)

A typical cluster of subjective and objective signs and symptoms gathered during the nutrition assessment process that provide evidence that a problem exists; quantify the problem and describe its severity. (See the next page for the nutrition assessment category and potential indicators.)

Excessive Mineral Intake

Nutrition Assessment Category	Potential Indicators of This Nutrition Diagnosis (one or more must be present)
Biochemical Data, Medical Tests and Procedures	Changes in appropriate laboratory values, such as: • ↑ TSH (excessive iodine intake) • ↓ HDL (excessive zinc intake) • ↑ Serum ferritin and transferrin saturation (iron overload or excessive intake) • ↑ Phosphorus, serum • ↑ Magnesium, serum • ↓ Copper, serum (excessive zinc intake) • ↑ Fluoride, plasma • ↑ Selenium, serum • ↑ Manganese, serum • ↑ Molybdenum, serum • ↑ Boron, serum or plasma
Anthropometric Measurements	
Physical Exam Findings	• Hair and nail changes • Extraskeletal calcifications, affecting vasculature or skin • Pruritis • Anorexia • GI disturbances • Enamel or skeletal fluorosis • Central nervous system effects • Verbalizes inaccurate or incomplete knowledge • Verbalizes unsupported beliefs and attitudes
Food/Nutrition-Related History	Reports or observations of estimated intake containing high amounts of mineral compared to reference intake standard (eg, DRIs)
Client History*	• Heart failure • Kidney disease • Liver damage • Parenteral nutrition
Assessment, Monitoring, and Evaluation Tools	
Comparative Standards	• Estimated calcium needs in 24 hours • Estimated chloride needs in 24 hours • Estimated iron needs in 24 hours • Estimated magnesium needs in 24 hours • Estimated potassium needs in 24 hours • Estimated phosphorus needs in 24 hours

Continued on next page

Excessive Mineral Intake

Continued from previous page

Nutrition Assessment Category	Potential Indicators of This Nutrition Diagnosis (one or more must be present)
Comparative Standards (continued)	• Estimated sodium needs in 24 hours • Estimated zinc needs in 24 hours • Estimated sulfate needs in 24 hours • Estimated fluoride needs in 24 hours • Estimated copper needs in 24 hours • Estimated iodine needs in 24 hours • Estimated selenium needs in 24 hours • Estimated manganese needs in 24 hours • Estimated chromium needs in 24 hours • Estimated molybdenum needs in 24 hours • Estimated boron needs in 24 hours • Estimated cobalt needs in 24 hours • Method for estimating 24 hour mineral needs

Arrows used with laboratory values: ↑ represents above reference standard and ↓ represents below reference standard.
** Client History terms are used for Nutrition Assessment but not for Nutrition Monitoring and Evaluation.*

Progress Evaluation

Communicate the progress toward the resolution of a nutrition diagnosis by selecting the appropriate nutrition diagnosis status value from the Nutrition Assessment, Monitoring, and Evaluation terms.

NCP Term	ANDUID
New nutrition diagnosis	14586
Active nutrition diagnosis	14587
Resolved nutrition diagnosis	14588
Discontinued nutrition diagnosis	14589

For details on these terms, visit the Nutrition Diagnosis Status reference sheet on page 200.

Predicted Inadequate Nutrient Intake

Definition

Future intake of one or more nutrients that is anticipated, based on observation, experience, or scientific reason, to fall short of estimated nutrient requirements, established reference standards, or recommendations based on physiological needs.

Etiology (Cause/Contributing Risk Factors)

Factors gathered during the nutrition assessment process that contribute to the existence or the maintenance of pathophysiological, psychosocial, situational, developmental, cultural, and/or environmental problems:

- Scheduled or planned medical therapy or medication that is predicted to increase nutrient requirements
- Scheduled or planned medical therapy or medication that is predicted to decrease ability to consume sufficient nutrients
- Physiological condition associated with increased need for a nutrient due to altered metabolism
- Cultural or religious practices that will affect nutrient intake
- Anticipated isolated living/housing situation without routine access to a variety of nutritious foods
- Danger for environmental emergency or catastrophe/disaster

Etiology Category

Etiologies are grouped by the type of cause or contributing risk factor. Communicate the etiology category by selecting the appropriate Nutrition Assessment, Monitoring, and Evaluation term.

NCP Term	ANDUID
Beliefs attitudes etiology	14567
Cultural etiology	14568
Knowledge etiology	14569
Physical function etiology	14570
Physiologic metabolic etiology	14571
Psychological etiology	14572
Social personal etiology	14573
Treatment etiology	14574
Access etiology	14575
Behavior etiology	14576

Visit the Nutrition Diagnosis Etiology Category Identification reference sheet on page 185 for more details on etiology categories. An additional useful resource to determine the etiology category is the Nutrition Diagnosis Matrix on page 528.

Signs/Symptoms (Defining Characteristics)

A typical cluster of subjective and objective signs and symptoms gathered during the nutrition assessment process that provide evidence that a problem exists; quantify the problem and describe its severity.

Predicted Inadequate Nutrient Intake

Nutrition Assessment Category	Potential Indicators of This Nutrition Diagnosis (one or more must be present)
Biochemical Data, Medical Tests and Procedures	Population-based biochemical parameters indicating inadequate nutrient intake
Anthropometric Measurements	Population-based anthropometric data indicating inadequate nutrient intake
Physical Exam Findings	Population-based data on acute and chronic disease prevalence indicating inadequate nutrient intake
Food/Nutrition-Related History	Reports or observations of: • Estimated nutrient(s) intake from all sources less than projected needs • History of marginal or inadequate nutrient(s) intake • Projected change in ability to shop, prepare, and/or consume sufficient nutrient(s) • Medications that decrease appetite and/or affect ability to consume sufficient nutrient(s) • No prior knowledge of need for food- and nutrition-related recommendations • Religious or cultural practices that will affect nutrient intake • Low supplies in home in preparation for environmental emergency or catastrophe/disaster
Client History*	• Scheduled surgical procedure or medical therapy known to increase nutrient(s) need or change ability to consume sufficient nutrient(s) • History or presence of a condition for which research shows an increased prevalence of insufficient nutrient(s) intake in a similar population • Isolated living/housing situation • Geographic location of home in location with danger for environmental emergency or catastrophe/disaster
Assessment, Monitoring, and Evaluation Tools	
Comparative Standards	

** Client History terms are used for Nutrition Assessment but not for Nutrition Monitoring and Evaluation.*

Progress Evaluation

Communicate the progress toward the resolution of a nutrition diagnosis by selecting the appropriate nutrition diagnosis status value from the Nutrition Assessment, Monitoring, and Evaluation terms.

NCP Term	ANDUID
New nutrition diagnosis	14586
Active nutrition diagnosis	14587
Resolved nutrition diagnosis	14588
Discontinued nutrition diagnosis	14589

For details on these terms, visit the Nutrition Diagnosis Status reference sheet on page 200.

Predicted Excessive Nutrient Intake

Definition

Future intake of one or more nutrients that is anticipated, based on observation, experience, or scientific reason, to be more than estimated nutrient requirements, established reference standards, or recommendations based on physiological needs.

Etiology (Cause/Contributing Risk Factors)

Factors gathered during the nutrition assessment process that contribute to the existence or the maintenance of pathophysiological, psychosocial, situational, developmental, cultural, and/or environmental problems:

- Scheduled or planned medical therapy or medication that is predicted to decrease nutrient requirements
- Anticipated physiological condition associated with reduced need for or altered metabolism of nutrients
- Scheduled or planned medical therapy or medication that is predicted to alter metabolism of nutrients

Etiology Category

Etiologies are grouped by the type of cause or contributing risk factor. Communicate the etiology category by selecting the appropriate Nutrition Assessment, Monitoring, and Evaluation term.

NCP Term	ANDUID
Beliefs attitudes etiology	14567
Cultural etiology	14568
Knowledge etiology	14569
Physical function etiology	14570
Physiologic metabolic etiology	14571
Psychological etiology	14572
Social personal etiology	14573
Treatment etiology	14574
Access etiology	14575
Behavior etiology	14576

Visit the Nutrition Diagnosis Etiology Category Identification reference sheet on page 185 for more details on etiology categories. An additional useful resource to determine the etiology category is the Nutrition Diagnosis Matrix on page 528.

Signs/Symptoms (Defining Characteristics)

A typical cluster of subjective and objective signs and symptoms gathered during the nutrition assessment process that provide evidence that a problem exists; quantify the problem and describe its severity.

Predicted Excessive Nutrient Intake

Nutrition Assessment Category	Potential Indicators of This Nutrition Diagnosis (one or more must be present)
Biochemical Data, Medical Tests and Procedures	Population-based biochemical parameters indicating excessive nutrient intake
Anthropometric Measurements	Population-based anthropometric data indicating excessive nutrient intake
Physical Exam Findings	Population-based data on acute and chronic disease prevalence indicating excessive nutrient
Food/Nutrition-Related History	Reports or observations of: • Estimated nutrient(s) intake from all sources more than projected needs • History of excessive nutrient(s) intake • No prior knowledge of need for food- and nutrition-related recommendations
Client History*	• Scheduled surgical procedure or medical therapy known to reduce nutrient(s) need or alter metabolism of a nutrient(s) • History or presence of a condition for which research shows an increased prevalence of excessive nutrient(s) intake in a similar population
Assessment, Monitoring, and Evaluation Tools	
Comparative Standards	

** Client History terms are used for Nutrition Assessment but not for Nutrition Monitoring and Evaluation.*

Progress Evaluation

Communicate the progress toward the resolution of a nutrition diagnosis by selecting the appropriate nutrition diagnosis status value from the Nutrition Assessment, Monitoring, and Evaluation terms.

NCP Term	ANDUID
New nutrition diagnosis	14586
Active nutrition diagnosis	14587
Resolved nutrition diagnosis	14588
Discontinued nutrition diagnosis	14589

For details on these terms, visit the Nutrition Diagnosis Status reference sheet on page 200.

Swallowing Difficulty

Definition

Impaired or difficult movement of food and liquid within the oral cavity to the stomach

Etiology (Cause/Contributing Risk Factors)

Factors gathered during the nutrition assessment process that contribute to the existence or the maintenance of pathophysiological, psychosocial, situational, developmental, cultural, and/or environmental problems:

- Mechanical causes, eg, inflammation, surgery, stricture; oral, pharyngeal, and esophageal tumors; prior mechanical ventilation
- Motor causes, eg, neurological or muscular disorders, such as cerebral palsy, stroke, multiple sclerosis, scleroderma; prematurity, altered suck/swallow, breath patterns

Etiology Category

Etiologies are grouped by the type of cause or contributing risk factor. Communicate the etiology category by selecting the appropriate Nutrition Assessment, Monitoring, and Evaluation term.

NCP Term	ANDUID
Beliefs attitudes etiology	14567
Cultural etiology	14568
Knowledge etiology	14569
Physical function etiology	14570
Physiologic metabolic etiology	14571
Psychological etiology	14572
Social personal etiology	14573
Treatment etiology	14574
Access etiology	14575
Behavior etiology	14576

Visit the Nutrition Diagnosis Etiology Category Identification reference sheet on page 185 for more details on etiology categories. An additional useful resource to determine the etiology category is the Nutrition Diagnosis Matrix on page 528.

Signs/Symptoms (Defining Characteristics)

A typical cluster of subjective and objective signs and symptoms gathered during the nutrition assessment process that provide evidence that a problem exists; quantify the problem and describe its severity.

Nutrition Assessment Category	Potential Indicators of This Nutrition Diagnosis (one or more must be present)
Biochemical Data, Medical Tests and Procedures	Radiological findings, eg, swallow study consistent with dysphagia
Anthropometric Measurements	

Continued on next page

Swallowing Difficulty

Continued from previous page

Nutrition Assessment Category	Potential Indicators of This Nutrition Diagnosis (one or more must be present)
Physical Exam Findings	• Evidence of dehydration, eg, dry mucous membranes, poor skin turgor • Findings in cranial nerves (CN VII) and muscles of facial expression (nerve IX), gag reflex, swallow (nerve X) and tongue range of motions (nerve XII), and cough reflex, with evidence of, eg, drooling, facial weakness, and ability to perform, and wet and dry swallow • Coughing, choking, prolonged chewing, pouching of food, regurgitation, facial expression changes during eating, drooling, noisy wet upper airway sounds, feeling of "food getting stuck," pain while swallowing
Food/Nutrition-Related History	Reports or observations of: • Prolonged eating time • Decreased estimated food intake • Reluctance to consume specific foods • Mealtime/eating occasion resistance
Client History*	• Conditions associated with a diagnosis or treatment, eg, dysphagia, achalasia • Repeated upper respiratory infections and or pneumonia
Assessment, Monitoring, and Evaluation Tools	• International Dysphagia Diet Standardisation Initiative Framework drinks level • International Dysphagia Diet Standardisation Initiative Framework food level • International Dysphagia Diet Standardisation Initiative Functional Diet Scale score
Comparative Standards	

** Client History terms are used for Nutrition Assessment but not for Nutrition Monitoring and Evaluation.*

Progress Evaluation

Communicate the progress toward the resolution of a nutrition diagnosis by selecting the appropriate nutrition diagnosis status value from the Nutrition Assessment, Monitoring, and Evaluation terms.

NCP Term	ANDUID
New nutrition diagnosis	14586
Active nutrition diagnosis	14587
Resolved nutrition diagnosis	14588
Discontinued nutrition diagnosis	14589

For details on these terms, visit the Nutrition Diagnosis Status reference sheet on page 200.

Difficulty Chewing

Definition

Impaired ability chew food in preparation for swallowing.

Etiology (Cause/Contributing Risk Factors)

Factors gathered during the nutrition assessment process that contribute to the existence or the maintenance of pathophysiological, psychosocial, situational, developmental, cultural, and/or environmental problems:

- Craniofacial malformations
- Oral surgery
- Neuromuscular dysfunction
- Partial or complete edentulism
- Soft tissue disease (primary or oral manifestations of a systemic disease)
- Xerostomia

Etiology Category

Etiologies are grouped by the type of cause or contributing risk factor. Communicate the etiology category by selecting the appropriate Nutrition Assessment, Monitoring, and Evaluation term.

NCP Term	ANDUID
Beliefs attitudes etiology	14567
Cultural etiology	14568
Knowledge etiology	14569
Physical function etiology	14570
Physiologic metabolic etiology	14571
Psychological etiology	14572
Social personal etiology	14573
Treatment etiology	14574
Access etiology	14575
Behavior etiology	14576

Visit the Nutrition Diagnosis Etiology Category Identification reference sheet on page 185 for more details on etiology categories. An additional useful resource to determine the etiology category is the Nutrition Diagnosis Matrix on page 528.

Signs/Symptoms (Defining Characteristics)

A typical cluster of subjective and objective signs and symptoms gathered during the nutrition assessment process that provide evidence that a problem exists; quantify the problem and describe its severity.

Difficulty Chewing

Nutrition Assessment Category	Potential Indicators of This Nutrition Diagnosis (one or more must be present)
Biochemical Data, Medical Tests and Procedures	Results of modified barium swallow, barium swallow, videofluoroscopic swallowing study
Anthropometric Measurements	• Weight change, especially weight loss • Growth less than expected in children
Physical Exam Findings	• Partial or complete edentulism • Alterations in cranial nerve function (V, VII, IX, X, XII) • Dry mouth • Oral lesions interfering with eating ability • Impaired tongue movement • Ill-fitting dentures or broken dentures • Dysphagia
Food/Nutrition-Related History	Reports or observations of: • Decreased estimated food intake • Alterations in estimated food intake from usual • Decreased estimated intake or avoidance of food difficult to form into a bolus, eg, nuts, whole pieces of meat, poultry, fish, fibrous, fruits, and vegetables • Avoidance of foods of age-appropriate texture • Spitting food out or prolonged eating time • Preference for easy to chew food
Client History*	• Conditions associated with a diagnosis or treatment, eg, alcoholism; Alzheimer disease; head, neck, or pharyngeal cancer; cerebral palsy; cleft lip; cleft palate; oral soft tissue infections (eg, candidiasis, leukoplakia); limited developmental readiness; oral manifestations of systemic disease (eg, rheumatoid arthritis, lupus, Crohn's disease, pemphigus vulgaris, HIV, diabetes); Sjögren syndrome • Recent major oral surgery • Wired jaw • Chemotherapy with oral side effects • Radiation therapy to oral cavity
Assessment, Monitoring, and Evaluation Tools	• Subjective Global Assessment (SGA) rating • Subjective global assessment (SGA) score • Patient-Generated Subjective Global Assessment (PG-SGA) rating • Patient generated subjective global assessment (PG-SGA score • Mini Nutritional Assessment Long Form (MNA-LF) rating • Mini nutritional assessment long form (MNA-LF score • Subjective Global Nutritional Assessment (SGNA) for children rating • Subjective global nutritional assessment (SGNA for children score
Comparative Standards	

** Client History terms are used for Nutrition Assessment but not for Nutrition Monitoring and Evaluation.*

Difficulty Chewing

Progress Evaluation

Communicate the progress toward the resolution of a nutrition diagnosis by selecting the appropriate nutrition diagnosis status value from the Nutrition Assessment, Monitoring, and Evaluation terms.

NCP Term	ANDUID
New nutrition diagnosis	14586
Active nutrition diagnosis	14587
Resolved nutrition diagnosis	14588
Discontinued nutrition diagnosis	14589

For details on these terms, visit the Nutrition Diagnosis Status reference sheet on page 200.

Breastfeeding* Difficulty

Definition

Inability to sustain infant nutrition through breastfeeding.

Etiology (Cause/Contributing Risk Factors)

Factors gathered during the nutrition assessment process that contribute to the existence or the maintenance of pathophysiological, psychosocial, situational, developmental, cultural, and/or environmental problems:

Infant:

- Difficulty latching on
- Poor sucking ability
- Oral pain
- Malnutrition/malabsorption
- Lethargy, sleepiness
- Irritability
- Introduction of feeding via bottle or other route that may affect breastfeeding
- Swallowing difficulty

Mother†:

- Painful breast tissue with lactating capability, nipples
- Breast or nipple abnormality
- Mastitis
- Perception of or actual inadequate breastmilk‡ supply
- Limited social or environmental support
- Limited food and nutrition related skill
- Cultural practices that may affect the ability to breastfeed
- Introduction of feeding via bottle or other route that may affect breastfeeding

Etiology Category

Etiologies are grouped by the type of cause or contributing risk factor. Communicate the etiology category by selecting the appropriate Nutrition Assessment, Monitoring, and Evaluation term.

NCP Term	ANDUID
Beliefs attitudes etiology	14567
Cultural etiology	14568
Knowledge etiology	14569
Physical function etiology	14570
Physiologic metabolic etiology	14571
Psychological etiology	14572
Social personal etiology	14573
Treatment etiology	14574
Access etiology	14575
Behavior etiology	14576

Visit the Nutrition Diagnosis Etiology Category Identification reference sheet on page 185 for more details on etiology categories. An additional useful resource to determine the etiology category is the Nutrition Diagnosis Matrix on page 528.

* If a synonym for the term "breastfeeding" is helpful or needed, an approved alternate is "chestfeeding."

† If a synonym for the term "mother" is helpful or needed, an approved alternate is "lactating parent."

‡ If a synonym for the term "breastmilk" is helpful or needed, an approved alternate is "human milk."

Breastfeeding Difficulty

Signs/Symptoms (Defining Characteristics)

A typical cluster of subjective and objective signs and symptoms gathered during the nutrition assessment process that provide evidence that a problem exists; quantify the problem and describe its severity.

Nutrition Assessment Category	Potential Indicators of This Nutrition Diagnosis (one or more must be present)
Biochemical Data, Medical Tests and Procedures	• Laboratory evidence of dehydration (infant) • Fewer than reference standard, eg, six wet diapers in 24 hours (infant)
Anthropometric Measurements	Any weight loss or limited weight gain (infant)
Physical Exam Findings	• Frenulum abnormality (infant) • Vomiting or diarrhea (infant) • Hunger, limited satiety after feeding (infant)
Food/Nutrition-Related History	Reports or observations of (infant): • Coughing • Crying, latching on and off, pounding on breasts • Decreased feeding frequency/duration, early cessation of feeding, and/or feeding resistance • Lethargy Reports or observations of (mother): • Small amount of breastmilk when pumping • Limited confidence in ability to breastfeed • Doesn't hear infant swallowing • Limited support of mother's choice to breastfeed • Limited knowledge of breastfeeding • Limited knowledge of infant hunger/satiety signals • Limited support for engaging employer in discussions about breastfeeding facilities • Limited facilities or accommodations at place of employment or in community for breastfeeding • Feeding via bottle or other route
Client History*	• Conditions associated with a diagnosis or treatment (infant), eg, cleft lip/palate, thrush, premature birth, malabsorption, infection • Conditions associated with a diagnosis or treatment (mother), eg, mastitis, candidiasis, engorgement, history of breast surgery • Social or personal considerations of the mother
Assessment, Monitoring, and Evaluation Tools	
Comparative Standards	

** Client History terms are used for Nutrition Assessment but not for Nutrition Monitoring and Evaluation.*

Breastfeeding Difficulty

Progress Evaluation

Communicate the progress toward the resolution of a nutrition diagnosis by selecting the appropriate nutrition diagnosis status value from the Nutrition Assessment, Monitoring, and Evaluation terms.

NCP Term	ANDUID
New nutrition diagnosis	14586
Active nutrition diagnosis	14587
Resolved nutrition diagnosis	14588
Discontinued nutrition diagnosis	14589

For details on these terms, visit the Nutrition Diagnosis Status reference sheet on page 200.

Altered Gastrointestinal (GI) Function

Definition

Changes in digestion, absorption, or elimination.

Etiology (Cause/Contributing Risk Factors)

Factors gathered during the nutrition assessment process that contribute to the existence or the maintenance of pathophysiological, psychosocial, situational, developmental, cultural, and/or environmental problems:

- Alteration in GI tract structure and/or function
- Changes in the GI tract motility, eg, gastroparesis
- Compromised exocrine function of related GI organs, eg, pancreas, liver
- Decreased functional length of the GI tract, eg, short bowel syndrome

Etiology Category

Etiologies are grouped by the type of cause or contributing risk factor. Communicate the etiology category by selecting the appropriate Nutrition Assessment, Monitoring, and Evaluation term.

NCP Term	ANDUID
Beliefs attitudes etiology	14567
Cultural etiology	14568
Knowledge etiology	14569
Physical function etiology	14570
Physiologic metabolic etiology	14571
Psychological etiology	14572
Social personal etiology	14573
Treatment etiology	14574
Access etiology	14575
Behavior etiology	14576

Visit the Nutrition Diagnosis Etiology Category Identification reference sheet on page 185 for more details on etiology categories. An additional useful resource to determine the etiology category is the Nutrition Diagnosis Matrix on page 528.

Signs/Symptoms (Defining Characteristics)

A typical cluster of subjective and objective signs and symptoms gathered during the nutrition assessment process that provide evidence that a problem exists; quantify the problem and describe its severity.

Nutrition Assessment Category	Potential Indicators of This Nutrition Diagnosis (one or more must be present)
Biochemical Data, Medical Tests and Procedures	• Abnormal digestive enzyme and fecal studies • Abnormal hydrogen breath test, d-xylose test, stool culture, and gastric emptying and/or bowel transit time • Endoscopic or colonoscopy examination, abdominal scan, biopsy results • Abnormal pH, sphincter, motility, morphology or reflux studies

Continued on next page

Altered Gastrointestinal (GI) Function

Continued from previous page

Nutrition Assessment Category	Potential Indicators of This Nutrition Diagnosis (one or more must be present)
Biochemical Data, Medical Tests and Procedures (continued)	• Abnormal anemia profile • Abnormal vitamin, mineral, fatty acid, trace element, and PTH results • Abnormal tissue transglutaminase antibodies (IgA/IgG)
Anthropometric Measurements	• Weight loss of ≥ 5% in 1 month, ≥ 10% in 6 months • Growth stunting or failure in children • Abnormal bone mineral density tests
Physical Exam Findings	• Abdominal distension • Increased (or sometimes decreased) bowel sounds • Wasting due to malnutrition in severe cases • Anorexia, nausea, vomiting, diarrhea, steatorrhea, constipation, abdominal pain, reflux, gas, belching, flatus, bloating, fecal incontinence • Evidence of vitamin and/or mineral deficiency, eg, glossitis, cheilosis, mouth lesions, skin rashes, hair loss
Food/Nutrition-Related History	Reports or observations of avoidance or limitation of estimated total intake or intake of specific foods/food groups due to GI symptoms, eg, bloating, cramping, pain, diarrhea, steatorrhea (greasy, floating, foul-smelling stools) especially following ingestion of food
Client History*	• Conditions associated with a diagnosis or treatment, eg, malabsorption, maldigestion, steatorrhea, obstruction, constipation, diverticulitis, Crohn's disease, inflammatory bowel disease, cystic fibrosis, celiac disease, cancers, irritable bowel syndrome, infection, dumping syndrome • Surgical procedures, eg, esophagectomy, dilatation, fundoplication, gastrectomy, vagotomy, gastric bypass, bowel resections
Assessment, Monitoring, and Evaluation Tools	
Comparative Standards	

** Client History terms are used for Nutrition Assessment but not for Nutrition Monitoring and Evaluation.*

Progress Evaluation

Communicate the progress toward the resolution of a nutrition diagnosis by selecting the appropriate nutrition diagnosis status value from the Nutrition Assessment, Monitoring, and Evaluation terms.

NCP Term	ANDUID
New nutrition diagnosis	14586
Active nutrition diagnosis	14587
Resolved nutrition diagnosis	14588
Discontinued nutrition diagnosis	14589

For details on these terms, visit the Nutrition Diagnosis Status reference sheet on page 200.

Predicted Breastfeeding* Difficulty

Definition

Future hindrance to breastfeeding, or lactation, is anticipated, based on observation, experience, or scientific reason.

Etiology (Cause/Contributing Risk Factors)

Factors gathered during the nutrition assessment process that contribute to the existence or the maintenance of pathophysiological, psychosocial, situational, developmental, cultural, and/or environmental problems:

- Scheduled or planned procedure, therapy, or medication (mother[s]† or infant[s])
- Condition (mother[s] or infant[s]) that may hinder breastfeeding
- Cultural or religious norms or practices that may hinder breastfeeding
- Presence or absence of organizational, community, and/or societal procedure or policy that may hinder breastfeeding
- Anticipated increased psychological/life stress
- Food and nutrition knowledge deficit
- Belief finding that hinders food and/or nutrition behavior change
- Attitude finding that hinders food and/or nutrition behavior change
- Lack of social support for breastfeeding
- Limited food and nutrition related skill

Etiology Category

Etiologies are grouped by the type of cause or contributing risk factor. Communicate the etiology category by selecting the appropriate Nutrition Assessment, Monitoring, and Evaluation term.

NCP Term	ANDUID
Beliefs attitudes etiology	14567
Cultural etiology	14568
Knowledge etiology	14569
Physical function etiology	14570
Physiologic metabolic etiology	14571
Psychological etiology	14572
Social personal etiology	14573
Treatment etiology	14574
Access etiology	14575
Behavior etiology	14576

Visit the Nutrition Diagnosis Etiology Category Identification reference sheet on page 185 for more details on etiology categories. An additional useful resource to determine the etiology category is the Nutrition Diagnosis Matrix on page 528.

* If a synonym for the term "breastfeeding" is helpful or needed, an approved alternate is "chestfeeding."

† If a synonym for the term "mother" is helpful or needed, an approved alternate is "lactating parent."

Predicted Breastfeeding Difficulty

Signs/Symptoms (Defining Characteristics)

A typical cluster of subjective and objective signs and symptoms gathered during the nutrition assessment process that provide evidence that a problem exists; quantify the problem and describe its severity.

Nutrition Assessment Category	Potential Indicators of This Nutrition Diagnosis (one or more must be present)
Biochemical Data, Medical Tests and Procedures	Population-based biochemical data that may hinder breastfeeding
Anthropometric Measurements	Population-based anthropometric data that may hinder breastfeeding
Physical Exam Findings	Population-based data anticipated physical exam finding that may hinder breastfeeding
Food/Nutrition-Related History	Reports or observations of: • History of impediment to breastfeeding or breastfeeding difficulty • Medications that may hinder breastfeeding • Inaccurate or incomplete food and nutrition knowledge • Unsupported food and nutrition beliefs and attitudes • Limited numeracy skill
Client History*	• Anticipated procedure or therapy for which research shows a hindrance to breastfeeding • History or presence of a condition for which research shows a hindrance to breastfeeding • Presence or absence of a policy that may hinder breastfeeding • Cultural or religious norms or practices • Absent or limited family and/or social breastfeeding support • Anticipated life stress or change • Social or personal considerations of the mother
Assessment, Monitoring, and Evaluation Tools	
Comparative Standards	

** Client History terms are used for Nutrition Assessment but not for Nutrition Monitoring and Evaluation.*

Progress Evaluation

Communicate the progress toward the resolution of a nutrition diagnosis by selecting the appropriate nutrition diagnosis status value from the Nutrition Assessment, Monitoring, and Evaluation terms.

NCP Term	ANDUID
New nutrition diagnosis	14586
Active nutrition diagnosis	14587
Resolved nutrition diagnosis	14588
Discontinued nutrition diagnosis	14589

For details on these terms, visit the Nutrition Diagnosis Status reference sheet on page 200.

Sarcopenia

Definition

A syndrome characterized by low muscle strength, low muscle mass and low physical performance, which is linked to negative clinical outcomes. Sarcopenia could be primary (ie, related to ageing) or secondary (ie, related to disease, low physical activity, and/or poor nutrition).

Etiology (Cause/Contributing Risk Factors)

Factors gathered during the nutrition assessment process that contribute to the existence or the maintenance of pathophysiological, psychosocial, situational, developmental, cultural, and/or environmental problems:

- Physiological causes increasing nutrient needs due to illness and/or condition
- Physiological causes increasing nutrient needs due to treatment(s)
- Physiological causes resulting in reduced ability to ingest sufficient protein
- Physiological causes resulting in reduced ability to ingest sufficient energy
- Alteration in gastrointestinal tract structure and/or function
- Physiological causes related to a loss of muscle mass, decreased strength, and/or decreased physical performance related to aging, hormonal balance, and/or inflammation
- Limited physical activity resulting in low muscle mass, strength, and/or function
- Psychological factors leading to inadequate intake and/or limited physical activity
- Inadequate knowledge of nutritional and/or physical activity recommendations
- Beliefs and/or attitudes leading to inadequate intake and/or limited physical activity
- Social–personal factors leading to inadequate intake and/or limited physical activity
- Food insecurity leading to inadequate intake and/or limited physical activity
- Physical function factors leading to inadequate intake and/or limited physical activity
- Treatment for health and medical conditions leading to inadequate intake and/or limited physical activity

Etiology Category

Etiologies are grouped by the type of cause or contributing risk factor. Communicate the etiology category by selecting the appropriate Nutrition Assessment, Monitoring, and Evaluation term.

NCP Term	ANDUID
Beliefs attitudes etiology	14567
Cultural etiology	14568
Knowledge etiology	14569
Physical function etiology	14570
Physiologic metabolic etiology	14571
Psychological etiology	14572
Social personal etiology	14573
Treatment etiology	14574
Access etiology	14575
Behavior etiology	14576

Visit the Nutrition Diagnosis Etiology Category Identification reference sheet on page 185 for more details on etiology categories. An additional useful resource to determine the etiology category is the Nutrition Diagnosis Matrix on page 528.

Sarcopenia

Signs/Symptoms (Defining Characteristics)

A typical cluster of subjective and objective signs and symptoms gathered during the nutrition assessment process that provide evidence that a problem exists; quantify the problem and describe its severity.

Nutrition Assessment Category	Potential Indicators of This Nutrition Diagnosis (one or more must be present)
Biochemical Data, Medical Tests and Procedures	
Anthropometric Measurements	• Mid upper arm muscle circumference • Left calf circumference • Right calf circumference • Thigh circumference • Appendicular skeletal muscle mass (ASM or ASMM) • Appendicular muscle mass index (ASMI) • Skeletal muscle mass • Skeletal muscle mass index (SMI) • Lean soft tissue mass • Fat free mass • Fat free mass index • Lumbar muscle cross section area • Muscle thickness • Method for assessing muscle mass (eg, bioelectrical impedance analysis [BIA], dual-energy x-ray absorptiometry [DXA], computed tomography [CT]) (necessary for interpretation of the measures)
Physical Exam Findings	• Abnormal muscle function • Asthenia (also called abnormal physical weakness) • Decreased functional residual capacity • Diaphragmatic weakness (also called diaphragmatic muscle weakness; diaphragmatic paresis) • Lethargy • Loss of muscle function • Loss of physical performance • Low muscle function • Muscle weakness (also called decreased muscle strength) • Obesity (also called adiposity) • Skeletal muscle problem • Skeletal muscle power problem • Muscle atrophy (eg, quadriceps muscle atrophy, gastrocnemius muscle atrophy)

Continued on next page

Sarcopenia

Continued from previous page

Nutrition Assessment Category	Potential Indicators of This Nutrition Diagnosis (one or more must be present)
Food/Nutrition-Related History	Reports or observations of: • Food intake less than needs • Energy intake less than energy needs • Protein intake less than protein needs • Limited ability to perform shopping activities • Limited ability to prepare food • Limited ability to self-feed • Limited ability to self-administer enteral nutrition • Limited ability to self-administer parenteral nutrition • Limited availability of shopping facilities • Limited ability to procure safe food • Individual food security, marginal, low, or very low • Household food security, marginal, low, or very low • Presence of situational food insecurity • Presence of chronic food insecurity • Limited participation in physical activity • Reduced handgrip strength (kg of force)* • Prolonged time for chair stand test (seconds for five rises) (also called chair rise test)* • Reduced gait speed test (meters per second)* • Low Short Physical Performance Battery (SPPB) score (score)* • Prolonged time for Timed Up and Go test (TUG) (seconds)* • Prolonged time for 400-meter walk test (minutes)*
Client History†	• Age • Sex • Gender • Ethnicity • Physical disability • Mobility • Literacy factors • Education • Any coexisting health condition that might contribute to activity-related, disease-related, or nutrition-related sarcopenia • Medical treatment/therapy • Surgical treatment • Palliative/end of life care • Occupation • Socioeconomic factors

Continued on next page

Sarcopenia

Continued from previous page

Nutrition Assessment Category	Potential Indicators of This Nutrition Diagnosis (one or more must be present)
Assessment, Monitoring, and Evaluation Tools	
Comparative Standards	• Total energy estimated needs in 24 hours • Total protein estimated needs in 24 hours

** Refer to local practice standard and/or organization guideline for cutoff point.*
† Client History terms are used for Nutrition Assessment but not for Nutrition Monitoring and Evaluation.

Progress Evaluation

Communicate the progress toward the resolution of a nutrition diagnosis by selecting the appropriate nutrition diagnosis status value from the Nutrition Assessment, Monitoring, and Evaluation terms.

NCP Term	ANDUID
New nutrition diagnosis	14586
Active nutrition diagnosis	14587
Resolved nutrition diagnosis	14588
Discontinued nutrition diagnosis	14589

For details on these terms, visit the Nutrition Diagnosis Status reference sheet on page 200.

Impaired Nutrient Utilization

Definition

Changes in ability to metabolize nutrients and bioactive substances.

Etiology (Cause/Contributing Risk Factors)

Factors gathered during the nutrition assessment process that contribute to the existence or the maintenance of pathophysiological, psychosocial, situational, developmental, cultural, and/or environmental problems:

- Compromised endocrine function of related gastrointestinal organs, eg, pancreas, liver, pituitary, parathyroid
- Metabolic disorders, including inborn errors of metabolism
- Medications that affect nutrient metabolism
- Alcohol or drug addiction

Etiology Category

Etiologies are grouped by the type of cause or contributing risk factor. Communicate the etiology category by selecting the appropriate Nutrition Assessment, Monitoring, and Evaluation term.

NCP Term	ANDUID
Beliefs attitudes etiology	14567
Cultural etiology	14568
Knowledge etiology	14569
Physical function etiology	14570
Physiologic metabolic etiology	14571
Psychological etiology	14572
Social personal etiology	14573
Treatment etiology	14574
Access etiology	14575
Behavior etiology	14576

Visit the Nutrition Diagnosis Etiology Category Identification reference sheet on page 185 for more details on etiology categories. An additional useful resource to determine the etiology category is the Nutrition Diagnosis Matrix on page 528.

Signs/Symptoms (Defining Characteristics)

A typical cluster of subjective and objective signs and symptoms gathered during the nutrition assessment process that provide evidence that a problem exists; quantify the problem and describe its severity.

Impaired Nutrient Utilization

Nutrition Assessment Category	Potential Indicators of This Nutrition Diagnosis (one or more must be present)
Biochemical Data, Medical Tests and Procedures	• Abnormal protein, fatty acid, or carbohydrate metabolism profile tests • Abnormal LFTs • Abnormal anemia profile • Abnormal pituitary hormones (growth hormone [GH], adrenocorticotropic hormone [ACTH], luteinizing hormone [LH] and follicle stimulating hormone [FSH]) • Vitamin and/or mineral deficiency • Hypoglycemia, hyperglycemia • Abnormal parathyroid hormone (PTH) • Positive result for urine porphyrins
Anthropometric Measurements	• Weight loss of ≥ 5% in 1 month, ≥ 10% in 6 months • Growth stunting or failure in children • Abnormal bone mineral density tests
Physical Exam Findings	• Evidence of vitamin and/or mineral deficiency, eg, glossitis, cheilosis, mouth lesions • Thin, wasted appearance
Food/Nutrition-Related History	Reports or observations of: • Avoidance or limitation of intake of specific foods/food groups due to physical symptoms • Alcohol or drug use
Client History*	Conditions associated with a diagnosis or treatment, eg, cystic fibrosis, celiac disease, Crohn's disease, infection, radiation therapy, inborn errors of metabolism, endocrine disorders, pituitary disorders, renal failure, liver failure, acute or inherited porphyria, short bowel syndrome
Assessment, Monitoring, and Evaluation Tools	
Comparative Standards	

** Client History terms are used for Nutrition Assessment but not for Nutrition Monitoring and Evaluation.*

Progress Evaluation

Communicate the progress toward the resolution of a nutrition diagnosis by selecting the appropriate nutrition diagnosis status value from the Nutrition Assessment, Monitoring, and Evaluation terms.

NCP Term	ANDUID
New nutrition diagnosis	14586
Active nutrition diagnosis	14587
Resolved nutrition diagnosis	14588
Discontinued nutrition diagnosis	14589

For details on these terms, visit the Nutrition Diagnosis Status reference sheet on page 200.

Altered Nutrition Related Laboratory Values

Definition

Changes in lab values due to body composition, medications, body system changes or genetics, or changes in ability to eliminate byproducts of digestive and metabolic processes.

Etiology (Cause/Contributing Risk Factors)

Factors gathered during the nutrition assessment process that contribute to the existence or the maintenance of pathophysiological, psychosocial, situational, developmental, cultural, and/or environmental problems:

- Kidney, liver, cardiac, endocrine, neurologic, and/or pulmonary dysfunction
- Prematurity
- Other organ dysfunction that leads to biochemical changes
- Metabolic disorders, including inborn errors of metabolism

Etiology Category

Etiologies are grouped by the type of cause or contributing risk factor. Communicate the etiology category by selecting the appropriate Nutrition Assessment, Monitoring, and Evaluation term.

NCP Term	ANDUID
Beliefs attitudes etiology	14567
Cultural etiology	14568
Knowledge etiology	14569
Physical function etiology	14570
Physiologic metabolic etiology	14571
Psychological etiology	14572
Social personal etiology	14573
Treatment etiology	14574
Access etiology	14575
Behavior etiology	14576

Visit the Nutrition Diagnosis Etiology Category Identification reference sheet on page 185 for more details on etiology categories. An additional useful resource to determine the etiology category is the Nutrition Diagnosis Matrix on page 528.

Signs/Symptoms (Defining Characteristics)

A typical cluster of subjective and objective signs and symptoms gathered during the nutrition assessment process that provide evidence that a problem exists; quantify the problem and describe its severity.

Nutrition Assessment Category	Potential Indicators of This Nutrition Diagnosis (one or more must be present)
Biochemical Data, Medical Tests and Procedures	• ↑ AST, ALT, total bilirubin, serum ammonia (liver disorders) • ↑ BUN, ↑ Cr, ↑ K, ↑ phosphorus, ↓ GFR (kidney disorders) • Altered pO_2 and pCO_2 (pulmonary disorders)

Continued on next page

Altered Nutrition Related Laboratory Values

Continued from previous page

Nutrition Assessment Category	Potential Indicators of This Nutrition Diagnosis (one or more must be present)
Biochemical Data, Medical Tests and Procedures (continued)	• ↑ Serum lipids • ↑ Plasma glucose and/or HbA1c levels • Inadequate blood glucose control • ↑ Urine microalbumin • Abnormal protein, fatty acid, or carbohydrate metabolism profile • Other findings of acute or chronic disorders that are abnormal and of nutritional origin or consequence
Anthropometric Measurements	• Rapid weight changes • Other anthropometric measures that are altered
Physical Exam Findings	• Jaundice, edema, ascites, pruritus (liver disorders) • Edema, shortness of breath (cardiac disorders) • Blue nail beds, clubbing (pulmonary disorders) • Anorexia, nausea, vomiting
Food/Nutrition-Related History	Reports or observations of: • Estimated intake of foods high in or overall excess intake of protein, potassium, phosphorus, sodium, fluid • Estimated intake of micronutrients less than recommendations • Food- and nutrition-related knowledge deficit, eg, lack of information, incorrect information • Limited adherence to modified diet
Client History*	Conditions associated with a diagnosis or treatment, eg, renal or liver disease, alcoholism, cardiopulmonary disorders, diabetes, inborn errors of metabolism
Assessment, Monitoring, and Evaluation Tools	
Comparative Standards	

Arrows used with laboratory values: ↑ represents above reference standard and ↓ represents below reference standard.
** Client History terms are used for Nutrition Assessment but not for Nutrition Monitoring and Evaluation.*

Progress Evaluation

Communicate the progress toward the resolution of a nutrition diagnosis by selecting the appropriate nutrition diagnosis status value from the Nutrition Assessment, Monitoring, and Evaluation terms.

NCP Term	ANDUID
New nutrition diagnosis	14586
Active nutrition diagnosis	14587
Resolved nutrition diagnosis	14588
Discontinued nutrition diagnosis	14589

For details on these terms, visit the Nutrition Diagnosis Status reference sheet on page 200.

Food Medication Interaction

Definition

Undesirable/harmful interaction(s) between food and over the counter (OTC) medications, prescribed medications, herbals, botanicals, and/or dietary supplements that diminishes, enhances, or alters the effect of nutrients and/or medications.

Etiology (Cause/Contributing Risk Factors)

Factors gathered during the nutrition assessment process that contribute to the existence or the maintenance of pathophysiological, psychosocial, situational, developmental, cultural, and/or environmental problems:

- Combined ingestion or administration of medication and food that results in undesirable/harmful interaction

Etiology Category

Etiologies are grouped by the type of cause or contributing risk factor. Communicate the etiology category by selecting the appropriate Nutrition Assessment, Monitoring, and Evaluation term.

NCP Term	ANDUID
Beliefs attitudes etiology	14567
Cultural etiology	14568
Knowledge etiology	14569
Physical function etiology	14570
Physiologic metabolic etiology	14571
Psychological etiology	14572
Social personal etiology	14573
Treatment etiology	14574
Access etiology	14575
Behavior etiology	14576

Visit the Nutrition Diagnosis Etiology Category Identification reference sheet on page 185 for more details on etiology categories. An additional useful resource to determine the etiology category is the Nutrition Diagnosis Matrix on page 528.

Signs/Symptoms (Defining Characteristics)

A typical cluster of subjective and objective signs and symptoms gathered during the nutrition assessment process that provide evidence that a problem exists; quantify the problem and describe its severity.

Food Medication Interaction

Nutrition Assessment Category	Potential Indicators of This Nutrition Diagnosis (one or more must be present)
Biochemical Data, Medical Tests and Procedures	Alterations of biochemical tests based on medication affect and client condition
Anthropometric Measurements	Alterations of anthropometric measurements based on medication effect and client conditions, eg, weight gain and corticosteroids
Physical Exam Findings	Changes in appetite or taste
Food/Nutrition-Related History	Reports or observations of: • Intake that is problematic or inconsistent with OTC, prescribed drugs, herbals, botanicals, or dietary supplements, such as: ○ fish oils and prolonged bleeding ○ coumadin and vitamin K–rich foods ○ high-fat diet while on cholesterol-lowering medications ○ iron supplements, constipation, and low-fiber diet • Intake that does not support replacement or mitigation of OTC, prescribed drugs, herbals, botanicals, and dietary supplements effects • Multiple drugs (OTC, prescribed drugs, herbals, botanicals, or dietary supplements) that are known to have food–medication interactions • Medications that require nutrient supplementation that cannot be accomplished via food intake, eg, isoniazid and vitamin B6
Client History*	
Assessment, Monitoring, and Evaluation Tools	
Comparative Standards	

** Client History terms are used for Nutrition Assessment but not for Nutrition Monitoring and Evaluation.*

Progress Evaluation

Communicate the progress toward the resolution of a nutrition diagnosis by selecting the appropriate nutrition diagnosis status value from the Nutrition Assessment, Monitoring, and Evaluation terms.

NCP Term	ANDUID
New nutrition diagnosis	14586
Active nutrition diagnosis	14587
Resolved nutrition diagnosis	14588
Discontinued nutrition diagnosis	14589

For details on these terms, visit the Nutrition Diagnosis Status reference sheet on page 200.

Predicted Food Medication Interaction

Definition

Potential undesirable/harmful interaction(s) between food and over the counter (OTC) medications, prescribed medications, herbals, botanicals, and/or dietary supplements that diminishes, enhances, or alters the effect of nutrients and/or medications.

Note: Appropriate nutrition diagnosis when food–medication interaction is predicted but has not yet occurred. This nutrition diagnosis is used when the practitioner wants to prevent a nutrient–medication interaction. Observed food–medication interactions should be documented using the Food Medication Interaction reference sheet on page 332.

Etiology (Cause/Contributing Risk Factors)

Factors gathered during the nutrition assessment process that contribute to the existence or the maintenance of pathophysiological, psychosocial, situational, developmental, cultural, and/or environmental problems:

- Combined ingestion or administration of medication and food that results in undesirable/harmful interaction.

Etiology Category

Etiologies are grouped by the type of cause or contributing risk factor. Communicate the etiology category by selecting the appropriate Nutrition Assessment, Monitoring, and Evaluation term.

NCP Term	ANDUID
Beliefs attitudes etiology	14567
Cultural etiology	14568
Knowledge etiology	14569
Physical function etiology	14570
Physiologic metabolic etiology	14571
Psychological etiology	14572
Social personal etiology	14573
Treatment etiology	14574
Access etiology	14575
Behavior etiology	14576

Visit the Nutrition Diagnosis Etiology Category Identification reference sheet on page 185 for more details on etiology categories. An additional useful resource to determine the etiology category is the Nutrition Diagnosis Matrix on page 528.

Signs/Symptoms (Defining Characteristics)

A typical cluster of subjective and objective signs and symptoms gathered during the nutrition assessment process that provide evidence that a problem exists; quantify the problem and describe its severity.

Predicted Food Medication Interaction

Nutrition Assessment Category	Potential Indicators of This Nutrition Diagnosis (one or more must be present)
Biochemical Data, Medical Tests and Procedures	
Anthropometric Measurements	
Physical Exam Findings	
Food/Nutrition-Related History	Reports or observations of: • Intake that is expected to be problematic or inconsistent with OTC medication, prescribed drugs, herbals, botanicals, or dietary supplements, such as: ○ fish oils and prolonged bleeding ○ coumadin and vitamin K–rich foods ○ high-fat diet while on cholesterol-lowering medications ○ iron supplements, constipation, and low-fiber diet • Intake that may not support replacement or mitigation of OTC medication, prescribed drugs, herbals, botanicals, and dietary supplements effects • Multiple drugs (OTC medication, prescribed drugs, herbals, botanicals, or dietary supplements) that are known to have food–medication interactions • Medications that require nutrient supplementation that cannot be accomplished via food intake, eg, isoniazid and vitamin B6
Client History*	
Assessment, Monitoring, and Evaluation Tools	
Comparative Standards	

** Client History terms are used for Nutrition Assessment but not for Nutrition Monitoring and Evaluation.*

Progress Evaluation

Communicate the progress toward the resolution of a nutrition diagnosis by selecting the appropriate nutrition diagnosis status value from the Nutrition Assessment, Monitoring, and Evaluation terms.

NCP Term	ANDUID
New nutrition diagnosis	14586
Active nutrition diagnosis	14587
Resolved nutrition diagnosis	14588
Discontinued nutrition diagnosis	14589

For details on these terms, visit the Nutrition Diagnosis Status reference sheet on page 200.

Underweight

Definition

Low body weight compared to established reference standards or recommendations.

Etiology (Cause/Contributing Risk Factors)

Factors gathered during the nutrition assessment process that contribute to the existence or the maintenance of pathophysiological, psychosocial, situational, developmental, cultural, and/or environmental problems:

- Disordered eating pattern
- Excessive physical activity
- Belief finding that hinders food and/or nutrition behavior change
- Attitude finding that hinders food and/or nutrition behavior change
- Inadequate energy intake
- Increased energy needs
- Food insecurity
- Small for gestational age, intrauterine growth retardation/restriction, and/or lack of progress/appropriate weight gain per day

Etiology Category

Etiologies are grouped by the type of cause or contributing risk factor. Communicate the etiology category by selecting the appropriate Nutrition Assessment, Monitoring, and Evaluation term.

NCP Term	ANDUID
Beliefs attitudes etiology	14567
Cultural etiology	14568
Knowledge etiology	14569
Physical function etiology	14570
Physiologic metabolic etiology	14571
Psychological etiology	14572
Social personal etiology	14573
Treatment etiology	14574
Access etiology	14575
Behavior etiology	14576

Visit the Nutrition Diagnosis Etiology Category Identification reference sheet on page 185 for more details on etiology categories. An additional useful resource to determine the etiology category is the Nutrition Diagnosis Matrix on page 528.

Signs/Symptoms (Defining Characteristics)

A typical cluster of subjective and objective signs and symptoms gathered during the nutrition assessment process that provide evidence that a problem exists; quantify the problem and describe its severity.

Underweight

Nutrition Assessment Category	Potential Indicators of This Nutrition Diagnosis (one or more must be present)
Biochemical Data, Medical Tests and Procedures	↑ Measured RMR higher than expected and/or estimated
Anthropometric Measurements	• Decreased skinfold thickness and mid-arm muscle circumference • BMI < 18.5 (adults) • BMI for older adults (older than 65 years) < 23 • Birth to 2 years ○ Weight for age < 5th percentile ○ Weight for length < 5th percentile • Ages 2 to 20 years ○ Weight for stature < 5th percentile ○ BMI < 5th percentile (for children 2 to 20) ○ Weight for age < 5th percentile
Physical Exam Findings	• Decreased muscle mass, muscle wasting (gluteal and temporal) • Hunger
Food/Nutrition-Related History	Reports or observations of: • Estimated intake of food less than estimated or measured needs • Limited supply of food in home • Dieting, food faddism • Refusal to eat • Physical activity more than recommended amount • Medications that affect appetite, eg, stimulants for ADHD
Client History*	• Malnutrition • Illness or physical disability • Mental illness, dementia, confusion • Athlete, dancer, gymnast • Vitamin/mineral deficiency
Assessment, Monitoring, and Evaluation Tools	
Comparative Standards	• Ideal/reference body weight (IBW) • Recommended body mass index (BMI) • Goal body weight • Goal body weight for length *z* score • Goal body mass index (BMI) for age *z* score

Arrows used with laboratory values: ↑ represents above reference standard and ↓ represents below reference standard.
** Client History terms are used for Nutrition Assessment but not for Nutrition Monitoring and Evaluation.*

Underweight

Progress Evaluation

Communicate the progress toward the resolution of a nutrition diagnosis by selecting the appropriate nutrition diagnosis status value from the Nutrition Assessment, Monitoring, and Evaluation terms.

NCP Term	ANDUID
New nutrition diagnosis	14586
Active nutrition diagnosis	14587
Resolved nutrition diagnosis	14588
Discontinued nutrition diagnosis	14589

For details on these terms, visit the Nutrition Diagnosis Status reference sheet on page 200.

Unintended* Weight Loss

Definition

Decrease in body weight that is not planned or desired.

Note: May not be an appropriate nutrition diagnosis when changes in body weight are due to fluid.

Etiology (Cause/Contributing Risk Factors)

Factors gathered during the nutrition assessment process that contribute to the existence or the maintenance of pathophysiological, psychosocial, situational, developmental, cultural, and/or environmental problems:

- Physiological causes increasing nutrient needs, eg, due to prolonged catabolic illness, trauma, malabsorption
- Decreased ability to consume sufficient energy
- Food insecurity
- Cultural practices that affect ability to access food
- Prolonged hospitalization
- Psychological causes such as depression and disordered eating
- Lack of self-feeding ability

Etiology Category

Etiologies are grouped by the type of cause or contributing risk factor. Communicate the etiology category by selecting the appropriate Nutrition Assessment, Monitoring, and Evaluation term.

NCP Term	ANDUID
Beliefs attitudes etiology	14567
Cultural etiology	14568
Knowledge etiology	14569
Physical function etiology	14570
Physiologic metabolic etiology	14571
Psychological etiology	14572
Social personal etiology	14573
Treatment etiology	14574
Access etiology	14575
Behavior etiology	14576

Visit the Nutrition Diagnosis Etiology Category Identification reference sheet on page 185 for more details on etiology categories. An additional useful resource to determine the etiology category is the Nutrition Diagnosis Matrix on page 528.

* If a *synonym*, or alternate word with the same meaning, for the term "unintended" is helpful or needed, an approved alternate is the word "involuntary."

Unintended Weight Loss

Signs/Symptoms (Defining Characteristics)

A typical cluster of subjective and objective signs and symptoms gathered during the nutrition assessment process that provide evidence that a problem exists; quantify the problem and describe its severity.

Nutrition Assessment Category	Potential Indicators of This Nutrition Diagnosis (one or more must be present)
Biochemical Data, Medical Tests and Procedures	
Anthropometric Measurements	• Adults: weight loss of ≥ 5% within 30 days, ≥ 7.5% in 90 days, or ≥ 10% in 180 days) • Pediatrics: not gaining weight as expected; 5% weight loss in 6 months and/or a shift downward in growth percentiles, crossing two or more percentile channels on reference growth standard charts
Physical Exam Findings	• Fever • Decreased senses, ie, smell, taste, vision • Increased heart rate • Increased respiratory rate • Loss of subcutaneous fat and muscle stores • Change in way clothes fit • Changes in mental status or function (eg, depression)
Food/Nutrition-Related History	Reports or observations of: • Normal or usual estimated intake in face of illness • Poor intake, change in eating habits, early satiety, skipped meals • Medications associated with weight loss, such as certain antidepressants
Client History*	• Conditions associated with a diagnosis or treatment, eg, AIDS/HIV, burns, chronic obstructive pulmonary disease, dysphagia, hip/long bone fracture, infection, surgery, trauma, hyperthyroidism (pre- or untreated), some types of cancer or metastatic disease, substance abuse • Cancer chemotherapy
Assessment, Monitoring, and Evaluation Tools	
Comparative Standards	• Ideal/reference body weight (IBW) • Recommended body mass index (BMI) • Goal body weight • Goal body weight for length *z* score • Goal body mass index (BMI) for age *z* score

** Client History terms are used for Nutrition Assessment but not for Nutrition Monitoring and Evaluation.*

Unintended Weight Loss

Progress Evaluation

Communicate the progress toward the resolution of a nutrition diagnosis by selecting the appropriate nutrition diagnosis status value from the Nutrition Assessment, Monitoring, and Evaluation terms.

NCP Term	ANDUID
New nutrition diagnosis	14586
Active nutrition diagnosis	14587
Resolved nutrition diagnosis	14588
Discontinued nutrition diagnosis	14589

For details on these terms, visit the Nutrition Diagnosis Status reference sheet on page 200.

Overweight/Obesity

Note: Specific nutrition diagnoses that are applicable: Overweight, adult or pediatric; Obesity, adult or pediatric; Obesity, pediatric; Obesity Class I; Obesity Class II; Obesity Class III.

Definition

Increased adiposity compared to established reference standards or recommendations, ranging from overweight to morbid obesity.

Etiology (Cause/Contributing Risk Factors)

Factors gathered during the nutrition assessment process that contribute to the existence or the maintenance of pathophysiological, psychosocial, situational, developmental, cultural, and/or environmental problems:

- Decreased energy needs
- Disordered eating pattern
- Excessive energy intake
- Food- and nutrition-related knowledge deficit
- Not ready for nutrition related behavior change
- Limited physical activity
- Increased psychological/life stress
- Limited food and nutrition related skill
- Food insecurity

Etiology Category

Etiologies are grouped by the type of cause or contributing risk factor. Communicate the etiology category by selecting the appropriate Nutrition Assessment, Monitoring, and Evaluation term.

NCP Term	ANDUID
Beliefs attitudes etiology	14567
Cultural etiology	14568
Knowledge etiology	14569
Physical function etiology	14570
Physiologic metabolic etiology	14571
Psychological etiology	14572
Social personal etiology	14573
Treatment etiology	14574
Access etiology	14575
Behavior etiology	14576

Visit the Nutrition Diagnosis Etiology Category Identification reference sheet on page 185 for more details on etiology categories. An additional useful resource to determine the etiology category is the Nutrition Diagnosis Matrix on page 528.

Overweight/Obesity

Signs/Symptoms (Defining Characteristics)

A typical cluster of subjective and objective signs and symptoms gathered during the nutrition assessment process that provide evidence that a problem exists; quantify the problem and describe its severity.

Nutrition Assessment Category	Potential Indicators of This Nutrition Diagnosis (one or more must be present)
Biochemical Data, Medical Tests and Procedures	↓ Measured RMR less than expected and/or estimated
Anthropometric Measurements	• BMI more than normative standard for age and sex: ○ Overweight: 25 to 29.9 (adults), 85th to 95th percentiles (pediatrics) ○ Obesity class I: 30 to 34.9 (adults) ○ Obesity class II: 35 to 39.9 (adults) ○ Obesity class III: 40+* (adults) ○ Obesity > 95th percentile (pediatrics) • Waist circumference more than normative standard for age and sex • Increased skinfold thickness • Body fat percentage > 25% for men and > 32% for women • Weight for height more than normative standard for age and sex
Physical Exam Findings	• Excess subcutaneous fat • Central adiposity • Acanthosis nigricans • Joint arthralgia
Food/Nutrition-Related History	Reports or observations of: • Consumption of energy-dense, nutrient-poor food or beverage • Limited intake of low-energy, high-nutrient foods • Large portions of food • Estimated excessive energy intake • Infrequent, low-duration and/or low-intensity physical activity, factors affecting physical activity access • Large amounts of sedentary activities, eg, TV watching, reading, computer use in both leisure and work/school • Uncertainty regarding nutrition-related recommendations • Limited ability to apply nutrition-related recommendations • Limited motivation to apply nutrition-related recommendations • Limited ability to lose a significant amount of excess weight through conventional weight loss intervention • Medications that impact RMR, eg, midazolam, propranolol, glipizide

Continued on next page

Overweight/Obesity

Continued from previous page

Nutrition Assessment Category	Potential Indicators of This Nutrition Diagnosis (one or more must be present)
Client History†	• Conditions associated with a diagnosis or treatment, eg, hypothyroidism, metabolic syndrome, eating disorder not otherwise specified, depression, diabetes mellitus, hypertension • Physical disability or limitation • History of familial obesity • History of childhood obesity • History of physical, sexual, or emotional abuse
Assessment, Monitoring, and Evaluation Tools	
Comparative Standards	• Ideal/reference body weight (IBW) • Recommended body mass index (BMI) • Goal body weight • Goal body weight for length *z* score • Goal body mass index (BMI) for age *z* score

Arrows used with laboratory values: ↑ represents above reference standard and ↓ represents below reference standard.
** If a synonym for the term "Obesity class III" is helpful or needed, an approved alternate is "morbid obesity."*
† Client History terms are used for Nutrition Assessment but not for Nutrition Monitoring and Evaluation.

Progress Evaluation

Communicate the progress toward the resolution of a nutrition diagnosis by selecting the appropriate nutrition diagnosis status value from the Nutrition Assessment, Monitoring, and Evaluation terms.

NCP Term	ANDUID
New nutrition diagnosis	14586
Active nutrition diagnosis	14587
Resolved nutrition diagnosis	14588
Discontinued nutrition diagnosis	14589

For details on these terms, visit the Nutrition Diagnosis Status reference sheet on page 200.

Unintended* Weight Gain

Definition

Body weight gain more than that which is desired or planned.

Etiology (Cause/Contributing Risk Factors)

Factors gathered during the nutrition assessment process that contribute to the existence or the maintenance of pathophysiological, psychosocial, situational, developmental, cultural, and/or environmental problems:

- Illnesses or conditions causing unexpected weight gain resulting from conditions like head trauma, immobility, paralysis or related condition, Cushing syndrome, hypothyroidism, or other endocrine disorders
- Chronic use of medications known to cause weight gain, such as use of certain antidepressants, antipsychotics, corticosteroids, and certain HIV medications
- Not ready for nutrition-related behavior change

Etiology Category

Etiologies are grouped by the type of cause or contributing risk factor. Communicate the etiology category by selecting the appropriate Nutrition Assessment, Monitoring, and Evaluation term.

NCP Term	ANDUID
Beliefs attitudes etiology	14567
Cultural etiology	14568
Knowledge etiology	14569
Physical function etiology	14570
Physiologic metabolic etiology	14571
Psychological etiology	14572
Social personal etiology	14573
Treatment etiology	14574
Access etiology	14575
Behavior etiology	14576

Visit the Nutrition Diagnosis Etiology Category Identification reference sheet on page 185 for more details on etiology categories. An additional useful resource to determine the etiology category is the Nutrition Diagnosis Matrix on page 528.

Signs/Symptoms (Defining Characteristics)

A typical cluster of subjective and objective signs and symptoms gathered during the nutrition assessment process that provide evidence that a problem exists; quantify the problem and describe its severity. (See the next page for the nutrition assessment category and potential indicators.)

* If a *synonym*, or alternate word with the same meaning, for the term "unintended" is helpful or needed, an approved alternate is the word "involuntary."

Unintended Weight Gain

Nutrition Assessment Category	Potential Indicators of This Nutrition Diagnosis (one or more must be present)
Biochemical Data, Medical Tests and Procedures	• ↓ Serum albumin • ↓ Sodium, serum • ↑ Fasting serum lipid levels • ↑ Fasting glucose levels • Fluctuating hormone levels, eg, cortisol • ↑ Growth hormone • ↑ TSH • ↓ Thyroxine (T4)
Anthropometric Measurements	• Increased weight, any increase in weight more than planned or desired • Weight gain of > 5% within 30 days, > 7.5% in 90 days, or > 10% in 180 days (adults)
Physical Exam Findings	• Fat accumulation, excessive subcutaneous fat stores, noticeable change in body fat distribution • Extreme hunger with or without palpitations, tremor, and sweating • Edema • Shortness of breath • Muscle weakness • Fatigue
Food/Nutrition-Related History	Reports or observations of: • Estimated intake inconsistent with estimated or measured energy needs • Changes in recent estimated food intake level • Fluid administration more than requirements • Use of alcohol, narcotics • Medications associated with increased appetite • Physical inactivity or change in physical activity level
Client History*	Conditions associated with a diagnosis or treatment of asthma, psychiatric illnesses, rheumatic conditions, Cushing syndrome, obesity, Prader-Willi syndrome, Down syndrome, spina bifida, hypothyroidism, pituitary conditions
Assessment, Monitoring, and Evaluation Tools	
Comparative Standards	• Ideal/reference body weight (IBW) • Recommended body mass index (BMI) • Goal body weight • Goal body weight for length *z* score • Goal body mass index (BMI) for age *z* score

Arrows used with laboratory values: ↑ represents above reference standard and ↓ represents below reference standard.
** Client History terms are used for Nutrition Assessment but not for Nutrition Monitoring and Evaluation.*

Unintended Weight Gain

Progress Evaluation

Communicate the progress toward the resolution of a nutrition diagnosis by selecting the appropriate nutrition diagnosis status value from the Nutrition Assessment, Monitoring, and Evaluation terms.

NCP Term	ANDUID
New nutrition diagnosis	14586
Active nutrition diagnosis	14587
Resolved nutrition diagnosis	14588
Discontinued nutrition diagnosis	14589

For details on these terms, visit the Nutrition Diagnosis Status reference sheet on page 200.

Growth Rate Below Expected

Definition

Rate of growth or growth velocity slower than expected, or weight gain that is suboptimal in comparison with goal or reference standard.

Etiology (Cause/Contributing Risk Factors)

Factors gathered during the nutrition assessment process that contribute to the existence or the maintenance of pathophysiological, psychosocial, situational, developmental, cultural, and/or environmental problems:

- Physiological impetus for increased nutrient needs (eg, critical illness or trauma; pregnancy; metabolic illness, eg, type 1 diabetes; malabsorption)
- Decreased ability to consume sufficient energy
- Food insecurity
- Psychological causes, such as depression or disordered eating pattern
- Limited food acceptance
- Food and nutrition-related knowledge deficit
- Limited food and nutrition related skill
- Belief finding that hinders food and/or nutrition behavior change
- Attitude finding that hinders food and/or nutrition behavior change
- Small for gestational age, intrauterine growth restriction/retardation, lack of appropriate weight gain, hyperemesis gravidarum

Etiology Category

Etiologies are grouped by the type of cause or contributing risk factor. Communicate the etiology category by selecting the appropriate Nutrition Assessment, Monitoring, and Evaluation term.

NCP Term	ANDUID
Beliefs attitudes etiology	14567
Cultural etiology	14568
Knowledge etiology	14569
Physical function etiology	14570
Physiologic metabolic etiology	14571
Psychological etiology	14572
Social personal etiology	14573
Treatment etiology	14574
Access etiology	14575
Behavior etiology	14576

Visit the Nutrition Diagnosis Etiology Category Identification reference sheet on page 185 for more details on etiology categories. An additional useful resource to determine the etiology category is the Nutrition Diagnosis Matrix on page 528.

Growth Rate Below Expected

Signs/Symptoms (Defining Characteristics)

A typical cluster of subjective and objective signs and symptoms gathered during the nutrition assessment process that provide evidence that a problem exists; quantify the problem and describe its severity.

Nutrition Assessment Category	Potential Indicators of This Nutrition Diagnosis (one or more must be present)
Biochemical Data, Medical Tests and Procedures	• Positive urine ketones, ↑ fasting (or postprandial) glucose level • Fluctuating hormone levels during pregnancy • Zinc deficiency • Iron deficiency • Abnormal protein, fatty acid or carbohydrate metabolism profile
Anthropometric Measurements	• Weight-for-age decrease in two or more percentile channels • Weight gain velocity less than expected, based on established reference standard and/or guideline • Length- or height-for-age decrease in two or more percentile channels • Length or height gain velocity less than expected, based on established reference standard and/or guideline
Physical Exam Findings	• Decreased muscle mass, muscle wasting (eg, gluteal, temporal) • Hunger • Decreased fat mass
Food/Nutrition-Related History	Reports or observations of: • Estimated energy intake inconsistent with estimated or measured needs • Restricted fluids decreasing ability to meet nutritional needs • Difficulty breastfeeding, eg, poor latch • Limited food acceptance, eg, not progressing to foods as expected or recommended • Medications associated with decreased appetite or weight loss • Use of alcohol or narcotics during pregnancy • Increase in physical activity levels • Normal or usual intake in presence of illness • Poor intake, change in eating habits, early satiety, or skipped meals
Client History*	• Conditions associated with a diagnosis or treatment impacting growth, including AIDS/HIV, burns, pulmonary disease, dysphagia, long bone fracture, infection, surgery, trauma, hyperthyroid, hypothyroid, substance abuse, some types of cancer or metastatic disease, inborn errors of metabolism • Food insecurity
Assessment, Monitoring, and Evaluation Tools	

Continued on next page

Growth Rate Below Expected

Continued from previous page

Nutrition Assessment Category	Potential Indicators of This Nutrition Diagnosis (one or more must be present)
Comparative Standards	• Ideal/reference body weight (IBW) • Recommended body mass index (BMI) • Goal body weight • Goal body weight for length *z* score • Goal body mass index (BMI) for age *z* score

Arrows used with laboratory values: ↑ represents above reference standard and ↓ represents below reference standard.
** Client History terms are used for Nutrition Assessment but not for Nutrition Monitoring and Evaluation.*

Progress Evaluation

Communicate the progress toward the resolution of a nutrition diagnosis by selecting the appropriate nutrition diagnosis status value from the Nutrition Assessment, Monitoring, and Evaluation terms.

NCP Term	ANDUID
New nutrition diagnosis	14586
Active nutrition diagnosis	14587
Resolved nutrition diagnosis	14588
Discontinued nutrition diagnosis	14589

For details on these terms, visit the Nutrition Diagnosis Status reference sheet on page 200.

Excessive Growth Rate

Definition

Rate of growth or growth velocity, during a period of growth (childhood, adolescence, pregnancy), that is higher in comparison with a goal, reference standard, or physiological needs.

Etiology (Cause/Contributing Risk Factors)

Factors gathered during the nutrition assessment process that contribute to the existence or the maintenance of pathophysiological, psychosocial, situational, developmental, cultural, and/or environmental problems:

- Physiological change resulting in decreased energy needs or unexpected growth rate
- Excessive energy intake
- Frequent intake of energy-dense foods
- Food and nutrition-related knowledge deficit
- Physical inactivity
- Not ready for nutrition related behavior change
- Chronic use of medications, eg, antidepressants, antipsychotics, and corticosteroids
- Limited food and nutrition related skill

Etiology Category

Etiologies are grouped by the type of cause or contributing risk factor. Communicate the etiology category by selecting the appropriate Nutrition Assessment, Monitoring, and Evaluation term.

NCP Term	ANDUID
Beliefs attitudes etiology	14567
Cultural etiology	14568
Knowledge etiology	14569
Physical function etiology	14570
Physiologic metabolic etiology	14571
Psychological etiology	14572
Social personal etiology	14573
Treatment etiology	14574
Access etiology	14575
Behavior etiology	14576

Visit the Nutrition Diagnosis Etiology Category Identification reference sheet on page 185 for more details on etiology categories. An additional useful resource to determine the etiology category is the Nutrition Diagnosis Matrix on page 528.

Excessive Growth Rate

Signs/Symptoms (Defining Characteristics)

A typical cluster of subjective and objective signs and symptoms gathered during the nutrition assessment process that provide evidence that a problem exists; quantify the problem and describe its severity.

Nutrition Assessment Category	Potential Indicators of This Nutrition Diagnosis (one or more must be present)
Biochemical Data, Medical Tests and Procedures	• ↑ Cortisol • ↑ Growth hormone • ↑ Thyroid stimulating hormone (TSH) • ↓ Thyroxine (T4)
Anthropometric Measurements	• Body weight gain greater than expected based on reference standard, recommendations, or understanding of growth pattern • Weight gain velocity greater than expected, based on reference standard and/or guidelines • Weight-for-length or BMI-for-age increase greater than expected • Rate of weight gain during pregnancy greater than expected • Fundal height greater than number of weeks of gestation
Physical Exam Findings	
Food/Nutrition-Related History	Reports or observations of: • Estimated energy intake inconsistent with estimated or measured needs • Medications associated with increased appetite or weight gain • Decrease in physical activity • Beliefs, attitudes, and behaviors that do not represent readiness to change
Client History*	Conditions associated with a diagnosis or treatment impacting growth, eg, Prader-Willi syndrome, Down syndrome, spina bifida, giantism, pituitary tumor, Cushing syndrome, hypothyroidism, and neurological conditions that impact satiety
Assessment, Monitoring, and Evaluation Tools	
Comparative Standards	• Ideal/reference body weight (IBW) • Recommended body mass index (BMI) • Goal body weight • Goal body weight for length *z* score • Goal body mass index (BMI) for age *z* score

Arrows used with laboratory values: ↑ represents above reference standard and ↓ represents below reference standard.
** Client History terms are used for Nutrition Assessment but not for Nutrition Monitoring and Evaluation.*

Excessive Growth Rate

Progress Evaluation

Communicate the progress toward the resolution of a nutrition diagnosis by selecting the appropriate nutrition diagnosis status value from the Nutrition Assessment, Monitoring, and Evaluation terms.

NCP Term	ANDUID
New nutrition diagnosis	14586
Active nutrition diagnosis	14587
Resolved nutrition diagnosis	14588
Discontinued nutrition diagnosis	14589

For details on these terms, visit the Nutrition Diagnosis Status reference sheet on page 200.

Malnutrition (Undernutrition)

Definition

Inadequate intake of protein and/or energy sufficient to negatively impact growth/development, and/or to result in loss of fat and or muscle stores.

Note for adult malnutrition: There is an ongoing international effort to harmonize the definitions of adult malnutrition.[1] At present, the NCPT malnutrition indicator criteria provided in the adult malnutrition reference sheets reflect the malnutrition clinical characteristics (MCC) Academy/ASPEN Adult Malnutrition Consensus Statement.[2] Three additional validated nutrition assessment approaches, the Subjective Global Assessment, the Scored Patient-Generated Subjective Global Assessment (PG-SGA), and the Mini Nutritional Assessment Long Form (MNA-LF), to identify malnutrition are also in a chart that follows the MCC in the adult malnutrition reference sheets and may be used to identify malnutrition*.

The Academy/ASPEN Adult Malnutrition Consensus Statement recommends a minimum of two clinical characteristics or indicators be present for diagnosis of malnutrition. For additional information please see the reference: White JV, Guenter P, Jensen G, Malone A, Schofield M. Consensus statement: Academy of Nutrition and Dietetics and American Society for Parenteral and Enteral Nutrition: characteristics recommended for the identification and documentation of adult malnutrition (undernutrition). *J Parenter Enteral Nutr.* May 2012;36(3):275-83. doi:10.1177/0148607112440285

Note for pediatric malnutrition: The Academy/ASPEN Pediatric Malnutrition Consensus Statement recommends specific indicators when only one indicator is present and additional indicators when two or more indicators are present for diagnosis of malnutrition.

Etiology (Cause/Contributing Risk Factors)

Factors gathered during the nutrition assessment process that contribute to the existence or the maintenance of pathophysiological, psychosocial, situational, developmental, cultural, and/or environmental problems.

Please refer to the reference sheets for the type and severity of adult or pediatric malnutrition (undernutrition) etiologies.

Etiology Category

Etiologies are grouped by the type of cause or contributing risk factor. Communicate the etiology category by selecting the appropriate Nutrition Assessment, Monitoring, and Evaluation term.

NCP Term	ANDUID
Beliefs attitudes etiology	14567
Cultural etiology	14568
Knowledge etiology	14569
Physical function etiology	14570
Physiologic metabolic etiology	14571
Psychological etiology	14572
Social personal etiology	14573
Treatment etiology	14574
Access etiology	14575
Behavior etiology	14576

Visit the Nutrition Diagnosis Etiology Category Identification reference sheet on page 185 for more details on etiology categories. An additional useful resource to determine the etiology category is the Nutrition Diagnosis Matrix on page 528.

Malnutrition (Undernutrition)

Signs/Symptoms (Defining Characteristics)

A typical cluster of subjective and objective signs and symptoms gathered during the nutrition assessment process that provide evidence that a problem exists; quantify the problem and describe its severity.

Nutrition Assessment Category	Potential Indicators of This Nutrition Diagnosis (one or more must be present)
Biochemical Data, Medical Tests and Procedures	
Anthropometric Measurements	Please refer to the reference sheets for the type and severity of adult or pediatric malnutrition (undernutrition) indicators.
Physical Exam Findings	Please refer to the reference sheets for the type and severity of adult or pediatric malnutrition (undernutrition) indicators.
Food/Nutrition-Related History	Please refer to the reference sheets for the type and severity of adult or pediatric malnutrition (undernutrition) indicators.
Client History	Please refer to the reference sheets for the type and severity of adult or pediatric malnutrition (undernutrition) indicators.
Assessment, Monitoring, and Evaluation Tools	Please refer to the reference sheets for the type and severity of adult or pediatric malnutrition (undernutrition) indicators.
Comparative Standards	Please refer to the reference sheets for the type and severity of adult or pediatric malnutrition (undernutrition) indicators.

Progress Evaluation

Communicate the progress toward the resolution of a nutrition diagnosis by selecting the appropriate nutrition diagnosis status value from the Nutrition Assessment, Monitoring, and Evaluation terms.

NCP Term	ANDUID
New nutrition diagnosis	14586
Active nutrition diagnosis	14587
Resolved nutrition diagnosis	14588
Discontinued nutrition diagnosis	14589

For details on these terms, visit the Nutrition Diagnosis Status reference sheet on page 200.

Starvation Related Malnutrition (Undernutrition)

Definition

Inadequate intake of protein and/or energy over a period of time sufficient to result in loss of fat and/or muscle mass without apparent inflammation and in the context of environmental and/or social circumstances. Indicators for identifying Moderate (non severe) and Severe starvation related malnutrition characteristics are included here.

Note: There is an ongoing international effort to harmonize the definitions of adult malnutrition. At present, the NCPT malnutrition indicator criteria provided reflect the malnutrition clinical characteristics (MCC) Academy/ASPEN Adult Malnutrition Consensus Statement. Three additional validated nutrition assessment approaches, the Subjective Global Assessment (SGA), the Scored Patient-Generated Subjective Global Assessment (PG-SGA), and the Mini Nutritional Assessment Long Form (MNA-LF), to identify malnutrition are also in a chart that follows the MCC and may be used to identify malnutrition.

The Academy/ASPEN Adult Malnutrition Consensus Statement recommends a minimum of two clinical characteristics or indicators be present for diagnosis of malnutrition. For additional information please see the reference: White JV, Guenter P, Jensen G, Malone A, Schofield M. Consensus statement: Academy of Nutrition and Dietetics and American Society for Parenteral and Enteral Nutrition: characteristics recommended for the identification and documentation of adult malnutrition (undernutrition). *J Parenter Enteral Nutr.* May 2012;36(3):275-283. doi:10.1177/0148607112440285

Etiology (Cause/Contributing Risk Factors)

Factors gathered during the nutrition assessment process that contribute to the existence or the maintenance of pathophysiological, psychosocial, situational, developmental, cultural, and/or environmental problems:

- Alteration in gastrointestinal tract structure and/or function
- Food insecurity
- Cultural or religious practices that affect the ability to access food
- Food and nutrition related knowledge deficit concerning amount of energy and amount and type of dietary protein
- Behavioral/psychological causes, eg, depression or eating disorders
- Oral health limitations
- Impaired sensory perception impacting food consumption
- Limited food and nutrition related skill

Etiology Category

Etiologies are grouped by the type of cause or contributing risk factor. Communicate the etiology category by selecting the appropriate Nutrition Assessment, Monitoring, and Evaluation term.

Starvation Related Malnutrition (Undernutrition)

NCP Term	ANDUID
Beliefs attitudes etiology	14567
Cultural etiology	14568
Knowledge etiology	14569
Physical function etiology	14570
Physiologic metabolic etiology	14571
Psychological etiology	14572
Social personal etiology	14573
Treatment etiology	14574
Access etiology	14575
Behavior etiology	14576

Visit the Nutrition Diagnosis Etiology Category Identification reference sheet on page 185 for more details on etiology categories. An additional useful resource to determine the etiology category is the Nutrition Diagnosis Matrix on page 528.

Signs/Symptoms (Defining Characteristics)

A typical cluster of subjective and objective signs and symptoms gathered during the nutrition assessment process that provide evidence that a problem exists; quantify the problem and describe its severity.

Nutrition Assessment Category	Potential Indicators of This Nutrition Diagnosis (one or more must be present)
Biochemical Data, Medical Tests and Procedures	
Anthropometric Measurements	Malnutrition can occur at any body weight/BMI • Inadequate maternal weight gain • Moderate (non-severe) malnutrition (adults): unintentional weight loss of 20% in 1 year; 10% in 6 months; 7.5% in 3 months; 5% in 1 month • Severe malnutrition (adults): unintentional weight loss of > 20% in 1 year; > 10% in 6 months; > 7.5% in 3 months; or > 5% in 1 month
Physical Exam Findings	Moderate (non-severe) malnutrition • Mild loss of subcutaneous fat, eg, orbital, triceps, fat overlying the ribs • Mild muscle loss, eg, wasting of the temples (temporalis muscle), clavicles (pectoralis and deltoids), shoulders (deltoids), interosseous muscles, scapula (latissimus dorsi, trapezius, deltoids), thigh (quadriceps), and calf (gastrocnemius) • Mild localized or generalized fluid accumulation (extremities, vulvar/scrotal, ascites)

Continued on next page

Starvation Related Malnutrition (Undernutrition)

Continued from previous page

Nutrition Assessment Category	Potential Indicators of This Nutrition Diagnosis (one or more must be present)
Physical Exam Findings (continued)	Severe malnutrition • Severe loss of subcutaneous fat, eg, orbital, triceps, fat overlying the ribs • Severe muscle loss, eg, wasting of the temples (temporalis muscle), clavicles (pectoralis and deltoids), shoulders (deltoids), interosseous muscles, scapula (latissimus dorsi, trapezius, deltoids), thigh (quadriceps), and calf (gastrocnemius) • Severe localized or generalized fluid accumulation (extremities, vulvar/scrotal, ascites)

Food/Nutrition-Related History	Reports or observations of:
	• Moderate (non-severe) malnutrition
	  ○ Estimated energy intake < 75% of estimated energy requirement for ≥ 3 months
	• Severe malnutrition
	  ○ Estimated energy intake ≤ 50% of estimated energy requirement for ≥ 1 month
	    o Measurably reduced changes in grip strength or other functional indicators
	Note. Handgrip strength in adults: norms are device dependent; can identify presence of malnutrition but not quantify the degree of the deficit; may not be able to perform on certain clients. Please refer to the Academy/ASPEN Adult and Pediatric Malnutrition Consensus Statements for further information.

Client History*	Reports or observations of the following, for example: • Anorexia nervosa, benign esophageal stricture, abuse, neglect, poverty, frailty, and anything that results in limited access to food (associated with malnutrition in the context of environmental and social circumstances) • Existing medical diagnosis of malnutrition including malnutrition • Genetic or acquired conditions: cerebral palsy, cystic fibrosis, seizure disorders, metabolic disease, inflammatory bowel disease
Assessment, Monitoring, and Evaluation Tools	• Subjective global assessment (SGA) rating • Subjective global assessment (SGA) score • The scored patient generated subjective global assessment (PG-SGA) rating • The scored patient generated subjective global assessment (PG-SGA) score • Mini nutritional assessment long form (MNA-LF) rating • Mini nutritional assessment long form (MNA-LF) score
Comparative Standards	

** Client History terms are used for Nutrition Assessment but not for Nutrition Monitoring and Evaluation.*
In the past, hepatic transport protein measures (eg, albumin and prealbumin) were used as indicators of malnutrition. See the Evidence Analysis Library questions on this topic at (accessed June 3, 2025): https://www.andeal.org/topic.cfm?cat=4302

Starvation Related Malnutrition (Undernutrition)

Nutrition Assessment Tools for Identifying Malnutrition

Assessment Parameter	SGA	PG-SGA	MNA-LF	MCCs (this tool is not validated)
Name/author/year	Detsky AS et al. 1987[4]	Ottery F. 2015 http://pt-global.org/	Guigoz Y et al. 1994 http://mna-elderly.com/	AND/ASPEN Consensus Statement 2012
Weight loss/BMI±	X	X	X	X
Dietary intake±	X	X	X	X
GI symptoms	X	X		
Comorbidity		X	X	
Metabolic demand		X		
Functional capacity±	X	X	X	X
Fluid status (edema/ascites)	X	X		X
Fat stores±	X	X	Mid arm circumference, calf circumference	X
Muscle stores±	X	X		X
Neuropsychological			X	
Method of categorization	Rating: SGA A (well nourished) SGA B (mild-moderate malnutrition) SGA C (severe malnutrition)	Rating: SGA A/B/C (assessed per SGA) Scores for triaging nutrition interventions	Numerical score: No nutritional risk Risk of malnutrition Malnourished	Two or more characteristics demonstrated out of six identifies malnutrition Severity defined by specific thresholds
Validated: setting	Acute Rehabilitation Community Residential aged care	Acute	Acute Rehabilitation Community Long-term care	
Validated: client group	Surgery Geriatric Oncology Renal	Oncology Renal Stroke	Geriatric	
Validated: ages	Adults of all ages	Adults of all ages	Adults ≥ 65 years	

± Parameters that most influence the rating

Starvation Related Malnutrition (Undernutrition)

Progress Evaluation

Communicate the progress toward the resolution of a nutrition diagnosis by selecting the appropriate nutrition diagnosis status value from the Nutrition Assessment, Monitoring, and Evaluation terms.

NCP Term	ANDUID
New nutrition diagnosis	14586
Active nutrition diagnosis	14587
Resolved nutrition diagnosis	14588
Discontinued nutrition diagnosis	14589

For details on these terms, visit the Nutrition Diagnosis Status reference sheet on page 200.

Chronic Disease or Condition Related Malnutrition (Undernutrition)

Definition

Inadequate intake of protein and/or energy over a period of time sufficient to result in loss of fat and/or muscle mass with apparent mild to moderate inflammation and in the context of chronic illness or condition. Indicators for identifying Moderate (non severe) and Severe chronic disease or condition related malnutrition characteristics are included here.

Note: There is an ongoing international effort to harmonize the definitions of adult malnutrition. At present, the NCPT malnutrition indicator criteria provided reflect the malnutrition clinical characteristics (MCC) Academy/ASPEN Adult Malnutrition Consensus Statement. Three additional validated nutrition assessment approaches, the Subjective Global Assessment (SGA), the Scored Patient-Generated Subjective Global Assessment (PG-SGA), and the Mini Nutritional Assessment Long Form (MNA-LF), to identify malnutrition are also in a chart that follows the MCC and may be used to identify malnutrition.

The Academy/ASPEN Adult Malnutrition Consensus Statement recommends a minimum of two clinical characteristics or indicators be present for diagnosis of malnutrition. For additional information please see the reference: White JV, Guenter P, Jensen G, Malone A, Schofield M. Consensus statement: Academy of Nutrition and Dietetics and American Society for Parenteral and Enteral Nutrition: characteristics recommended for the identification and documentation of adult malnutrition (undernutrition). *J Parenter Enteral Nutr.* May 2012;36(3):275-283. doi:10.1177/0148607112440285

Etiology (Cause/Contributing Risk Factors)

Factors gathered during the nutrition assessment process that contribute to the existence or the maintenance of pathophysiological, psychosocial, situational, developmental, cultural, and/or environmental problems:

- Physiological causes increasing nutrient needs due to illness or condition
- Physiological causes resulting in anorexia or diminished intake
- Alteration in gastrointestinal tract structure and/or function

Etiology Category

Etiologies are grouped by the type of cause or contributing risk factor. Communicate the etiology category by selecting the appropriate Nutrition Assessment, Monitoring, and Evaluation term.

NCP Term	ANDUID
Beliefs attitudes etiology	14567
Cultural etiology	14568
Knowledge etiology	14569
Physical function etiology	14570
Physiologic metabolic etiology	14571
Psychological etiology	14572
Social personal etiology	14573

Continued on next page

Chronic Disease or Condition Related Malnutrition (Undernutrition)

Continued from previous page

NCP Term	ANDUID
Treatment etiology	14574
Access etiology	14575
Behavior etiology	14576

Visit the Nutrition Diagnosis Etiology Category Identification reference sheet on page 185 for more details on etiology categories. An additional useful resource to determine the etiology category is the Nutrition Diagnosis Matrix on page 528.

Signs/Symptoms (Defining Characteristics)

A typical cluster of subjective and objective signs and symptoms gathered during the nutrition assessment process that provide evidence that a problem exists; quantify the problem and describe its severity.

Nutrition Assessment Category	Potential Indicators of This Nutrition Diagnosis (one or more must be present)
Biochemical Data, Medical Tests and Procedures	
Anthropometric Measurements	Malnutrition can occur at any body weight/BMI • Inadequate maternal weight gain • Moderate (non severe) malnutrition: Unintentional weight loss, adults, of 20% in 1 year; 10% in 6 months; 7.5% in 3 months; 5% in 1 month • Severe malnutrition: Unintentional weight loss, adults, of > 20% in 1 year; > 10% in 6 months; > 7.5% in 3 months; or > 5% in 1 month
Physical Exam Findings	Moderate (non severe) malnutrition • Mild loss of subcutaneous fat, eg, orbital, triceps, fat overlying the ribs • Mild muscle loss, eg, wasting of the temples (temporalis muscle), clavicles (pectoralis and deltoids), shoulders (deltoids), interosseous muscles, scapula (latissimus dorsi, trapezius, deltoids), thigh (quadriceps) and calf (gastrocnemius) • Mild localized or generalized fluid accumulation (extremities, vulvar/scrotal, ascites) Severe malnutrition • Severe loss of subcutaneous fat, eg, orbital, triceps, fat overlying the ribs • Severe muscle loss, eg, wasting of the temples (temporalis muscle), clavicles (pectoralis and deltoids), shoulders (deltoids), interosseous muscles, scapula (latissimus dorsi, trapezius, deltoids), thigh (quadriceps) and calf (gastrocnemius) • Severe localized or generalized fluid accumulation (extremities, vulvar/scrotal, ascites)

Continued on next page

Chronic Disease or Condition Related Malnutrition (Undernutrition)

Continued from previous page

Nutrition Assessment Category	Potential Indicators of This Nutrition Diagnosis (one or more must be present)
Food/Nutrition-Related History	Reports or observations of: • Moderate (non severe) malnutrition ○ Estimated energy intake < 75% of estimated energy requirement for ≥ 1 month • Severe malnutrition ○ Estimated energy intake < 75% of estimated energy requirement for ≥ 1 month ○ Measurably reduced changes in grip strength or other functional indicators *Note. Handgrip strength in adults: norms are device dependent; can identify presence of malnutrition but not quantify the degree of the deficit; may not be able to perform on certain clients. Please refer to the Academy/ASPEN Adult and Pediatric Malnutrition Consensus Statements for further information.*
Client History*	Reports or observations of the following, for example: • Organ failure, malignancies, rheumatoid diseases, gastrointestinal diseases, sarcopenic obesity, malabsorptive syndromes, and other etiologies including but not limited to diabetes, congestive heart failure, chronic kidney disease, and chronic obstructive pulmonary disease (associated with malnutrition in the context of chronic disease/condition) • Existing medical diagnosis of malnutrition including malnutrition • Genetic or acquired conditions, eg, cerebral palsy, cystic fibrosis, seizure disorders, metabolic disease, irritable bowel disease
Assessment, Monitoring, and Evaluation Tools	• Subjective global assessment (SGA) rating • Subjective global assessment (SGA) score • The scored patient generated subjective global assessment (PG-SGA) rating • The scored patient generated subjective global assessment (PG-SGA) score • Mini nutritional assessment long form (MNA-LF) rating • Mini nutritional assessment long form (MNA-LF) score
Comparative Standards	

** Client History terms are used for Nutrition Assessment but not for Nutrition Monitoring and Evaluation.*
In the past, hepatic transport protein measures (eg, albumin and prealbumin) were used as indicators of malnutrition. See the Evidence Analysis Library questions on this topic (accessed June 3, 2025): https://www.andeal.org/topic.cfm?cat=4302

Chronic Disease or Condition Related Malnutrition (Undernutrition)

Nutrition Assessment Tools for Identifying Malnutrition

Assessment parameter	SGA	PG-SGA	MNA-LFF	MCPs (this tool is not validated)
Name/author/year	Detsky AS et al. 1987[4]	Ottery F. 2015 http://pt-global.org/[18]	Guigoz Y et al. 1994 http://mna-elderly.com/[19,20]	AND/ASPEN Consensus Statement 2012[2]
Weight loss/BMI±	X	X	X	X
Dietary intake±	X	X	X	X
GI symptoms	X	X		
Comorbidity		X	X	
Metabolic demand		X		
Functional capacity±	X	X	X	X
Fluid status (edema/ ascites)	X	X		X
Fat stores±	X	X	Mid arm circumference, calf circumference	X
Muscle stores±	X	X		X
Neuropsychological			X	
Method of categorization	Rating: SGA A (well nourished) SGA B (mild-moderate malnutrition) SGA C (severe malnutrition)	Rating: SGA A/B/C (assessed per SGA) Scores for triaging nutrition interventions	Numerical score: No nutritional risk Risk of malnutrition Malnourished	Two or more characteristics demonstrated out of six identifies malnutrition Severity defined by specific thresholds
Validated: setting	Acute Rehabilitation Community Residential aged care	Acute	Acute Rehabilitation Community Long-term care	
Validated: client group	Surgery Geriatric Oncology Renal	Oncology Renal Stroke	Geriatric	
Validated: ages	Adults of all ages	Adults of all ages	Adults ≥ 65 years	

± Parameters that most influence the rating

Chronic Disease or Condition Related Malnutrition (Undernutrition)

Progress Evaluation

Communicate the progress toward the resolution of a nutrition diagnosis by selecting the appropriate nutrition diagnosis status value from the Nutrition Assessment, Monitoring, and Evaluation terms.

NCP Term	ANDUID
New nutrition diagnosis	14586
Active nutrition diagnosis	14587
Resolved nutrition diagnosis	14588
Discontinued nutrition diagnosis	14589

For details on these terms, visit the Nutrition Diagnosis Status reference sheet on page 200.

Acute Disease or Injury Related Malnutrition (Undernutrition)

Definition

Inadequate intake of protein and/or energy resulting in loss of fat and/or muscle mass with apparent marked inflammatory response and in the context of acute illness or injury. Indicators for identifying Moderate (non severe) and Severe acute disease or injury related malnutrition are included here.

Note: There is an ongoing international effort to harmonize the definitions of adult malnutrition. At present, the NCPT malnutrition indicator criteria provided reflect the malnutrition clinical characteristics (MCC) Academy/ASPEN Adult Malnutrition Consensus Statement. Three additional validated nutrition assessment approaches, the Subjective Global Assessment (SGA), the Scored Patient-Generated Subjective Global Assessment (PG-SGA), and the Mini Nutritional Assessment Long Form (MNA-LF), to identify malnutrition are also in a chart that follows the MCC and may be used to identify malnutrition.

The Academy/ASPEN Adult Malnutrition Consensus Statement recommends a minimum of two clinical characteristics or indicators be present for diagnosis of malnutrition. For additional information please see the reference: White JV, Guenter P, Jensen G, Malone A, Schofield M. Consensus statement: Academy of Nutrition and Dietetics and American Society for Parenteral and Enteral Nutrition: characteristics recommended for the identification and documentation of adult malnutrition (undernutrition). *J Parenter Enteral Nutr.* May 2012;36(3):275-283. doi:10.1177/0148607112440285

Etiology (Cause/Contributing Risk Factors)

Factors gathered during the nutrition assessment process that contribute to the existence or the maintenance of pathophysiological, psychosocial, situational, developmental, cultural, and/or environmental problems:

- Physiological causes increasing nutrient needs due to acute illness or injury/trauma
- Physiological causes resulting in anorexia or diminished intake
- Food and nutrition related knowledge deficit concerning amount of energy and amount and type of dietary protein
- Limited food- and nutrition- related skill

Etiology Category

Etiologies are grouped by the type of cause or contributing risk factor. Communicate the etiology category by selecting the appropriate Nutrition Assessment, Monitoring, and Evaluation term.

NCP Term	ANDUID
Beliefs attitudes etiology	14567
Cultural etiology	14568
Knowledge etiology	14569
Physical function etiology	14570
Physiologic metabolic etiology	14571
Psychological etiology	14572
Social personal etiology	14573

Acute Disease or Injury Related Malnutrition (Undernutrition)

NCP Term	ANDUID
Treatment etiology	14574
Access etiology	14575
Behavior etiology	14576

Visit the Nutrition Diagnosis Etiology Category Identification reference sheet on page 185 for more details on etiology categories. An additional useful resource to determine the etiology category is the Nutrition Diagnosis Matrix on page 528.

Signs/Symptoms (Defining Characteristics)

A typical cluster of subjective and objective signs and symptoms gathered during the nutrition assessment process that provide evidence that a problem exists; quantify the problem and describe its severity.

Nutrition Assessment Category	Potential Indicators of This Nutrition Diagnosis (one or more must be present)
Biochemical Data, Medical Tests and Procedures	
Anthropometric Measurements	Malnutrition can occur at any body weight/BMI • Inadequate maternal weight gain • Moderate (non-severe) malnutrition: Unintentional weight loss, adults, of 7.5% in 3 months; 5% in 1 month; or 1% to 2% in 1 week • Severe malnutrition: Unintentional weight loss, adults, of >7.5% in 3 months; or >5% in 1 month; or > 2% in 1 week
Physical Exam Findings	Moderate (non severe) malnutrition • Mild loss of subcutaneous fat, eg, orbital, triceps, fat overlying the ribs • Mild muscle loss, eg, wasting of the temples (temporalis muscle), clavicles (pectoralis and deltoids), shoulders (deltoids), interosseous muscles, scapula (latissimus dorsi, trapezius, deltoids), thigh (quadriceps) and calf (gastrocnemius) • Mild localized or generalized fluid accumulation (extremities, vulvar/scrotal, ascites) Severe malnutrition • Moderate loss of subcutaneous fat, eg, orbital, triceps, fat overlying the ribs • Moderate muscle loss, eg, wasting of the temples (temporalis muscle), clavicles (pectoralis and deltoids), shoulders (deltoids), interosseous muscles, scapula (latissimus dorsi, trapezius, deltoids), thigh (quadriceps) and calf (gastrocnemius) • Moderate to severe localized or generalized fluid accumulation (extremities, vulvar/scrotal, ascites)

Continued on next page

Acute Disease or Injury Related Malnutrition (Undernutrition)

Continued from previous page

Nutrition Assessment Category	Potential Indicators of This Nutrition Diagnosis (one or more must be present)
Food/Nutrition-Related History	Reports or observations of: • Moderate (non severe) malnutrition ○ Estimated energy intake < 75% of estimated energy requirement for > 7 days • Severe malnutrition ○ Estimated energy intake ≤ 50% of estimated energy requirement for ≥ 5 days ○ Measurably reduced changes in grip strength or other functional indicators *Note. Handgrip strength in adults: norms are device dependent; can identify presence of malnutrition but not quantify the degree of the deficit; may not be able to perform on certain clients. Please refer to the Academy/ASPEN Adult and Pediatric Malnutrition Consensus Statements for further information.*
Client History*	Reports or observations of the following, for example: • Major infections such as sepsis, pneumonia, peritonitis, and wound infections, major burns, trauma, closed head injury, acute lung injury, adult respiratory distress syndrome, and selected major surgeries (associated with malnutrition in the context of acute injury/illness) • Preexisting medical diagnosis of malnutrition
Assessment, Monitoring, and Evaluation Tools	• Subjective global assessment (SGA) rating • The scored patient generated subjective global assessment (PG-SGA) rating • The scored patient generated subjective global assessment (PG-SGA) score • Mini nutritional assessment long form (MNA-LF) score
Comparative Standards	

** Client History terms are used for Nutrition Assessment but not for Nutrition Monitoring and Evaluation.*
In the past, hepatic transport protein measures (eg, albumin and prealbumin) were used as indicators of malnutrition. See the Evidence Analysis Library questions on this topic (accessed June 3, 2025): https://www.andeal.org/topic.cfm?cat=4302

Acute Disease or Injury Related Malnutrition (Undernutrition)

Nutrition Assessment Tools for Identifying Malnutrition

Assessment parameter	SGA	PG-SGA	MNA-LFF	MCPs (this tool is not validated)
Name/author/year	Detsky AS et al. 1987[4]	Ottery F. 2015 http://pt-global.org/[18]	Guigoz Y et al. 1994 http://mna-elderly.com/[19,20]	AND/ASPEN Consensus Statement 2012[2]
Weight loss/BMI±	X	X	X	X
Dietary intake±	X	X	X	X
GI symptoms	X	X		
Comorbidity		X	X	
Metabolic demand		X		
Functional capacity±	X	X	X	X
Fluid status (edema/ascites)	X	X		X
Fat stores±	X	X	Mid arm circumference, calf circumference	X
Muscle stores±	X	X		X
Neuropsychological			X	
Method of categorization	Rating: SGA A (well nourished) SGA B (mild-moderate malnutrition) SGA C (severe malnutrition)	Rating: SGA A/B/C (assessed per SGA) Scores for triaging nutrition interventions	Numerical score: No nutritional risk Risk of malnutrition Malnourished	Two or more characteristics demonstrated out of six identifies malnutrition Severity defined by specific thresholds
Validated: setting	Acute Rehabilitation Community Residential aged care	Acute	Acute Rehabilitation Community Long-term care	
Validated: client group	Surgery Geriatric Oncology Renal	Oncology Renal Stroke	Geriatric	
Validated: ages	Adults of all ages	Adults of all ages	Adults ≥ 65 years	

± Parameters that most influence the rating

Acute Disease or Injury Related Malnutrition (Undernutrition)

Progress Evaluation

Communicate the progress toward the resolution of a nutrition diagnosis by selecting the appropriate nutrition diagnosis status value from the Nutrition Assessment, Monitoring, and Evaluation terms.

NCP Term	ANDUID
New nutrition diagnosis	14586
Active nutrition diagnosis	14587
Resolved nutrition diagnosis	14588
Discontinued nutrition diagnosis	14589

For details on these terms, visit the Nutrition Diagnosis Status reference sheet on page 200.

Non Illness Related Pediatric Malnutrition (Undernutrition)

Definition

Inadequate nutrient intake due to environmental or behavioral factors which may negatively affect growth, development, and/or other outcomes. Indicators for identifying Mild, Moderate, and Severe non illness related pediatric malnutrition are included here.

Note: The Academy/ASPEN Pediatric Malnutrition Consensus Statement recommends specific indicators when only one indicator is present and additional indicators when two or more indicators are present for diagnosis of malnutrition.

The Academy/ASPEN Adult Malnutrition Consensus Statement recommends a minimum of two clinical characteristics or indicators be present for diagnosis of malnutrition. For additional information please see the reference: White JV, Guenter P, Jensen G, Malone A, Schofield M. Consensus statement: Academy of Nutrition and Dietetics and American Society for Parenteral and Enteral Nutrition: characteristics recommended for the identification and documentation of adult malnutrition (undernutrition). *J Parenter Enteral Nutr.* May 2012;36(3):275-283. doi:10.1177/0148607112440285

Etiology (Cause/Contributing Risk Factors)

Factors gathered during the nutrition assessment process that contribute to the existence or the maintenance of pathophysiological, psychosocial, situational, developmental, cultural, and/or environmental problems:

- Food insecurity
- Interruptions of or intolerance to feedings
- Social, economic, behavioral, cultural, or religious practices that affect the ability to access food

Etiology Category

Etiologies are grouped by the type of cause or contributing risk factor. Communicate the etiology category by selecting the appropriate Nutrition Assessment, Monitoring, and Evaluation term.

NCP Term	ANDUID
Beliefs attitudes etiology	14567
Cultural etiology	14568
Knowledge etiology	14569
Physical function etiology	14570
Physiologic metabolic etiology	14571
Psychological etiology	14572
Social personal etiology	14573
Treatment etiology	14574
Access etiology	14575
Behavior etiology	14576

Visit the Nutrition Diagnosis Etiology Category Identification reference sheet on page 185 for more details on etiology categories. An additional useful resource to determine the etiology category is the Nutrition Diagnosis Matrix on page 528.

Non Illness Related Pediatric Malnutrition (Undernutrition)

Signs/Symptoms (Defining Characteristics)

A typical cluster of subjective and objective signs and symptoms gathered during the nutrition assessment process that provide evidence that a problem exists; quantify the problem and describe its severity.

Nutrition Assessment Category	Potential Indicators of This Nutrition Diagnosis (one or more must be present)
Biochemical Data, Medical Tests and Procedures	
Anthropometric Measurements	When a single data point is available: • Mild malnutrition ○ −1 to −1.9 body weight for length *z* score ○ −1 to −1.9 body mass index for age *z* score ○ −1 to −1.9 mid upper arm circumference *z* score • Moderate malnutrition ○ −2 to −2.9 body weight for length z score ○ −2 to −2.9 body mass index for age z score ○ −2 to −2.9 mid upper arm circumference *z* score • Severe malnutrition ○ −3 body weight for length *z* score or below ○ −3 body mass index for age *z* score or below ○ −3 length/height for age *z* score or below ○ −3 mid upper arm circumference *z* score or below *Note: For further information on z score data interpretation refer to:* https://apps.who.int/iris/bitstream/handle/10665/43601/9789241595070_C_eng.pdf?sequence=3&isAllowed=y When two or more data points are available the following additional indicators may then be assessed: • Mild malnutrition ○ Less than 75% of the norm for expected weight gain velocity (< 2 y of age) ○ 5% usual body weight loss (2 to 20 y of age) ○ Decline of 1 *z* score in weight for length or BMI for age *z* score • Moderate malnutrition ○ Less than 50% of the norm for expected weight gain velocity (< 2 y of age) ○ 7.5% usual body weight loss (2 to 20 y of age) ○ Decline of 2 *z* score in weight for length or BMI for age *z* score

Continued on next page

Non Illness Related Pediatric Malnutrition (Undernutrition)

Continued from previous page

Nutrition Assessment Category	Potential Indicators of This Nutrition Diagnosis (one or more must be present)

Anthropometric Measurements (continued)	• Severe malnutrition
	  ○ Less than 25% of the norm for expected weight gain velocity (< 2 y of age)
	  ○ 10% usual body weight loss (2 to 20 y of age)
	  ○ Decline of 3 *z* score in weight for length or BMI for age *z* score
	Note: Proxy measures described in the Academy/ASPEN Pediatric Malnutrition Consensus Statement can be used when typical anthropometric measures cannot be obtained.

Physical Exam Findings	• Stagnation in Tanner staging Moderate malnutrition • Mild loss of subcutaneous fat, eg, orbital, triceps, fat overlying the ribs • Mild muscle loss, eg, wasting of the temples (temporalis muscle), clavicles (pectoralis and deltoids), shoulders (deltoids), interosseous muscles, scapula (latissimus dorsi, trapezius, deltoids), thigh (quadriceps) and calf (gastrocnemius) • Mild localized or generalized fluid accumulation (extremities, vulvar/scrotal, ascites) Severe malnutrition • Severe loss of subcutaneous fat, eg, orbital, triceps, fat overlying the ribs • Severe muscle loss, eg, wasting of the temples (temporalis muscle), clavicles (pectoralis and deltoids), shoulders (deltoids), interosseous muscles, scapula (latissimus dorsi, trapezius, deltoids), thigh (quadriceps) and calf (gastrocnemius) • Severe localized or generalized fluid accumulation (extremities, vulvar/scrotal, ascites)
Food/Nutrition-Related History	Reports or observations of change in functional indicators, eg, handgrip strength or other measures of physical activity and/or strength *Note: Handgrip strength in children older than 6 years of age: norms are device dependent; can identify presence of malnutrition but not quantify the degree of the deficit; may not be able to perform on certain client. Please refer to the Academy/ASPEN Pediatric Malnutrition Consensus Statement for further information.*

Continued on next page

Non Illness Related Pediatric Malnutrition (Undernutrition)

Continued from previous page

Nutrition Assessment Category	Potential Indicators of This Nutrition Diagnosis (one or more must be present)
Food/Nutrition-Related History (continued)	When two or more data points are available: • Mild malnutrition: inadequate nutrient intake of 51% to 75% estimated energy/protein need • Moderate malnutrition: inadequate nutrient intake 26% to 50% estimated energy/protein need • Severe malnutrition: inadequate nutrient intake of ≤ 25% estimated energy/protein need
Client History*	Reports or observations of the following, for example: • Anorexia nervosa, abuse, neglect, poverty, frailty, and anything that results in limited access to food (associated with malnutrition in the context of environmental and social circumstances) • Existing medical diagnosis of malnutrition
Assessment, Monitoring, and Evaluation Tools	• Subjective global nutritional assessment (SGNA) for children rating⁺ • Subjective global nutritional assessment (SGNA) for children score⁺
Comparative Standards	

In the past, hepatic transport protein measures (eg, albumin and prealbumin) were used as indicators of malnutrition. See the Evidence Analysis Library questions on this topic at (accessed June 3, 2025): www.andeal.org/topic.cfm?cat=4302

** Client History terms are used for Nutrition Assessment but not for Nutrition Monitoring and Evaluation.*

⁺ Alternate approaches to interpretation of anthropometric measurements are recommended for children. Therefore, this tool should be used in conjunction with the evidence-based anthropometric measurement assessment criteria.

Progress Evaluation

Communicate the progress toward the resolution of a nutrition diagnosis by selecting the appropriate nutrition diagnosis status value from the Nutrition Assessment, Monitoring, and Evaluation terms.

NCP Term	ANDUID
New nutrition diagnosis	14586
Active nutrition diagnosis	14587
Resolved nutrition diagnosis	14588
Discontinued nutrition diagnosis	14589

For details on these terms, visit the Nutrition Diagnosis Status reference sheet on page 200.

Illness Related Pediatric Malnutrition (Undernutrition)

Definition

Nutrient deficit or imbalance due to disease or injury which may negatively affect growth, development, and/or other outcomes. Indicators for identifying Mild, Moderate, and Severe illness related pediatric malnutrition are included here.

Note: The Academy/ASPEN Pediatric Malnutrition Consensus Statement recommends specific indicators when only one indicator is present and additional indicators when two or more indicators are present for diagnosis of malnutrition.

The Academy/ASPEN Adult Malnutrition Consensus Statement recommends a minimum of two clinical characteristics or indicators be present for diagnosis of malnutrition. For additional information please see the reference: White JV, Guenter P, Jensen G, Malone A, Schofield M. Consensus statement: Academy of Nutrition and Dietetics and American Society for Parenteral and Enteral Nutrition: characteristics recommended for the identification and documentation of adult malnutrition (undernutrition). *J Parenter Enteral Nutr.* May 2012;36(3):275-283. doi:10.1177/0148607112440285

Etiology (Cause/Contributing Risk Factors)

Factors gathered during the nutrition assessment process that contribute to the existence or the maintenance of pathophysiological, psychosocial, situational, developmental, cultural, and/or environmental problems:

- Physiological causes increasing nutrient needs due to prematurity, genetic/congenital disorders, illness, injury, or trauma
- Inadequate intake related to anorexia or feeding intolerance
- Alteration in gastrointestinal tract structure and/or function
- Altered utilization of nutrients
- Food and nutrition related knowledge deficit concerning amount of energy and amount and type of dietary protein
- Psychological causes, eg, depression or eating disorders
- Limited food and nutrition related skill

Etiology Category

Etiologies are grouped by the type of cause or contributing risk factor. Communicate the etiology category by selecting the appropriate Nutrition Assessment, Monitoring, and Evaluation term.

NCP Term	ANDUID
Beliefs attitudes etiology	14567
Cultural etiology	14568
Knowledge etiology	14569
Physical function etiology	14570
Physiologic metabolic etiology	14571

Continued on next page

Illness Related Pediatric Malnutrition (Undernutrition)

Continued from previous page

NCP Term	ANDUID
Psychological etiology	14572
Social personal etiology	14573
Treatment etiology	14574
Access etiology	14575
Behavior etiology	14576

Visit the Nutrition Diagnosis Etiology Category Identification reference sheet on page 185 for more details on etiology categories. An additional useful resource to determine the etiology category is the Nutrition Diagnosis Matrix on page 528.

Signs/Symptoms (Defining Characteristics)

A typical cluster of subjective and objective signs and symptoms gathered during the nutrition assessment process that provide evidence that a problem exists; quantify the problem and describe its severity.

Nutrition Assessment Category	Potential Indicators of This Nutrition Diagnosis (one or more must be present)
Biochemical Data, Medical Tests and Procedures	
Anthropometric Measurements	When a single data point is available: • Mild malnutrition ○ −1 to −1.9 body weight for length z score ○ −1 to −1.9 body mass index for age z score ○ −1 to −1.9 mid upper arm circumference z score • Moderate malnutrition ○ −2 to −2.9 body weight for length z score ○ −2 to −2.9 body mass index for age z score ○ −2 to −2.9 mid upper arm circumference z score • Severe malnutrition ○ −3 body weight for length z score or below ○ −3 body mass index for age z score or below ○ −3 length/height for age z score or below ○ −3 mid upper arm circumference z score or below *Note: For further information on z score data interpretation refer to: https://apps.who.int/iris/bitstream/handle/10665/43601/9789241595070_C_eng.pdf?sequence=3&isAllowed=y* When two or more data points are available, the following additional indicators may then be assessed: • Mild malnutrition ○ Less than 75% of the norm for expected weight gain velocity (< 2 y of age)

Continued on next page

Illness Related Pediatric Malnutrition (Undernutrition)

Continued from previous page

Nutrition Assessment Category	Potential Indicators of This Nutrition Diagnosis (one or more must be present)
Anthropometric Measurements (continued)	○ 5% usual body weight loss (2 to 20 y of age) ○ Decline of 1 z score in weight for length or BMI for age z score When two or more data points are available, the following additional indicators may then be assessed: • Mild malnutrition ○ Less than 75% of the norm for expected weight gain velocity (< 2 y of age) ○ 5% usual body weight loss (2 to 20 y of age) ○ Decline of 1 z score in weight for length or BMI for age z score • Moderate malnutrition ○ Less than 50 % of the norm for expected weight gain velocity (< 2 y of age) ○ 7.5% usual body weight loss (2 to 20 y of age) ○ Decline of 2 z score in weight for length or BMI for age z score • Severe malnutrition ○ Less than 25% of the norm for expected weight gain velocity (< 2 y of age) ○ 10% usual body weight loss (2 to 20 y of age) ○ Decline of 3 z score in weight for length or BMI for age z score *Note: Proxy measures described in the Academy/ASPEN Pediatric Malnutrition Consensus Statement can be used when typical anthropometric measures cannot be obtained.*
Physical Exam Findings	• Stagnation in Tanner staging Moderate malnutrition • Mild loss of subcutaneous fat, eg, orbital, triceps, fat overlying the ribs • Mild muscle loss, eg, wasting of the temples (temporalis muscle), clavicles (pectoralis and deltoids), shoulders (deltoids), interosseous muscles, scapula (latissimus dorsi, trapezius, deltoids), thigh (quadriceps) and calf (gastrocnemius) • Mild localized or generalized fluid accumulation (extremities, vulvar/scrotal, ascites) Severe malnutrition • Severe loss of subcutaneous fat, eg, orbital, triceps, fat overlying the ribs

Continued on next page

Illness Related Pediatric Malnutrition (Undernutrition)

Continued from previous page

Nutrition Assessment Category	Potential Indicators of This Nutrition Diagnosis (one or more must be present)
Physical Exam Findings (continued)	• Severe muscle loss, eg, wasting of the temples (temporalis muscle), clavicles (pectoralis and deltoids), shoulders (deltoids), interosseous muscles, scapula (latissimus dorsi, trapezius, deltoids), thigh (quadriceps) and calf (gastrocnemius) • Severe localized or generalized fluid accumulation (extremities, vulvar/scrotal, ascites)
Food/Nutrition-Related History (continued)	Reports or observations of change in functional indicators, eg, handgrip strength or other measures of physical activity and/or strength *Note: Handgrip strength in children older than 6 years of age: norms are device dependent; can identify presence of malnutrition but not quantify the degree of the deficit; may not be able to perform on certain clients. Please refer to the Academy/ASPEN Pediatric Malnutrition Consensus Statement for further information.* When two or more data points are available • Mild malnutrition: inadequate nutrient intake of 51% to 75% estimated energy/protein need • Moderate malnutrition: inadequate nutrient intake 26% to 50% estimated energy/protein need • Severe malnutrition: inadequate nutrient intake of ≤ 25% estimated energy/protein need
Client History*	Reports or observations of the following, for example: • Organ failure, malignancies, rheumatoid diseases, gastrointestinal diseases, growth failure, malabsorptive syndromes, and other etiologies including but not limited to congenital birth defects, genetic anomalies such as spinal muscular atrophy • Sepsis, pneumonia, peritonitis, and wound infections, burns, trauma, closed head injury, acute lung injury, respiratory distress syndrome, and surgeries • Existing medical diagnosis of malnutrition • History of prematurity, congenital birth defects (cardiac/renal/gastrointestinal/neurological/pulmonary) • Genetic or acquired conditions: cerebral palsy, cystic fibrosis, seizure disorders, metabolic disease, irritable bowel syndrome • Feeding difficulty, food allergy, eosinophilic enteritis
Assessment, Monitoring, and Evaluation Tools	• Subjective global nutritional assessment (SGNA) for children rating[+] • Subjective global nutritional assessment (SGNA) for children score[+]
Comparative Standards	

In the past, hepatic transport protein measures (eg, albumin and prealbumin) were used as indicators of malnutrition. See the Evidence Analysis Library questions on this topic at (accessed June 3, 2025): www.andeal.org/topic.cfm?cat=4302

** Client History terms are used for Nutrition Assessment but not for Nutrition Monitoring and Evaluation.*

[+] Alternate approaches to interpretation of anthropometric measurements are recommended for children. Therefore, this tool should be used in conjunction with the evidence-based anthropometric measurement assessment criteria.

Illness Related Pediatric Malnutrition (Undernutrition)

Progress Evaluation

Communicate the progress toward the resolution of a nutrition diagnosis by selecting the appropriate nutrition diagnosis status value from the Nutrition Assessment, Monitoring, and Evaluation terms.

NCP Term	ANDUID
New nutrition diagnosis	14586
Active nutrition diagnosis	14587
Resolved nutrition diagnosis	14588
Discontinued nutrition diagnosis	14589

For details on these terms, visit the Nutrition Diagnosis Status reference sheet on page 200.

Food and Nutrition Related Knowledge Deficit*

Definition

Incomplete and/or inaccurate knowledge about food, nutrition, or nutrition related information and guidelines.

Etiology (Cause/Contributing Risk Factors)

Factors gathered during the nutrition assessment process that contribute to the existence or the maintenance of pathophysiological, psychosocial, situational, developmental, cultural, and/or environmental problems:

- Belief finding that hinders food and/or nutrition behavior change
- Attitude finding that hinders food and/or nutrition behavior change
- Limited prior nutrition-related education
- Limited literacy
- Limited numeracy
- Cultural beliefs that may affect access to and receptivity of information
- Impaired cognitive ability, eg, learning disabilities, neurological or sensory impairment, and/or dementia
- Prior exposure to misinformation, disinformation, and/or contradictory information
- Limited prioritization for learning food and nutrition information
- Limited self-efficacy for learning food and nutrition information
- Recent medical diagnosis or change in health or disease status
- Change in life course stage or responsibility for self or others
- Limited access to sources of reliable food and nutrition information

Etiology Category

Etiologies are grouped by the type of cause or contributing risk factor. Communicate the etiology category by selecting the appropriate Nutrition Assessment, Monitoring, and Evaluation term.

NCP Term	ANDUID
Beliefs attitudes etiology	14567
Cultural etiology	14568
Knowledge etiology	14569
Physical function etiology	14570
Physiologic metabolic etiology	14571
Psychological etiology	14572
Social personal etiology	14573
Treatment etiology	14574
Access etiology	14575
Behavior etiology	14576

Visit the Nutrition Diagnosis Etiology Category Identification reference sheet on page 185 for more details on etiology categories. An additional useful resource to determine the etiology category is the Nutrition Diagnosis Matrix on page 528.

* If a synonym for the term "Food and nutrition related knowledge deficit" is helpful or needed, an approved alternate is "Limited food and nutrition related knowledge."

Food and Nutrition Related Knowledge Deficit

Signs/Symptoms (Defining Characteristics)

A typical cluster of subjective and objective signs and symptoms gathered during the nutrition assessment process that provide evidence that a problem exists; quantify the problem and describe its severity.

Nutrition Assessment Category	Potential Indicators of This Nutrition Diagnosis (one or more must be present)
Biochemical Data, Medical Tests and Procedures	Altered laboratory value
Anthropometric Measurements	• Body weight above or below expected body weight • Body weight change • Growth parameters inconsistent with expected
Physical Exam Findings	
Food/Nutrition-Related History	Reports or observations of: • Nutrition knowledge level (none to intermediate) of community, supportive individuals, and/or individual client • No prior awareness of need for food- and nutrition-related information • Nutrition- related education is not considered a priority • Information conflicts with individual client's values • Information conflicts with client's supportive individuals • Information conflicts with client's supportive structures • Information conflicts with client's stakeholder's value system • Limited readiness to change nutrition-related behavior • Presence of limited self-efficacy for learning information • Relates difficulties about previous attempts to learn information • Disinterest in learning information • Low perceived susceptibility of nutrition related health problems score • Low perceived severity of risk to health score • Low perceived benefit of nutrition related change score • High perceived barrier to nutrition related behavior change score • Low food and/or nutrition literacy score • Limited numeracy understanding • Questions relating to nutrition and food • Limited previous food and nutrition education • Limited experience related to food and nutrition need • Limited relevant food and nutrition knowledge • Limited adherence to food and nutrition recommendations • Limited support for behavior change • Cultural belief that may impact engagement in learning information

Continued on next page

Food and Nutrition Related Knowledge Deficit

Continued from previous page

Nutrition Assessment Category	Potential Indicators of This Nutrition Diagnosis (one or more must be present)
Client History*	• Conditions associated with a diagnosis or treatment • New medical diagnosis or change in existing diagnosis or condition • Change in life course stage and responsibilities (eg, transition to independent living, change marital status, becoming parent, loss of spouse) • Socio economic factors that present barriers • Unfavorable social and/or economic conditions of community • Inequities in access to health care or insurance
Assessment, Monitoring, and Evaluation Tools	
Comparative Standards	

** Client History terms are used for Nutrition Assessment but not for Nutrition Monitoring and Evaluation.*

Progress Evaluation

Communicate the progress toward the resolution of a nutrition diagnosis by selecting the appropriate nutrition diagnosis status value from the Nutrition Assessment, Monitoring, and Evaluation terms.

NCP Term	ANDUID
New nutrition diagnosis	14586
Active nutrition diagnosis	14587
Resolved nutrition diagnosis	14588
Discontinued nutrition diagnosis	14589

For details on these terms, visit the Nutrition Diagnosis Status reference sheet on page 200.

Belief Finding That Hinders Food and/or Nutrition Behavior Change

Definition

Belief (an acceptance that something exists or is true) about food, nutrition, and/or nutrition-related topics that impedes food and/or nutrition behavior change (excluding disordered eating patterns and eating disorders).

Etiology (Cause/Contributing Risk Factors)

Factors gathered during the nutrition assessment process that contribute to the existence or the maintenance of pathophysiological, psychosocial, situational, developmental, cultural, and/or environmental problems:

- Exposure to misinformation, disinformation, or contradictory information about the food and/or nutrition behavior
- Perceived risk of a disease
- Perceived benefits of adopting a food and/or nutrition behavior
- Perceived barriers to adopting a food and/or nutrition behavior (eg, personal, social, cultural, environmental, economic)
- Exposure to cues to action to adopt a food and/or nutrition behavior, such as internal cues (eg, experiencing signs or symptoms of illness) or external cues (eg, recommendation of a health care provider, access to food and/or nutrition information)
- Perceived confidence in the ability to perform a food and/or nutrition behavior (self-efficacy)
- Perceived control about adopting the food and/or nutrition behavior (eg, beliefs about what makes it easier or harder to adopt the behavior)
- Perceived norms about the approval or disapproval of the client's food and/or nutrition behavior by supportive individuals (eg, family, caregivers) and/or supportive structures (eg, social service agencies, faith-based organizations) (injunctive norm)
- Belief that supportive individuals (eg, family, caregivers) and/or supportive structures (eg, social service agencies, faith-based organizations) do or do not adopt the food and/or nutrition behavior (descriptive norm)
- Limited motivation to adopt the food and/or nutrition behavior
- Limited literacy
- Limited numeracy

Etiology Category

Etiologies are grouped by the type of cause or contributing risk factor. Communicate the etiology category by selecting the appropriate Nutrition Assessment, Monitoring, and Evaluation term.

NCP Term	ANDUID
Beliefs attitudes etiology	14567
Cultural etiology	14568
Knowledge etiology	14569
Physical function etiology	14570
Physiologic metabolic etiology	14571

Continued on next page

Belief Finding That Hinders Food and/or Nutrition Behavior Change

Continued from previous page

NCP Term	ANDUID
Psychological etiology	14572
Social personal etiology	14573
Treatment etiology	14574
Access etiology	14575
Behavior etiology	14576

Visit the Nutrition Diagnosis Etiology Category Identification reference sheet on page 185 for more details on etiology categories. An additional useful resource to determine the etiology category is the Nutrition Diagnosis Matrix on page 528.

Signs/Symptoms (Defining Characteristics)

A typical cluster of subjective and objective signs and symptoms gathered during the nutrition assessment process that provide evidence that a problem exists; quantify the problem and describe its severity.

Nutrition Assessment Category	Potential Indicators of This Nutrition Diagnosis (one or more must be present)
Biochemical Data, Medical Tests and Procedures	
Anthropometric Measurements	
Physical Exam Findings	
Food/Nutrition-Related History	Reports or observations of: • Estimated intake that reflects an unbalanced diet • Avoiding foods/food groups (eg, sugar, wheat, cooked foods) for which there is limited scientific support about the benefits of avoiding craving for nonfood item • Evidence of nutrition information–seeking behavior • Nutrition priority of individual client inconsistent with identified food and/or nutrition needs • Conflict with individual client's value system present • Conflict with client's supportive individual's value system present • Conflict with client's supportive structures' value system present • Conflict with stakeholder's value system present • Presence of negative nutrition self talk • Absence of positive nutrition self talk • Low perceived susceptibility to nutrition related health problems score • Low perceived severity of risk to health score • High perceived benefit of nutrition related change score when scientific evidence for the client's belief appears limited

Continued on next page

Belief Finding That Hinders Food and/or Nutrition Behavior Change

Continued from previous page

Nutrition Assessment Category	Potential Indicators of This Nutrition Diagnosis (one or more must be present)
Food/Nutrition-Related History (continued)	• Low perceived benefit of nutrition related change score • Low likelihood of performing nutrition related behavior score • Low nutrition self efficacy score • High perceived barrier to nutrition related behavior score • Limited food and/or nutrition knowledge • Low food and/or nutrition literacy score • Limited numeracy understanding • Nutrition related goals that may not be viable • Avoidance of foods and/or social gatherings with food that interferes with quality of life and/or nutrition related concern • Inclusion of foods (eg, coconut oil) in intake that appear inconsistent with science-based evidence • Use of therapies, dietary supplements, or other approaches for which there is limited scientific support about the benefits of their use • Intake of food and/or supplements influenced by cultural factors that appear to have limited scientific support
Client History*	• Conditions associated with a diagnosis or treatment, eg, obesity, diabetes, cancer, cardiovascular disease, mental illness, end of life care • Pica
Assessment, Monitoring, and Evaluation Tools	
Comparative Standards	

** Client History terms are used for Nutrition Assessment but not for Nutrition Monitoring and Evaluation.*

Progress Evaluation

Communicate the progress toward the resolution of a nutrition diagnosis by selecting the appropriate nutrition diagnosis status value from the Nutrition Assessment, Monitoring, and Evaluation terms.

NCP Term	ANDUID
New nutrition diagnosis	14586
Active nutrition diagnosis	14587
Resolved nutrition diagnosis	14588
Discontinued nutrition diagnosis	14589

For details on these terms, visit the Nutrition Diagnosis Status reference sheet on page 200.

Not Ready for Nutrition Related Behavior Change

Definition

Lack of perceived value of nutrition-related behavior change compared to costs (consequences or effort required to make changes); conflict with personal value system; preceding event, condition or cause to behavior change.

Etiology (Cause/Contributing Risk Factors)

Factors gathered during the nutrition assessment process that contribute to the existence or the maintenance of pathophysiological, psychosocial, situational, developmental, cultural, and/or environmental problems:

- Belief finding that hinders food and/or nutrition behavior change
- Attitude finding that hinders food and/or nutrition behavior change
- Limited social support for implementing changes
- Limited cognitive ability, including learning disabilities, neurological or sensory impairment, and/or dementia
- Limited acceptance of need to change
- Perception that time, interpersonal, or financial constraints prevent changes
- Limited interest in learning information
- Limited interest in applying skill
- Limited self-efficacy for making change or demoralization from previous challenges associated with change

Etiology Category

Etiologies are grouped by the type of cause or contributing risk factor. Communicate the etiology category by selecting the appropriate Nutrition Assessment, Monitoring, and Evaluation term.

NCP Term	ANDUID
Beliefs attitudes etiology	14567
Cultural etiology	14568
Knowledge etiology	14569
Physical function etiology	14570
Physiologic metabolic etiology	14571
Psychological etiology	14572
Social personal etiology	14573
Treatment etiology	14574
Access etiology	14575
Behavior etiology	14576

Visit the Nutrition Diagnosis Etiology Category Identification reference sheet on page 185 for more details on etiology categories. An additional useful resource to determine the etiology category is the Nutrition Diagnosis Matrix on page 528.

Not Ready for Nutrition Related Behavior Change

Signs/Symptoms (Defining Characteristics)

A typical cluster of subjective and objective signs and symptoms gathered during the nutrition assessment process that provide evidence that a problem exists; quantify the problem and describe its severity.

Nutrition Assessment Category	Potential Indicators of This Nutrition Diagnosis (one or more must be present)
Biochemical Data, Medical Tests and Procedures	
Anthropometric Measurements	
Physical Exam Findings	Body language that may suggest discomfort with interaction (eg, frowning, crossed arms, limited eye contact) (Note: body language varies by culture)
Food/Nutrition-Related History	Reports or observations of: • Limited acceptance of need for food- and nutrition-related changes • Limited ability to understand required changes • Low nutrition encounter ratio • Precontemplation stage or contemplation stage identified • Previous challenges effectively changing target behavior • Resistance to change • Limited self-efficacy to make change or to overcome barriers to change • Factors affecting physical activity access
Client History*	
Assessment, Monitoring, and Evaluation Tools	
Comparative Standards	

** Client History terms are used for Nutrition Assessment but not for Nutrition Monitoring and Evaluation.*

Progress Evaluation

Communicate the progress toward the resolution of a nutrition diagnosis by selecting the appropriate nutrition diagnosis status value from the Nutrition Assessment, Monitoring, and Evaluation terms.

NCP Term	ANDUID
New nutrition diagnosis	14586
Active nutrition diagnosis	14587
Resolved nutrition diagnosis	14588
Discontinued nutrition diagnosis	14589

For details on these terms, visit the Nutrition Diagnosis Status reference sheet on page 200.

Self Monitoring Deficit*

Definition

Lack of data recording to track personal progress.

Etiology (Cause/Contributing Risk Factors)

Factors gathered during the nutrition assessment process that contribute to the existence or the maintenance of pathophysiological, psychosocial, situational, developmental, cultural, and/or environmental problems:

- Food and nutrition related knowledge deficit concerning self-monitoring
- Limited social support for implementing changes
- Limited value for behavior change or competing values
- Perception that limited resources (eg, time, financial, or interpersonal) prevent self-monitoring
- Cultural practices that affect the ability to track personal progress
- Belief finding that hinders food and/or nutrition behavior change
- Attitude finding that hinders food and/or nutrition behavior change
- Prior exposure to incompatible information
- Impaired cognitive ability, including learning disabilities, neurological or sensory impairment, and/or dementia
- Not ready for nutrition related behavior change
- Limited interest in tracking progress
- Limited focus and attention to detail, difficulty with time management and/or organization
- Limited food and nutrition related skill

Etiology Category

Etiologies are grouped by the type of cause or contributing risk factor. Communicate the etiology category by selecting the appropriate Nutrition Assessment, Monitoring, and Evaluation term.

NCP Term	ANDUID
Beliefs attitudes etiology	14567
Cultural etiology	14568
Knowledge etiology	14569
Physical function etiology	14570
Physiologic metabolic etiology	14571
Psychological etiology	14572
Social personal etiology	14573
Treatment etiology	14574
Access etiology	14575
Behavior etiology	14576

Visit the Nutrition Diagnosis Etiology Category Identification reference sheet on page 185 for more details on etiology categories. An additional useful resource to determine the etiology category is the Nutrition Diagnosis Matrix on page 528.

* If a *synonym* for the term "Self-monitoring deficit" is helpful or needed, an approved alternate is "Limited self-monitoring."

Self Monitoring Deficit

Signs/Symptoms (Defining Characteristics)

A typical cluster of subjective and objective signs and symptoms gathered during the nutrition assessment process that provide evidence that a problem exists; quantify the problem and describe its severity.

Nutrition Assessment Category	Potential Indicators of This Nutrition Diagnosis (one or more must be present)
Biochemical Data, Medical Tests and Procedures	Recorded data inconsistent with biochemical data, eg, estimated dietary intake is not consistent with biochemical data
Anthropometric Measurements	
Physical Exam Findings	
Food/Nutrition-Related History	Reports or observations of: • Incomplete self-monitoring records, eg, glucose, food, fluid intake, weight, physical activity, ostomy output records • Estimated food intake data inconsistent with weight status or growth pattern data • Embarrassment or anger regarding need for self-monitoring • Uncertainty of how to complete monitoring records • Uncertainty regarding changes that could/should be made in response to data in self-monitoring records • No self-management equipment, eg, no blood glucose monitor, pedometer • Verbalizes inaccurate or incomplete knowledge • Cultural or religious practices that affect intake
Client History*	• Diagnoses associated with self-monitoring, eg, diabetes mellitus, obesity, new ostomy • New medical diagnosis or change in existing diagnosis or condition • Limited social and/or familial support
Assessment, Monitoring, and Evaluation Tools	
Comparative Standards	

** Client History terms are used for Nutrition Assessment, but not for Nutrition Monitoring and Evaluation.*

Progress Evaluation

Communicate the progress toward the resolution of a nutrition diagnosis by selecting the appropriate nutrition diagnosis status value from the Nutrition Assessment, Monitoring, and Evaluation terms.

NCP Term	ANDUID
New nutrition diagnosis	14586
Active nutrition diagnosis	14587
Resolved nutrition diagnosis	14588
Discontinued nutrition diagnosis	14589

For details on these terms, visit the Nutrition Diagnosis Status reference sheet on page 200.

Disordered Eating Pattern

Definition

Beliefs, attitudes, thoughts, and behaviors related to food, eating, body composition and weight, including classic eating disorders as well as similar conditions that negatively impact health or quality of life.

Note: May not be an appropriate nutrition diagnosis for individuals with Limited food acceptance.

A resource that may be helpful for classification of eating disorders is the *Diagnostic and Statistical Manual of Mental Disorders*, 5th Edition (DSM-5).

Etiology (Cause/Contributing Risk Factors)

Factors gathered during the nutrition assessment process that contribute to the existence or the maintenance of pathophysiological, psychosocial, situational, developmental, cultural, and/or environmental problems:

- Cultural, societal, biological/genetic, and/or environmental-related fear of weight gain
- Weight regulation/preoccupation
- Obsessive desire to be healthy or have a specific body shape
- Physiological causes that put emphasis on food, weight, or shape
- Psychological causes that put emphasis on food, weight, or shape
- Personality characteristics or temperament associated with eating disorders
- Traumatic event(s) that causes a physical or psychological stress reaction

Etiology Category

Etiologies are grouped by the type of cause or contributing risk factor. Communicate the etiology category by selecting the appropriate Nutrition Assessment, Monitoring, and Evaluation term.

NCP Term	ANDUID
Beliefs attitudes etiology	14567
Cultural etiology	14568
Knowledge etiology	14569
Physical function etiology	14570
Physiologic metabolic etiology	14571
Psychological etiology	14572
Social personal etiology	14573
Treatment etiology	14574
Access etiology	14575
Behavior etiology	14576

Visit the Nutrition Diagnosis Etiology Category Identification reference sheet on page 185 for more details on etiology categories. An additional useful resource to determine the etiology category is the Nutrition Diagnosis Matrix on page 528.

Disordered Eating Pattern

Signs/Symptoms (Defining Characteristics)

A typical cluster of subjective and objective signs and symptoms gathered during the nutrition assessment process that provide evidence that a problem exists; quantify the problem and describe its severity.

Nutrition Assessment Category	Potential Indicators of This Nutrition Diagnosis (one or more must be present)
Biochemical Data, Medical Tests and Procedures	• ↓ or ↑ Cholesterol, abnormal lipid profiles • Hypoglycemia • Hyperglycemia, ↑ HgbA1c • Hypokalemia and hypochloremic alkalosis • Hypophosphatemia • Hypomagnesemia • ↓ Serum vitamin D • Hyponatremia • Hypothyroid • ↑ BUN • ↑ carbon dioxide (CO_2) • Urine positive for ketones • Laboratory data indicating anemia • Abnormal ECG • ↑ LFTs • Hyperosmolarity, hypoosmolarity • Low luteinizing hormone, FSH, estradiol, or testosterone levels • Low bone mineralization findings
Anthropometric Measurements	• BMI < 17.5 • Arrested growth and development • Failure to gain weight according to predicted growth trajectory, weight less than 85% of expected • Significant weight fluctuation • Significant weight loss or significant weight gain • Frequent weighing or measuring of oneself
Physical Exam Findings	• Normal or depleted adipose and somatic protein stores • Cachexia • Lethargy • Lanugo hair formation • Brittle, listless hair • Dry skin • Damaged tooth enamel • Enlarged parotid glands

Continued on next page

Disordered Eating Pattern

Continued from previous page

Nutrition Assessment Category	Potential Indicators of This Nutrition Diagnosis (one or more must be present)
Physical Exam Findings (continued)	• Peripheral and central edema • Skeletal muscle loss • Low body temperature • Inability to concentrate • Reports of always feeling cold • Bradycardia (heart rate < 60 beats/min for adults, < 50 beats/min pediatrics) • Hypotension (systolic blood pressure < 90 mm HG) • Orthostatic hypotension • Postural tachycardia • Cyanosis of hands and feet • Delayed capillary refill • Self-induced vomiting • Positive Russell's sign, callous on back of hand from self-induced vomiting • Gastroesophageal reflux disease • Diarrhea • Bloating, flatulence • Constipation • Blood in vomit • Blood in stool • Muscle weakness • Muscle or joint pain • Dry mucus membranes • Absence of hunger cues • Acanthosis nigricans • Amenorrhea or disruption of menstrual cycle • Delay in sexual development and/or puberty
Food/Nutrition-Related History	Reports or observations of: • Body image disturbance • Limited recognition of low body weight • Self-evaluation is based upon body shape and/or weight • Avoidance of food or energy-containing beverages • Avoidance of social events at which food is served • Fear of foods or dysfunctional thoughts regarding food or food experiences • Food and weight preoccupation

Continued on next page

Disordered Eating Pattern

Continued from previous page

Nutrition Assessment Category	Potential Indicators of This Nutrition Diagnosis (one or more must be present)
Food/Nutrition-Related History (continued)	• Conflict with individual client value system • Conflict with client's supportive individuals value system • Preoccupation with energy or nutrient content of foods • Avoidance of specific food textures or consistencies • Knowledgeable about current diet fads • Fasting for long periods of time during typical eating hours • Estimated intake of larger quantity of food in a defined time period, a sense of limited control over eating • Ritualized eating behavior • Excessive physical activity • Eating much more rapidly than normal, until feeling uncomfortably full • Consuming large amounts of food when not feeling physically hungry • Eating more slowly than usual to delay eating • Hiding food • Distorted perception of appropriate amounts to eat • Eating alone because of embarrassment • Eats in private • Feeling unpleasant emotions after eating, such as guilt, disgust, shame, anger, or depression • Pattern of chronic dieting • Previous food restriction (intentional or unintentional) • Recent change in food or nutrient intake pattern • Excessive reliance on nutrition terming, including placing labels on foods that rank the superiority of one food over another • Inflexibility with food selection • Use of laxatives, enemas, diuretics, stimulants, metabolic enhancers, medications, performance enhancing products • In clients with diabetes, purposeful omission of insulin • Night eating • Perceived control around nutrition intake through calorie counting, macronutrient monitoring, record keeping • Chewing and spitting of food • Persistent behavior that interferes with weight gain • Persistent use of a mirror • Excessive time spent sourcing food • Excessive time spent preparing food • Avoidance of food deemed to be too processed or unhealthy • Excessive use of condiments and food mixing

Continued on next page

Disordered Eating Pattern

Continued from previous page

Nutrition Assessment Category	Potential Indicators of This Nutrition Diagnosis (one or more must be present)
Client History*	• Diagnosis, eg, anorexia nervosa, bulimia nervosa, binge eating disorder, other specified feeding or eating disorder • History of mental health condition, depression, anxiety, OCD, personality disorders, substance abuse disorders, self-injury • Family history of mental health condition, eating disorder, depression, OCD, anxiety disorders • Osteoporosis, osteopenia • Social isolation • Sexual abuse • Previous traumatic event(s) • Infertility • Gall bladder disease • Competitive or professional athlete • Bariatric surgery • Cardiac arrhythmias, bradycardia
Assessment, Monitoring, and Evaluation Tools	
Comparative Standards	

Arrows used with laboratory values: ↑ represents above reference standard and ↓ represents below reference standard.
** Client History terms are used for Nutrition Assessment but not for Nutrition Monitoring and Evaluation.*

Progress Evaluation

Communicate the progress toward the resolution of a nutrition diagnosis by selecting the appropriate nutrition diagnosis status value from the Nutrition Assessment, Monitoring, and Evaluation terms.

NCP Term	ANDUID
New nutrition diagnosis	14586
Active nutrition diagnosis	14587
Resolved nutrition diagnosis	14588
Discontinued nutrition diagnosis	14589

For details on these terms, visit the Nutrition Diagnosis Status reference sheet on page 200.

Limited Adherence to Nutrition Related Recommendations

Definition

Lack of nutrition related changes as per intervention agreed on by client.

Etiology (Cause/Contributing Risk Factors)

Factors gathered during the nutrition assessment process that contribute to the existence or the maintenance of pathophysiological, psychosocial, situational, developmental, cultural, and/or environmental problems:

- Limited social support for implementing changes
- Limited value for behavior change or competing values
- Limited confidence in ability to change
- Perception that limited resources (eg, time, financial, or interpersonal) prevent changes
- Previous limited success in making health-related changes
- Food and nutrition related knowledge deficit concerning how to make nutrition related changes
- Limited interest in applying/learning information
- Belief finding that hinders food and/or nutrition behavior change
- Attitude finding that hinders food and/or nutrition behavior change
- Limited food and nutrition related skill

Etiology Category

Etiologies are grouped by the type of cause or contributing risk factor. Communicate the etiology category by selecting the appropriate Nutrition Assessment, Monitoring, and Evaluation term.

NCP Term	ANDUID
Beliefs attitudes etiology	14567
Cultural etiology	14568
Knowledge etiology	14569
Physical function etiology	14570
Physiologic metabolic etiology	14571
Psychological etiology	14572
Social personal etiology	14573
Treatment etiology	14574
Access etiology	14575
Behavior etiology	14576

Visit the Nutrition Diagnosis Etiology Category Identification reference sheet on page 185 for more details on etiology categories. An additional useful resource to determine the etiology category is the Nutrition Diagnosis Matrix on page 528.

Limited Adherence to Nutrition Related Recommendations

Signs/Symptoms(Defining Characteristics)

A typical cluster of subjective and objective signs and symptoms gathered during the nutrition assessment process that provide evidence that a problem exists; quantify the problem and describe its severity.

Nutrition Assessment Category	Potential Indicators of This Nutrition Diagnosis (one or more must be present)
Biochemical Data, Medical Tests and Procedures	Expected laboratory outcomes are not achieved
Anthropometric Measurements	Expected anthropometric outcomes are not achieved
Physical Exam Findings	Negative body language, eg, frowning, limited eye contact, fidgeting, defensive posture, crying (Note: body language varies by culture)
Food/Nutrition-Related History	Reports or observations of: • Expected food/nutrition-related outcomes are not achieved • Limited ability to recall changes agreed upon • Limited adherence completing any agreed upon homework • Limited or inconsistent adherence with plan • Challenges keeping appointments or scheduling follow-up appointments • Limited understanding of the importance of making recommended nutrition-related changes • Uncertainty as to how to consistently apply food/nutrition information • Verbalizes frustration with attempts to apply food/nutrition information • Verbalizes previous challenges effectively changing target behavior • Presence of a limited self-efficacy or confidence to make changes • Notes internal and/or external barriers to change
Client History*	Limited social and/or familial support
Assessment, Monitoring, and Evaluation Tools	
Comparative Standards	

** Client History terms are used for Nutrition Assessment but not for Nutrition Monitoring and Evaluation.*

Progress Evaluation

Communicate the progress toward the resolution of a nutrition diagnosis by selecting the appropriate nutrition diagnosis status value from the Nutrition Assessment, Monitoring, and Evaluation terms.

NCP Term	ANDUID
New nutrition diagnosis	14586
Active nutrition diagnosis	14587
Resolved nutrition diagnosis	14588
Discontinued nutrition diagnosis	14589

For details on these terms, visit the Nutrition Diagnosis Status reference sheet on page 200.

Limited Food Acceptance

Definition

Response to food (ie, solid, liquid) that unfavorably impacts ability to meet nutrition needs through intake.

Note: May not be an appropriate nutrition diagnosis for individuals with anorexia nervosa, bulimia nervosa, binge eating disorder, or other eating disorder. Please consider using Disordered Eating Pattern.

Etiology (Cause/Contributing Risk Factors)

Factors gathered during the nutrition assessment process that contribute to the existence or the maintenance of pathophysiological, psychosocial, situational, developmental, cultural, and/or environmental problems:

- Physiological causes, eg, pain, discomfort, or functional issues in the GI tract, developmental delay, neurological disorders, side effect of treatment
- Aversion to food (ie, solid, liquid)
- Self-limitation of foods/food groups
- Behavioral issues including caregiver issues and eating behavior that serves a purpose other than nourishment
- Belief findings that hinder food and/or nutrition behavior change
- Attitude findings that hinder food and/or nutrition behavior change
- Food allergy, food intolerance
- Limited motivation and/or readiness to apply or support systems change
- Limited interest in learning information and/or applying skills
- Cultural belief that contributes to limited food acceptance

Etiology Category

Etiologies are grouped by the type of cause or contributing risk factor. Communicate the etiology category by selecting the appropriate Nutrition Assessment, Monitoring, and Evaluation term.

NCP Term	ANDUID
Beliefs attitudes etiology	14567
Cultural etiology	14568
Knowledge etiology	14569
Physical function etiology	14570
Physiologic metabolic etiology	14571
Psychological etiology	14572
Social personal etiology	14573
Treatment etiology	14574
Access etiology	14575
Behavior etiology	14576

Visit the Nutrition Diagnosis Etiology Category Identification reference sheet on page 185 for more details on etiology categories. An additional useful resource to determine the etiology category is the Nutrition Diagnosis Matrix on page 528.

Limited Food Acceptance

Signs/Symptoms (Defining Characteristics)

A typical cluster of subjective and objective signs and symptoms gathered during the nutrition assessment process that provide evidence that a problem exists; quantify the problem and describe its severity.

Nutrition Assessment Category	Potential Indicators of This Nutrition Diagnosis (one or more must be present)
Biochemical Data, Medical Tests and Procedures	↑ and/or ↓ micronutrient levels
Anthropometric Measurements	Body weight loss, insufficient growth velocity, body weight gain due
Physical Exam Findings	• Clinical evidence of vitamin/mineral deficiency • Erratic appetite
Food/Nutrition-Related History	Reports or observations of: • Limited food (ie, solid, liquid) intake consistent with nutrition reference standards for type, variety, diet quality • Less than optimal reliance on foods, food groups, supplements, or nutrition support • Negative emotions about food and nutrition • Shortened meal duration • Low percentage of typical eating occasion spent consuming food • Refusing food • Limited readiness to consume new food • Sensory aversion to food • Aversion to particular food • Aversion to particular beverage • Distracted during eating • Limited readiness to change nutrition related behavior score • Precontemplation state for readiness to change
Client History*	Conditions associated with a diagnosis or treatment that might contribute to limited food acceptance
Assessment, Monitoring, and Evaluation Tools	Low minimum dietary diversity for women (MDD-W) score
Comparative Standards	• Ideal/reference body weight (IBW) • Recommended body mass index (BMI) • Goal body weight • Goal body weight for length *z* score • Goal body mass index (BMI) for age *z* score • Percent median body mass index (BMI)

** Client History terms are used for Nutrition Assessment but not for Nutrition Monitoring and Evaluation.*

Limited Food Acceptance

Progress Evaluation

Communicate the progress toward the resolution of a nutrition diagnosis by selecting the appropriate nutrition diagnosis status value from the Nutrition Assessment, Monitoring, and Evaluation terms.

NCP Term	ANDUID
New nutrition diagnosis	14586
Active nutrition diagnosis	14587
Resolved nutrition diagnosis	14588
Discontinued nutrition diagnosis	14589

For details on these terms, visit the Nutrition Diagnosis Status reference sheet on page 200.

Limited Food and Nutrition Related Skill

Definition

Incomplete ability to perform food, nutrition, or nutrition related activities.

Etiology (Cause/Contributing Risk Factors)

Factors gathered during the nutrition assessment process that contribute to the existence or the maintenance of pathophysiological, psychosocial, situational, developmental, cultural, and/or environmental problems:

- Limited food and nutrition literacy
- Limited numeracy
- Limited prior food and nutrition skill education
- Limited prior application of food and nutrition skill
- Limited cognitive ability, eg, learning disabilities, neurological or sensory impairment, and/or dementia
- Limited emotional ability
- Impaired psychological ability
- Limited physical ability
- New skill requirement due to recent medical diagnosis or change in health or disease status
- New skill requirement due to change in life course stage or responsibility for self or others
- Limited prioritization of applying food and nutrition information
- Limited self-efficacy for acquiring or performing the skill
- Belief finding that hinders food and/or nutrition behavior change
- Attitude finding that hinders food and/or nutrition behavior change
- Limited access to resources (eg, food, supplies, equipment, money) to support skill acquisition
- Limited support system for developing and performing skill
- Limited training availability
- Cultural beliefs that may affect access to and receptivity to acquire and perform skill
- Limited ability to prepare food for eating

Signs/Symptoms (Defining Characteristics)

A typical cluster of subjective and objective signs and symptoms gathered during the nutrition assessment process that provide evidence that a problem exists; quantify the problem and describe its severity.

Nutrition Assessment Category	Potential Indicators of This Nutrition Diagnosis (one or more must be present)
Biochemical Data, Medical Tests and Procedures	Altered lab value
Anthropometric Measurements	Weight above or below expected weight, weight change, growth parameters below expected
Physical Exam Findings	

Continued on next page

Limited Food and Nutrition Related Skill

Continued from previous page

Nutrition Assessment Category	Potential Indicators of This Nutrition Diagnosis (one or more must be present)
Food/Nutrition-Related History	Reports or observations of: • Nutrition skill level (none to intermediate) of community, supportive individuals, and/or individual client eg, self-monitoring, self-management, nutrition support care and/or administration, select food consistent with goals, identify food energy sources, choose between food options • Inaccurate or incomplete responses to evaluation of food and nutrition related skill • Nutrition skill education and/or application of the skill is not considered a priority • Low food and/or nutrition literacy score • Limited numeracy skills ability • Limited readiness to change nutrition related skill behavior • Limited self-efficacy for learning new skill • Concern about previous attempts to learn and/or perform skill • Disinterest in learning and/or performing skill • Low perceived susceptibility of nutrition related health problems score • Low perceived severity of risk to health score • Low perceived benefit of nutrition related change score • High perceived barrier to nutrition related behavior change score • Food or nutrient intake not meeting needs • Limited experience related to food and nutrition need • Limited previous food and nutrition education and/or skill education • Limited relevant food and nutrition knowledge • Limited relevant food and nutrition skill • Limited support for skill behavior change • Limited participation in food and nutrition programs and services • Limited resources (eg, food, supplies, equipment) • Limited physical ability affecting food and meal preparation • Limited cognitive ability to develop and perform skill • Limited emotional and/or psychological ability to develop and perform skill
Client History*	• Conditions associated with a diagnosis or treatment • New medical diagnosis or change in existing diagnosis or condition • Change in life-course stage and responsibilities (eg, transition to independent living, change marital status, becoming parent, loss of spouse)

Continued on next page

Limited Food and Nutrition Related Skill

Continued from previous page

Nutrition Assessment Category	Potential Indicators of This Nutrition Diagnosis (one or more must be present)
Client History* (continued)	• Socioeconomic factors that present barriers to developing and performing skill • Unfavorable social and/or economic conditions of community • Inequities in access to health care or insurance • Cultural belief that may impact developing and performing food and nutrition skill
Assessment, Monitoring, and Evaluation Tools	
Comparative Standards	

Attitude Finding That Hinders Food and/or Nutrition Behavior Change

Definition

A way of thinking or feeling about food, nutrition, or nutrition-related behavior (may be favorable/positive, unfavorable/negative, or neutral) that impedes food and/or nutrition behavior change (excluding disordered eating patterns and eating disorders).

Etiology (Cause/Contributing Risk Factors)

Factors gathered during the nutrition assessment process that contribute to the existence or the maintenance of pathophysiological, psychosocial, situational, developmental, cultural, and/or environmental problems:

- Emotional response to adopting the food and/or nutrition behavior (how the client feels about the behavior, such as feeling anger, sadness, fear, ambivalence)
- Beliefs about the outcome of adopting the food and/or nutrition behavior (what the client perceives as the plusses or minuses of the behavioral outcome, such as weight loss or weight gain)

Etiology Category

Etiologies are grouped by the type of cause or contributing risk factor. Communicate the etiology category by selecting the appropriate Nutrition Assessment, Monitoring, and Evaluation term.

NCP Term	ANDUID
Beliefs attitudes etiology	14567
Cultural etiology	14568
Knowledge etiology	14569
Physical function etiology	14570
Physiologic metabolic etiology	14571
Psychological etiology	14572
Social personal etiology	14573
Treatment etiology	14574
Access etiology	14575
Behavior etiology	14576

Visit the Nutrition Diagnosis Etiology Category Identification reference sheet on page 185 for more details on etiology categories. An additional useful resource to determine the etiology category is the Nutrition Diagnosis Matrix on page 528.

Signs/Symptoms (Defining Characteristics)

A typical cluster of subjective and objective signs and symptoms gathered during the nutrition assessment process that provide evidence that a problem exists; quantify the problem and describe its severity. (See the next page for the nutrition assessment category and potential indicators.)

Attitude Finding That Hinders Food and/or Nutrition Behavior Change

Nutrition Assessment Category	Potential Indicators of This Nutrition Diagnosis (one or more must be present)
Biochemical Data, Medical Tests and Procedures	
Anthropometric Measurements	
Physical Exam Findings	
Food/Nutrition-Related History	Reports or observations of: • Evidence of nutrition information–seeking behavior • Nutrition-related goals that may not be viable • Low perceived susceptibility to nutrition related health problems score • Low perceived severity of risk to health score • Low likelihood of performing nutrition related behavior score • Low nutrition self efficacy score • High perceived barrier to nutrition related behavior score • Estimated intake that reflects unbalanced diet • Nutrition attitudes about use of complementary and alternative medicine, dietary supplements, or other approaches • Avoidance of foods/food groups that interfere with quality of life • Low food and/or nutrition literacy score • Limited numeracy understanding • Conflict with individual client's value system present • Conflict with client's supportive individual's value system present • Conflict with client's supportive structures' value system present • Conflict with stakeholder's value system present • Presence of negative nutrition self talk • Absence of positive nutrition self talk
Client History*	• Conditions associated with a diagnosis or treatment, eg, obesity, diabetes, cancer, cardiovascular disease, mental illness • Expression of diminished quality of life
Assessment, Monitoring, and Evaluation Tools	
Comparative Standards	

** Client History terms are used for Nutrition Assessment but not for Nutrition Monitoring and Evaluation.*

Attitude Finding That Hinders Food and/or Nutrition Behavior Change

Progress Evaluation

Communicate the progress toward the resolution of a nutrition diagnosis by selecting the appropriate nutrition diagnosis status value from the Nutrition Assessment, Monitoring, and Evaluation terms.

NCP Term	ANDUID
New nutrition diagnosis	14586
Active nutrition diagnosis	14587
Resolved nutrition diagnosis	14588
Discontinued nutrition diagnosis	14589

For details on these terms, visit the Nutrition Diagnosis Status reference sheet on page 200.

Physical Inactivity*

Definition

Low level of activity or sedentary behavior to the extent that it reduces energy expenditure and impacts health.

Etiology (Cause/Contributing Risk Factors)

Factors gathered during the nutrition assessment process that contribute to the existence or the maintenance of pathophysiological, psychosocial, situational, developmental, cultural, and/or environmental problems:

- Belief finding that hinders food and/or nutrition behavior change
- Attitude finding that hinders food and/or nutrition behavior change
- Injury, lifestyle change, condition (eg, advanced stages of cardiovascular disease, obesity, kidney disease), physical disability, or limitation that reduces physical activity or activities of daily living
- Food and nutrition related knowledge deficit concerning health benefits of physical activity
- Limited prior exposure to accurate nutrition-related information
- Limited role models, eg, for children
- Limited social support for implementing changes
- Limited or limited access to safe exercise environment and/or equipment
- Limited value for behavior change or competing values
- Time constraints
- Financial constraints that may prevent sufficient level of activity (eg, cost of equipment or shoes or club membership to gain access)

Etiology Category

Etiologies are grouped by the type of cause or contributing risk factor. Communicate the etiology category by selecting the appropriate Nutrition Assessment, Monitoring, and Evaluation term.

NCP Term	ANDUID
Beliefs attitudes etiology	14567
Cultural etiology	14568
Knowledge etiology	14569
Physical function etiology	14570
Physiologic metabolic etiology	14571
Psychological etiology	14572
Social personal etiology	14573
Treatment etiology	14574
Access etiology	14575
Behavior etiology	14576

Visit the Nutrition Diagnosis Etiology Category Identification reference sheet on page 185 for more details on etiology categories. An additional useful resource to determine the etiology category is the Nutrition Diagnosis Matrix on page 528.

* If a *synonym* for the term "Physical inactivity" is helpful or needed, an approved alternate is "Limited physical activity."

Physical Inactivity

Signs/Symptoms (Defining Characteristics)

A typical cluster of subjective and objective signs and symptoms gathered during the nutrition assessment process that provide evidence that a problem exists; quantify the problem and describe its severity.

Nutrition Assessment Category	Potential Indicators of This Nutrition Diagnosis (one or more must be present)
Biochemical Data, Medical Tests and Procedures	
Anthropometric Measurements	Obesity: BMI > 30 (adults), BMI > 95th percentile (pediatrics > 3 years)
Physical Exam Findings	Excessive subcutaneous fat and low muscle mass
Food/Nutrition-Related History	Reports or observations of: • Infrequent, low-duration, and/or low-intensity physical activity • Large amounts of sedentary activities, eg, TV watching, reading, computer use in both leisure and work/school • Low level of NEAT (non-exercise activity thermogenesis) expended by physical activities other than planned exercise, eg, sitting, standing, walking, fidgeting • Low cardiorespiratory fitness and/or low muscle strength • Medications that cause somnolence and decreased cognition • Factors affecting physical activity access
Client History*	• Medical diagnoses that may be associated with or result in decreased activity, eg, arthritis, chronic fatigue syndrome, morbid obesity, knee surgery • Psychological diagnosis, eg, depression, anxiety disorders
Assessment, Monitoring, and Evaluation Tools	
Comparative Standards	

** Client History terms are used for Nutrition Assessment but not for Nutrition Monitoring and Evaluation.*

Progress Evaluation

Communicate the progress toward the resolution of a nutrition diagnosis by selecting the appropriate nutrition diagnosis status value from the Nutrition Assessment, Monitoring, and Evaluation terms.

NCP Term	ANDUID
New nutrition diagnosis	14586
Active nutrition diagnosis	14587
Resolved nutrition diagnosis	14588
Discontinued nutrition diagnosis	14589

For details on these terms, visit the Nutrition Diagnosis Status reference sheet on page 200.

Excessive Physical Activity

Definition

Involuntary or voluntary physical activity or movement that interferes with energy needs, growth, or exceeds that which is necessary to achieve optimal health.

Etiology (Cause/Contributing Risk Factors)

Factors gathered during the nutrition assessment process that contribute to the existence or the maintenance of pathophysiological, psychosocial, situational, developmental, cultural, and/or environmental problems:

- Disordered eating
- Irrational beliefs/attitudes about food, nutrition, and fitness
- "Addictive" behaviors/personality

Etiology Category

Etiologies are grouped by the type of cause or contributing risk factor. Communicate the etiology category by selecting the appropriate Nutrition Assessment, Monitoring, and Evaluation term.

NCP Term	ANDUID
Beliefs attitudes etiology	14567
Cultural etiology	14568
Knowledge etiology	14569
Physical function etiology	14570
Physiologic metabolic etiology	14571
Psychological etiology	14572
Social personal etiology	14573
Treatment etiology	14574
Access etiology	14575
Behavior etiology	14576

Visit the Nutrition Diagnosis Etiology Category Identification reference sheet on page 185 for more details on etiology categories. An additional useful resource to determine the etiology category is the Nutrition Diagnosis Matrix on page 528.

Signs/Symptoms (Defining Characteristics)

A typical cluster of subjective and objective signs and symptoms gathered during the nutrition assessment process that provide evidence that a problem exists; quantify the problem and describe its severity.

Nutrition Assessment Category	Potential Indicators of This Nutrition Diagnosis (one or more must be present)
Biochemical Data, Medical Tests and Procedures	• ↑ Liver enzymes, eg, LDH, AST • Altered micronutrient status, eg, ↓ serum ferritin, zinc, and inslin-like growth factor-binding protein (IGFBP) • ↑ Hematocrit • Possibly ↑ cortisol levels

Continued on next page

Excessive Physical Activity

Continued from previous page

Nutrition Assessment Category	Potential Indicators of This Nutrition Diagnosis (one or more must be present)
Anthropometric Measurements	• Weight loss, arrested growth and development, failure to gain weight during period of expected growth (related usually to disordered eating)
Physical Exam Findings	• Depleted adipose and somatic protein stores (related usually to disordered eating) • Chronic muscle soreness
Food/Nutrition-Related History	Reports or observations of: • Continued/repeated high levels of exercise exceeding levels necessary to improve health and/or athletic performance • Exercise daily without rest/rehabilitation days • Exercise while injured/sick • Forsaking family, job, social responsibilities to exercise • Overtraining
Client History*	• Conditions associated with a diagnosis or treatment, eg, anorexia nervosa, bulimia nervosa, binge eating, eating disorder not otherwise specified, amenorrhea, stress fractures • Chronic fatigue • Evidence of addictive, obsessive, or compulsive tendencies • Suppressed immune function • Frequent and/or prolonged injuries and/or illnesses
Assessment, Monitoring, and Evaluation Tools	
Comparative Standards	

Arrows used with laboratory values: ↑ represents above reference standard and ↓ represents below reference standard.
** Client History terms are used for Nutrition Assessment but not for Nutrition Monitoring and Evaluation.*

Progress Evaluation

Communicate the progress toward the resolution of a nutrition diagnosis by selecting the appropriate nutrition diagnosis status value from the Nutrition Assessment, Monitoring, and Evaluation terms.

NCP Term	ANDUID
New nutrition diagnosis	14586
Active nutrition diagnosis	14587
Resolved nutrition diagnosis	14588
Discontinued nutrition diagnosis	14589

For details on these terms, visit the Nutrition Diagnosis Status reference sheet on page 200.

Inability to Manage Self Care*

Definition

Limited of capacity or willingness to implement methods to support healthful food and nutrition related behavior.

Etiology (Cause/Contributing Risk Factors)

Factors gathered during the nutrition assessment process that contribute to the existence or the maintenance of pathophysiological, psychosocial, situational, developmental, cultural, and/or environmental problems:

- Food and nutrition related knowledge deficit concerning self care
- Limited social support for implementing changes
- Limited developmental readiness to perform self management tasks, eg, pediatrics
- Limited value for behavior change or competing values
- Perception that limited resources (eg, time, financial, or interpersonal) prevent self care
- Cultural practices that affect ability to manage self care
- Belief finding that hinders food and/or nutrition behavior
- Attitude finding that hinders food and/or nutrition behavior change
- Impaired cognitive ability, including learning disabilities, neurological or sensory impairment, and/or dementia
- Prior exposure to incompatible information
- Not ready for nutrition related behavior change
- Limited interest in learning information and/or applying skills
- Limited access to self management tools or decision guides

Etiology Category

Etiologies are grouped by the type of cause or contributing risk factor. Communicate the etiology category by selecting the appropriate Nutrition Assessment, Monitoring and Evaluation term.

NCP Term	ANDUID
Beliefs attitudes etiology	14567
Cultural etiology	14568
Knowledge etiology	14569
Physical function etiology	14570
Physiologic metabolic etiology	14571
Psychological etiology	14572
Social personal etiology	14573
Treatment etiology	14574
Access etiology	14575
Behavior etiology	14576

Visit the Nutrition Diagnosis Etiology Category Identification reference sheet on page 185 for more details on etiology categories. An additional useful resource to determine the etiology category is the Nutrition Diagnosis Matrix on page 528.

* If a synonym for the term "Inability to manage self care" is helpful or needed, an approved alternate is "Limited ability to manage self care."

Inability to Manage Self Care

Signs/Symptoms (Defining Characteristics)

A typical cluster of subjective and objective signs and symptoms gathered during the nutrition assessment process that provide evidence that a problem exists; quantify the problem and describe its severity.

Nutrition Assessment Category	Potential Indicators of This Nutrition Diagnosis (one or more must be present)
Biochemical Data, Medical Tests and Procedures	
Anthropometric Measurements	
Physical Exam Findings	
Food/Nutrition-Related History	Reports or observations of: • Limited ability to interpret data or self management tools • Embarrassment or anger regarding need for self monitoring • Uncertainty regarding changes could/should be made in response to data in self monitoring records
Client History*	• Diagnoses that are associated with self management, eg, diabetes mellitus, obesity, cardiovascular disease, renal or liver disease • Conditions associated with a diagnosis or treatment, eg, cognitive or emotional impairment • New medical diagnosis or change in existing diagnosis or condition
Assessment, Monitoring, and Evaluation Tools	
Comparative Standards	

** Client History terms are used for Nutrition Assessment, but not for Nutrition Monitoring and Evaluation.*

Progress Evaluation

Communicate the progress toward the resolution of a nutrition diagnosis by selecting the appropriate nutrition diagnosis status value from the Nutrition Assessment, Monitoring, and Evaluation terms.

NCP Term	ANDUID
New nutrition diagnosis	14586
Active nutrition diagnosis	14587
Resolved nutrition diagnosis	14588
Discontinued nutrition diagnosis	14589

For details on these terms, visit the Nutrition Diagnosis Status reference sheet on page 200.

Limited Ability to Prepare Food for Eating

Definition

Limitation that hinders preparation of food (ie, solid and/or liquid food) for consumption.

Etiology (Cause/Contributing Risk Factors)

Factors gathered during the nutrition assessment process that contribute to the existence or the maintenance of pathophysiological, psychosocial, situational, developmental, cultural, and/or environmental problems:

- Limited cognitive ability, eg, learning differences, neurological or sensory impairment, brain injury and/or dementia
- Limited physical ability
- High level of fatigue or other side effects of therapy
- Food and nutrition related knowledge deficit
- Limited food and nutrition related skill

Etiology Category

Etiologies are grouped by the type of cause or contributing risk factor. Communicate the etiology category by selecting the appropriate Nutrition Assessment, Monitoring, and Evaluation term.

NCP Term	ANDUID
Beliefs attitudes etiology	14567
Cultural etiology	14568
Knowledge etiology	14569
Physical function etiology	14570
Physiologic metabolic etiology	14571
Psychological etiology	14572
Social personal etiology	14573
Treatment etiology	14574
Access etiology	14575
Behavior etiology	14576

Visit the Nutrition Diagnosis Etiology Category Identification reference sheet on page 185 for more details on etiology categories. An additional useful resource to determine the etiology category is the Nutrition Diagnosis Matrix on page 528.

Signs/Symptoms (Defining Characteristics)

A typical cluster of subjective and objective signs and symptoms gathered during the nutrition assessment process that provide evidence that a problem exists; quantify the problem and describe its severity.

Nutrition Assessment Category	Potential Indicators of This Nutrition Diagnosis (one or more must be present)
Biochemical Data, Medical Tests and Procedures	

Continued on next page

Limited Ability to Prepare Food for Eating

Continued from previous page

Nutrition Assessment Category	Potential Indicators of This Nutrition Diagnosis (one or more must be present)
Anthropometric Measurements	
Physical Exam Findings	• Lethargic • Muscle atrophy • Muscle weakness
Food/Nutrition-Related History	Reports or observations of: • Decreased overall estimated intake • Processed food intake, pre-prepared meal intake, and quick-service food intake that results in a limited ability to adhere to nutrition prescription • Uncertainty regarding foods to prepare based on nutrition prescription • Confusion regarding food preparation activities • Limited ability to procure and transport foods to one's place of residence • Low muscle strength • Low handgrip strength • Limited food and nutrition literacy • Limited food preparation ability • Limited ability to open and close containers
Client History*	Conditions associated with a diagnosis or treatment, eg, cognitive impairment, cerebral palsy, paraplegia, vision problems, rigorous therapy regimen, recent surgery, arthritis, autism, traumatic brain injury, chronic obstructive pulmonary disease, shortness of breath
Assessment, Monitoring, and Evaluation Tools	
Comparative Standards	

** Client History terms are used for Nutrition Assessment but not for Nutrition Monitoring and Evaluation.*

Progress Evaluation

Communicate the progress toward the resolution of a nutrition diagnosis by selecting the appropriate nutrition diagnosis status value from the Nutrition Assessment, Monitoring, and Evaluation terms.

NCP Term	ANDUID
New nutrition diagnosis	14586
Active nutrition diagnosis	14587
Resolved nutrition diagnosis	14588
Discontinued nutrition diagnosis	14589

For details on these terms, visit the Nutrition Diagnosis Status reference sheet on page 200.

Poor Food and/or Nutrition Quality of Life

Definition

Diminished client perception of quality of life in response to food and/or nutrition.

Etiology (Cause/Contributing Risk Factors)

Factors gathered during the nutrition assessment process that contribute to the existence or the maintenance of pathophysiological, psychosocial, situational, developmental, cultural, and/or environmental problems:

- Food and nutrition knowledge related deficit
- Not ready for nutrition related behavior change
- Belief finding that hinders food and/or nutrition behavior change
- Attitude finding that hinders food and/or nutrition behavior change
- Perceived and/or actual negative impact of current or previous MNT
- Limited self-efficacy
- Altered body image
- Food insecurity
- Lack of social support for implementing changes
- Limited food and nutrition related skill

Etiology Category

Etiologies are grouped by the type of cause or contributing risk factor. Communicate the etiology category by selecting the appropriate Nutrition Assessment, Monitoring, and Evaluation term.

NCP Term	ANDUID
Beliefs attitudes etiology	14567
Cultural etiology	14568
Knowledge etiology	14569
Physical function etiology	14570
Physiologic metabolic etiology	14571
Psychological etiology	14572
Social personal etiology	14573
Treatment etiology	14574
Access etiology	14575
Behavior etiology	14576

Visit the Nutrition Diagnosis Etiology Category Identification reference sheet on page 185 for more details on etiology categories. An additional useful resource to determine the etiology category is the Nutrition Diagnosis Matrix on page 528.

Signs/Symptoms (Defining Characteristics)

A typical cluster of subjective and objective signs and symptoms gathered during the nutrition assessment process that provide evidence that a problem exists; quantify the problem and describe its severity.

Poor Food and/or Nutrition Quality of Life

Nutrition Assessment Category	Potential Indicators of This Nutrition Diagnosis (one or more must be present)
Biochemical Data, Medical Tests and Procedures	
Anthropometric Measurements	
Physical Exam Findings	
Food/Nutrition-Related History	Reports or observations of: • Unfavorable food and/or nutrition quality of life response • Food and/or nutrition related concern with impact on quality of life • Unfavorable client-reported experience measure • Unfavorable client-reported outcome measure • Decreased confidence (self-efficacy) implementing food and/or nutrition plan • Food insecurity
Client History*	• New medical diagnosis or change in existing diagnosis or condition contributing to diminished quality of life • Recent lifestyle or life changes, eg, quit smoking, initiated exercise, work change, home relocation • Limited social and familial support • Limited access to economic resources (eg, underemployment, low wages, high cost of health care
Assessment, Monitoring, and Evaluation Tools	
Comparative Standards	

** Client History terms are used for Nutrition Assessment but not for Nutrition Monitoring and Evaluation.*

Progress Evaluation

Communicate the progress toward the resolution of a nutrition diagnosis by selecting the appropriate nutrition diagnosis status value from the Nutrition Assessment, Monitoring, and Evaluation terms.

NCP Term	ANDUID
New nutrition diagnosis	14586
Active nutrition diagnosis	14587
Resolved nutrition diagnosis	14588
Discontinued nutrition diagnosis	14589

For details on these terms, visit the Nutrition Diagnosis Status reference sheet on page 200.

Self Feeding Difficulty

Definition

Impaired actions to place food or beverages in mouth.

Etiology (Cause/Contributing Risk Factors)

Factors gathered during the nutrition assessment process that contribute to the existence or the maintenance of pathophysiological, psychosocial, situational, developmental, cultural, and/or environmental problems:

- Physiological difficulty causing inability to physically grasp cups and utensils, support and/or control head and neck, coordinate hand movement to mouth, close lips (or any other suckling issue), bend elbow or wrist, sit with hips square and back straight
- Limited physical strength or range of motion
- Limited access to foods and/or adaptive eating devices conducive for self-feeding
- Limited vision
- Impaired cognitive ability, including learning disabilities, neurological or sensory impairment, and/or dementia
- Reluctance or avoidance of self-feeding

Etiology Category

Etiologies are grouped by the type of cause or contributing risk factor. Communicate the etiology category by selecting the appropriate Nutrition Assessment, Monitoring, and Evaluation term.

NCP Term	ANDUID
Beliefs attitudes etiology	14567
Cultural etiology	14568
Knowledge etiology	14569
Physical function etiology	14570
Physiologic metabolic etiology	14571
Psychological etiology	14572
Social personal etiology	14573
Treatment etiology	14574
Access etiology	14575
Behavior etiology	14576

Visit the Nutrition Diagnosis Etiology Category Identification reference sheet on page 185 for more details on etiology categories. An additional useful resource to determine the etiology category is the Nutrition Diagnosis Matrix on page 528.

Signs/Symptoms (Defining Characteristics)

A typical cluster of subjective and objective signs and symptoms gathered during the nutrition assessment process that provide evidence that a problem exists; quantify the problem and describe its severity.

Self Feeding Difficulty

Nutrition Assessment Category	Potential Indicators of This Nutrition Diagnosis (one or more must be present)
Biochemical Data, Medical Tests and Procedures	
Anthropometric Measurements	Weight loss
Physical Exam Findings	• Dry mucous membranes, hoarse or wet voice, tongue extrusion • Poor lip closure, drooling • Shortness of breath
Food/Nutrition-Related History	Reports or observations of: • Being provided with foods that may not be conducive to self-feeding, eg, peas, broth-type soups • Dropping of cups, utensils • Emotional distress, anxiety, or frustration surrounding eating occasions • Challenges recognizing foods • Forgets to eat • Less than optimal use of food • Refusal to eat or chew • Dropping of food from utensil (splashing and spilling of food) on repeated attempts to feed • Limited strength or stamina to lift utensils and/or cup • Utensil biting • Absence of recommended adaptive eating devices
Client History*	• Conditions associated with a diagnosis or treatment, eg, neurological disorders, Parkinson disease, Alzheimer disease, tardive dyskinesia, multiple sclerosis, stroke, paralysis, developmental delay • Physical limitations, eg, fractured arms, traction, contractures • Surgery requiring recumbent position • Dementia/organic brain syndrome • Dysphagia • Tremors
Assessment, Monitoring, and Evaluation Tools	
Comparative Standards	

** Client History terms are used for Nutrition Assessment but not for Nutrition Monitoring and Evaluation.*

Self Feeding Difficulty

Progress Evaluation

Communicate the progress toward the resolution of a nutrition diagnosis by selecting the appropriate nutrition diagnosis status value from the Nutrition Assessment, Monitoring, and Evaluation terms.

NCP Term	ANDUID
New nutrition diagnosis	14586
Active nutrition diagnosis	14587
Resolved nutrition diagnosis	14588
Discontinued nutrition diagnosis	14589

For details on these terms, visit the Nutrition Diagnosis Status reference sheet on page 200.

Intake of Unsafe Food

Definition

Intake of food and/or fluids intentionally or unintentionally contaminated with toxins, poisonous products, infectious agents, microbial agents, additives, allergens, and/or agents of bioterrorism.

Etiology (Cause/Contributing Risk Factors)

Factors gathered during the nutrition assessment process that contribute to the existence or the maintenance of pathophysiological, psychosocial, situational, developmental, cultural, and/or environmental problems:

- Food and nutrition related knowledge deficit concerning potentially unsafe food
- Lack of knowledge about proper food/feeding, (infant and enteral formula, breastmilk*) storage, and preparation
- Exposure to contaminated water or food, eg, community outbreak of illness documented by surveillance and/or response agency
- Mental illness, confusion, or altered awareness
- Lack of or limited access to food storage equipment/facilities, eg, refrigerator
- Lack of or limited access to safe food supply, eg, inadequate markets with safe, uncontaminated food

Etiology Category

Etiologies are grouped by the type of cause or contributing risk factor. Communicate the etiology category by selecting the appropriate Nutrition Assessment, Monitoring, and Evaluation term.

NCP Term	ANDUID
Beliefs attitudes etiology	14567
Cultural etiology	14568
Knowledge etiology	14569
Physical function etiology	14570
Physiologic metabolic etiology	14571
Psychological etiology	14572
Social personal etiology	14573
Treatment etiology	14574
Access etiology	14575
Behavior etiology	14576

Visit the Nutrition Diagnosis Etiology Category Identification reference sheet on page 185 for more details on etiology categories. An additional useful resource to determine the etiology category is the Nutrition Diagnosis Matrix on page 528.

Signs/Symptoms (Defining Characteristics)

A typical cluster of subjective and objective signs and symptoms gathered during the nutrition assessment process that provide evidence that a problem exists; quantify the problem and describe its severity. (See the next page for the nutrition assessment category and potential indicators.)

* If a synonym for the term "breastmilk" is helpful or needed, an approved alternate is "human milk."

Intake of Unsafe Food

Nutrition Assessment Category	Potential Indicators of This Nutrition Diagnosis (one or more must be present)
Biochemical Data, Medical Tests and Procedures	• Positive stool culture for infectious causes, such as *Listeria*, *Salmonella*, hepatitis A, *E coli*, cyclospora • Toxicology reports for drugs, medicinals, poisons in blood or food samples
Anthropometric Measurements	
Physical Exam Findings	• Evidence of dehydration, eg, dry mucous membranes, damaged tissues • Diarrhea, cramping, bloating, fever, nausea, vomiting, vision problems, chills, dizziness, headache
Food/Nutrition-Related History	Reports or observations of: • Fish suspected to contain mercury (pregnant and lactating women) • Nonfood items (pregnant and lactating women) • Raw eggs, unpasteurized milk products, soft cheeses, undercooked meats (infants, children, immunocompromised persons, pregnant and lactating women, and elderly) • Wild plants, berries, mushrooms • Unsafely stored and prepared foods or products (enteral and infant formula, breastmilk) • Mislabeled or unlabeled foods • Verbalizes inaccurate or incomplete knowledge • Availability of suitable sanitation facilities • Ability to wash hands with soap and water
Client History*	• Conditions associated with a diagnosis or treatment, eg, foodborne illness such as bacterial, viral, or parasitic infection, mental illness, dementia • Poisoning by drugs, medicinals, and biological substances • Poisoning from poisonous food stuffs and poisonous plants • Cardiac, neurologic, respiratory changes
Assessment, Monitoring, and Evaluation Tools	
Comparative Standards	

** Client History terms are used for Nutrition Assessment but not for Nutrition Monitoring and Evaluation.*

Intake of Unsafe Food

Progress Evaluation

Communicate the progress toward the resolution of a nutrition diagnosis by selecting the appropriate nutrition diagnosis status value from the Nutrition Assessment, Monitoring, and Evaluation terms.

NCP Term	ANDUID
New nutrition diagnosis	14586
Active nutrition diagnosis	14587
Resolved nutrition diagnosis	14588
Discontinued nutrition diagnosis	14589

For details on these terms, visit the Nutrition Diagnosis Status reference sheet on page 200.

Food Insecurity

Definition

Uncertain, limited, or unstable access to food that is adequate in quantity and in nutritional quality; culturally acceptable; safe and acquired in socially acceptable ways.

Note: The definition is an outcome from the collaborative work of the Gravity Project, where the Academy was a terminology lead for the Food Insecurity data set.

Etiology (Cause/Contributing Risk Factors)

Factors gathered during the nutrition assessment process that contribute to the existence or the maintenance of pathophysiological, psychosocial, situational, developmental, cultural, and/or environmental problems:

- Social personal factors (includes utilization pillar of food security, eg, limited access to financial resources, limited health care coverage, social determinants of health, previous or current trauma or discrimination, rural or isolated location)
- Access factors (includes access and availability pillars of food security, eg, limited transportation; cost of food; limited availability of charitable food resources; limited availability of social programs; barriers to charitable food resources; barriers to social programs; disruption of food production, processing, and/or distribution network; food injustice; weather emergency; contaminated food supply; neighborhood and/or community barriers and/or safety concerns; residing in area that has limited food outlet options or one that has abundance of food outlets lacking nutrient-rich foods)
- Physical function conditions (eg, limited physical ability to access charitable food resources)
- Physiologic metabolic conditions (eg, health condition, cognitive ability)
- Psychological health factors
- Food and nutrition related knowledge deficit
- Limited food and nutrition related skill

Etiology Category

Etiologies are grouped by the type of cause or contributing risk factor. Communicate the etiology category by selecting the appropriate Nutrition Assessment, Monitoring, and Evaluation term.

NCP Term	ANDUID
Beliefs attitudes etiology	14567
Cultural etiology	14568
Knowledge etiology	14569
Physical function etiology	14570
Physiologic metabolic etiology	14571
Psychological etiology	14572
Social personal etiology	14573
Treatment etiology	14574
Access etiology	14575
Behavior etiology	14576

Visit the Nutrition Diagnosis Etiology Category Identification reference sheet on page 185 for more details on etiology categories. An additional useful resource to determine the etiology category is the Nutrition Diagnosis Matrix on page 528.

Food Insecurity

Signs/Symptoms (Defining Characteristics)

A typical cluster of subjective and objective signs and symptoms gathered during the nutrition assessment process that provide evidence that a problem exists; quantify the problem and describe its severity.

Nutrition Assessment Category	Potential Indicators of This Nutrition Diagnosis (one or more must be present)
Biochemical Data, Medical Tests and Procedures	
Anthropometric Measurements	
Physical Exam Findings	Hunger
Food/Nutrition-Related History	Reports or observations of: • Individual client food security level (marginal, low, or very low food security, may also be called mild, moderate, or severe food insecurity) • Household food security level (marginal, low, or very low food security, may also be called mild, moderate, or severe food insecurity) • Estimated inadequate intake of food and/or specific nutrients • Limited supply of food in place of residence • Limited variety of foods in place of residence • Limited resources for food • Limited transportation • None to intermediate knowledge of how to plan, procure, prepare, and/or store food • None to intermediate food preparation and/or storage skills • None to intermediate knowledge on how to apply and/or participate in food assistance programs • None to intermediate skills on how to apply and/or participate in food assistance programs • Limited eligibility for government nutrition programs • Limited enrollment in government nutrition programs • Limited eligibility for community nutrition programs • Limited enrollment in community nutrition programs • Limited awareness of programs offering food support and/or nutrition intervention • Limited ability to procure safe food • Limited access to food preparation equipment • Limited ability to store food safely • Limited availability of food refrigeration • Behaviors consistent with food insecurity (eg, skipping meals; buying low-cost food items; changes in eating patterns, rituals, or customs) • Conditions that contribute to food contamination

Continued on next page

Food Insecurity

Continued from previous page

Nutrition Assessment Category	Potential Indicators of This Nutrition Diagnosis (one or more must be present)
Food/Nutrition-Related History (continued)	• Fasting pattern changes because of food insecurity • Use of charitable food resources (eg, food pantry) • Living in an area with limited availability of shopping facilities/food outlets • Living in an area with an abundance of quick-serve restaurants • Food program supports with a limited amount and/or variety of appetizing, culturally acceptable, healthful foods • School-based programs with a limited amount and/or variety of appetizing, culturally acceptable, healthful foods • Time constraints affecting food acquisition • Limited ability to build and utilize social network • Concerns about neighborhood safety • Concerns about walkability of neighborhood
Client History*	• Limited access to economic resources (eg, underemployment, low wages, high cost of health care, rent) • Health conditions (eg, malnutrition, vitamin/mineral deficiency) • Mental health concerns • Cognitive delay, limited focus and attention in school (children) • Housing insufficiency • Limited access to transportation • Remote or isolated location • Member of marginalized community or group • Community constraints (eg, limited public transportation, limited sidewalks) • Supportive structure (eg, social service agencies and faith-based organizations) factors impacting food security and/or access • Supportive individual (eg, family and caregivers) factors impacting food security and/or access • History of food insecurity • Language barrier • Physical impairment
Assessment, Monitoring, and Evaluation Tools	• Score > 1 for US household food security module: six item short form raw score • Scale score > 2.86 for US household food security module: six item short form scale score • Food insecurity experience scale (FIES) raw score > 1 • Score < 5 for Minimum dietary diversity for women (MDD-W) indicator score

Continued on next page

Food Insecurity

Continued from previous page

Nutrition Assessment Category	Potential Indicators of This Nutrition Diagnosis (one or more must be present)
Assessment, Monitoring, and Evaluation Tools (continued)	• US Children's food security scale: 1 (marginal food security among children), 2 to 4 (low food security among children), 5 to 8 (very low food security among children) • Score > 1 for the Household Food Security Survey Module (HFSSM)
Comparative Standards	• Estimated energy needs • Estimated protein needs • Estimated vitamin needs • Estimated mineral needs

** Client History terms are used for Nutrition Assessment but not for Nutrition Monitoring and Evaluation.*

Progress Evaluation

Communicate the progress toward the resolution of a nutrition diagnosis by selecting the appropriate nutrition diagnosis status value from the Nutrition Assessment, Monitoring, and Evaluation terms.

NCP Term	ANDUID
New nutrition diagnosis	14586
Active nutrition diagnosis	14587
Resolved nutrition diagnosis	14588
Discontinued nutrition diagnosis	14589

For details on these terms, visit the Nutrition Diagnosis Status reference sheet on page 200.

Limited Access to Nutrition Related Supplies

Definition

Diminished ability to acquire nutrition related supplies based on identified needs.

Etiology (Cause/Contributing Risk Factors)

Factors gathered during the nutrition assessment process that contribute to the existence or the maintenance of pathophysiological, psychosocial, situational, developmental, cultural, and/or environmental problems:

- Caregiver intentionally or unintentionally not providing access to nutrition related supplies, eg, unmet needs, abuse/neglect
- Community and geographical constraints for shopping and transportation to obtain nutrition related supplies
- Food and nutrition related knowledge deficit concerning nutrition related supplies
- Limited financial resources or limited access to financial resources to purchase nutrition related supplies
- Reluctance to participate in community or other programs that provide access to nutrition related supplies
- Physical or psychological limitations that diminish ability to shop, eg, walking, sight, mental/emotional health

Etiology Category

Etiologies are grouped by the type of cause or contributing risk factor. Communicate the etiology category by selecting the appropriate Nutrition Assessment, Monitoring, and Evaluation term.

NCP Term	ANDUID
Beliefs attitudes etiology	14567
Cultural etiology	14568
Knowledge etiology	14569
Physical function etiology	14570
Physiologic metabolic etiology	14571
Psychological etiology	14572
Social personal etiology	14573
Treatment etiology	14574
Access etiology	14575
Behavior etiology	14576

Visit the Nutrition Diagnosis Etiology Category Identification reference sheet on page 185 for more details on etiology categories. An additional useful resource to determine the etiology category is the Nutrition Diagnosis Matrix on page 528.

Signs/Symptoms (Defining Characteristics)

A typical cluster of subjective and objective signs and symptoms gathered during the nutrition assessment process that provide evidence that a problem exists; quantify the problem and describe its severity.

Limited Access to Nutrition Related Supplies

Nutrition Assessment Category	Potential Indicators of This Nutrition Diagnosis (one or more must be present)
Biochemical Data, Medical Tests and Procedures	Abnormal biochemical findings consistent with vitamin/mineral deficiency
Anthropometric Measurements	• Growth failure, based on reference growth standards, eg National Center for Health Statistics (NCHS) • Underweight: BMI < 18.5 (adults) • Unintentional weight loss: adults, of > 10% in 6 months, > 5% in 1 month; any unintentional weight loss in children
Physical Exam Findings	• Findings consistent with vitamin/mineral deficiency • Hunger, thirst • Evidence of dehydration, eg, dry mucous membranes, poor skin turgor
Food/Nutrition-Related History	Reports or observations of: • Food faddism • Belief finding that hinders food and/or nutrition behavior change • Attitude finding that hinders food and/or nutrition behavior change • Limited supply of nutrition related supplies (eg, glucose testing strips, meter, assistive eating devices, assistive cooking devices) in home • Transportation or other community constraints limiting availability of nutrition related supplies • Limited knowledge or skills on how to use nutrition related supplies • Limited knowledge or skills on how to apply and/or participate in nutrition-related supply assistance programs
Client History*	• Malnutrition, vitamin/mineral deficiency • Illness or physical disability • Conditions associated with a diagnosis or treatment, eg, mental illness, dementia • Limited support systems • Resource constraints for obtaining nutrition related supplies
Assessment, Monitoring, and Evaluation Tools	
Comparative Standards	

** Client History terms are used for Nutrition Assessment but not for Nutrition Monitoring and Evaluation.*

Progress Evaluation

Communicate the progress toward the resolution of a nutrition diagnosis by selecting the appropriate nutrition diagnosis status value from the Nutrition Assessment, Monitoring, and Evaluation terms. (See the next page for the NCP terms and ANDUID.)

Limited Access to Nutrition Related Supplies

NCP Term	ANDUID
New nutrition diagnosis	14586
Active nutrition diagnosis	14587
Resolved nutrition diagnosis	14588
Discontinued nutrition diagnosis	14589

For details on these terms, visit the Nutrition Diagnosis Status reference sheet on page 200.

Limited Access to Potable Water

Definition

Diminished ability to acquire a sufficient quantity of safe drinking water based on dietary reference intake standards (eg, Dietary Reference Intakes), national food guidelines (eg, U.S. Dietary Guidelines, MyPlate) or as defined in the nutrition prescription.

Etiology (Cause/Contributing Risk Factors)

Factors gathered during the nutrition assessment process that contribute to the existence or the maintenance of pathophysiological, psychosocial, situational, developmental, cultural, and/or environmental problems:

- Caregiver intentionally or unintentionally not providing access to water, eg, unmet needs for food or eating assistance, abuse/neglect
- Community and geographical constraints for shopping and transportation
- Food and nutrition related knowledge deficit concerning safe drinking water
- Limited financial resources or limited access to financial resources to purchase a sufficient quantity of drinking water
- Schools lacking nutrition/wellness policies or application of policies ensuring access to potable water
- Physical or psychological limitations that diminish ability to shop, eg, walking, sight, mental/emotional health
- Factors contributing to a contaminated water supply
- Factors contributing to insufficient water access
- Belief finding that hinders food and/or nutrition behavior change
- Attitude finding that hinders food and/or nutrition behavior change

Etiology Category

Etiologies are grouped by the type of cause or contributing risk factor. Communicate the etiology category by selecting the appropriate Nutrition Assessment, Monitoring, and Evaluation term.

NCP Term	ANDUID
Beliefs attitudes etiology	14567
Cultural etiology	14568
Knowledge etiology	14569
Physical function etiology	14570
Physiologic metabolic etiology	14571
Psychological etiology	14572
Social personal etiology	14573
Treatment etiology	14574
Access etiology	14575
Behavior etiology	14576

Visit the Nutrition Diagnosis Etiology Category Identification reference sheet on page 185 for more details on etiology categories. An additional useful resource to determine the etiology category is the Nutrition Diagnosis Matrix on page 528.

Limited Access to Potable Water

Signs/Symptoms (Defining Characteristics)

A typical cluster of subjective and objective signs and symptoms gathered during the nutrition assessment process that provide evidence that a problem exists; quantify the problem and describe its severity.

Nutrition Assessment Category	Potential Indicators of This Nutrition Diagnosis (one or more must be present)
Biochemical Data, Medical Tests and Procedures	• ↓ Urine volume • Urine color reflecting concentration of urine • ↑ Urine specific gravity • Abnormal stool study results
Anthropometric Measurements	Weight loss
Physical Exam Findings	• Thirst • Evidence of dehydration, eg, dry mucous membranes, poor skin turgor, cognitive changes • Diarrhea, vomiting, abdominal pain
Food/Nutrition-Related History	Reports or observations of: • Belief findings that impact potable water access • Attitude findings that impact potable water access • Limited access to water • Limited resources for water • Limited transportation or other community constraints limiting availability of water • Limited knowledge or skills related to safe water • Limited knowledge or skills on how to apply and/or participate in water assistance programs • Conditions that contribute to water contamination • Geographic or other factors contributing to insufficient water access • Fasting pattern that restricts safe water access or a sufficient amount of water • Availability of suitable sanitation facilities • Ability to wash hands with soap and water
Client History*	• Malnutrition • Physical disability • Conditions associated with a diagnosis or treatment that impacts water intake • Limited support systems
Assessment, Monitoring, and Evaluation Tools	
Comparative Standards	

Arrows used with laboratory values: ↑ represents above reference standard and ↓ represents below reference standard.
** Client History terms are used for Nutrition Assessment but not for Nutrition Monitoring and Evaluation.*

Limited Access to Potable Water

Progress Evaluation

Communicate the progress toward the resolution of a nutrition diagnosis by selecting the appropriate nutrition diagnosis status value from the Nutrition Assessment, Monitoring, and Evaluation terms.

NCP Term	ANDUID
New nutrition diagnosis	14586
Active nutrition diagnosis	14587
Resolved nutrition diagnosis	14588
Discontinued nutrition diagnosis	14589

For details on these terms, visit the Nutrition Diagnosis Status reference sheet on page 200.

No Nutrition Diagnosis At This Time

Definition

Absence of a current nutrition problem warranting a nutrition intervention. This determination results from a nutrition assessment.

Note: This nutrition diagnostic term is not appropriate if additional information for the nutrition assessment is needed or pending.

Etiology (Cause/Contributing Risk Factors)

Factors gathered during the nutrition assessment process that contribute to the existence or the maintenance of pathophysiological, psychosocial, situational, developmental, cultural, and/or environmental problems:

- Not applicable

Etiology Category

Etiologies are grouped by the type of cause or contributing risk factor. Communicate the etiology category by selecting the appropriate Nutrition Assessment, Monitoring, and Evaluation term.

NCP Term	ANDUID
Beliefs attitudes etiology	14567
Cultural etiology	14568
Knowledge etiology	14569
Physical function etiology	14570
Physiologic metabolic etiology	14571
Psychological etiology	14572
Social personal etiology	14573
Treatment etiology	14574
Access etiology	14575
Behavior etiology	14576

Visit the Nutrition Diagnosis Etiology Category Identification reference sheet on page 185 for more details on etiology categories. An additional useful resource to determine the etiology category is the Nutrition Diagnosis Matrix on page 528.

Signs/Symptoms (Defining Characteristics)

A typical cluster of subjective and objective signs and symptoms gathered during the nutrition assessment process that provide evidence that a problem exists; quantify the problem and describe its severity.

Nutrition Assessment Category	Potential Indicators of This Nutrition Diagnosis (one or more must be present)
Biochemical Data, Medical Tests and Procedures	Not applicable

Continued on next page

No Nutrition Diagnosis At This Time

Continued from previous page

Nutrition Assessment Category	Potential Indicators of This Nutrition Diagnosis (one or more must be present)
Anthropometric Measurements	Not applicable
Physical Exam Findings	Not applicable
Food/Nutrition-Related History	Not applicable
Client History*	Conditions associated with a diagnosis or treatment, eg, palliative/ end-of-life care
Assessment, Monitoring, and Evaluation Tools	
Comparative Standards	Not applicable

** Client History terms are used for Nutrition Assessment but not for Nutrition Monitoring and Evaluation.*

Progress Evaluation

Communicate the progress toward the resolution of a nutrition diagnosis by selecting the appropriate nutrition diagnosis status value from the Nutrition Assessment, Monitoring, and Evaluation terms.

NCP Term	ANDUID
New nutrition diagnosis	14586
Active nutrition diagnosis	14587
Resolved nutrition diagnosis	14588
Discontinued nutrition diagnosis	14589

For details on these terms, visit the Nutrition Diagnosis Status reference sheet on page 200.

SNAPSHOT
NCP Step 3: Nutrition Intervention

Definition: A nutrition intervention is a purposely planned action(s) designed with the intent of changing a nutrition-related behavior, risk factor, environmental condition, or aspect of health status to resolve or improve the identified nutrition diagnosis(es) or nutrition problem(s). Nutrition interventions are selected and tailored to the client needs by planning and implementing appropriate interventions.

Determining a nutrition intervention: The nutrition diagnosis and its etiology drive the selection of a nutrition intervention.

Nutrition intervention strategies are directed toward resolving the nutrition diagnosis(es) by altering or eliminating the etiology(ies). Less often, it is directed at relieving the signs and symptoms of the nutrition problem(s). Nutrition intervention goals, developed collaboratively with the client, provide the basis for monitoring progress and measuring outcomes.

Terminology for Nutrition Intervention is organized in eight domains (categories). The first two terms are planning terms, while the last six terms are implementation.

Goal Planning	Customized approach to desired outcome development
Prescription Planning	Customized approach to care recommendations development
Food and/or Nutrient Delivery	Individualized approach for food/nutrient provision
Nutrition Education	A formal process to instruct or train a patient/client in a skill or to impart knowledge to help patients/clients voluntarily man- age or modify food, nutrition, and physical activity choices and behavior to maintain or improve health
Nutrition Counseling	A supportive process, characterized by a collaborative counselor–patient relationship, to establish food, nutrition, and physical activity priorities, goals, and individualized action plans that acknowledge and foster responsibility for self-care to treat an existing condition and promote health
Coordination of Nutrition Care	Consultation with, referral to, or coordination of nutrition care with other health care providers, institutions, or agencies that can assist in treating or managing nutrition-related problems
Population Based Nutrition Action	Interventions designed to improve the nutritional well-being of a population
Nutrition Intervention Encounter Context	Circumstances for nutrition intervention implementation

Use of nutrition intervention terminology: Nutrition intervention is accomplished in two distinct and interrelated steps: planning and implementing.

Planning the nutrition intervention involves:

- Prioritizing nutrition interventions based on urgency, impact, and available resources
- Collaborating with the client to identify goals of the intervention for each diagnosis
- Writing a nutrition prescription based on a client's tailored recommended intake based on current reference standards and evidence-based nutrition guidelines and related to the client's health condition, nutrition diagnosis, and/or client values
- Selecting specific nutrition intervention strategies that are focused on the etiology of the problem and that are known to be effective based on best current knowledge and evidence
- Defining the time and frequency of care, including intensity, duration, and follow-up

Implementation is the action phase and involves:

- Collaborating with the client to carry out the plan of care
- Communicating the nutrition care plan
- Modifying the plan of care as needed
- Following up and verifying that the plan is being implemented
- Revising strategies based on changes in condition or response to intervention

Critical Thinking Skills

- Setting goals and prioritizing
- Defining the nutrition prescription or basic plan
- Making interdisciplinary connections
- Matching nutrition intervention strategies with client needs, nutrition diagnosis(es), and values
- Choosing from among alternatives to determine a course of action
- Specifying the time and frequency of care

For more detailed information about the Nutrition Intervention step, log in as a subscriber to www.nutritioncareprocess.org.

NCP Step 3: Nutrition Intervention

The following is a quick reference outline of the Nutrition Intervention Step. This outline does not include all the terms in this step.

Key: ◆ = NCP Domain; ▲ = NCP Class; ● = NCP Subclass; □ = NCP Term

Each term is designated with a a five-digit (eg, 99999) Academy unique identifier (ANDUID). This should not be used in nutrition documentation. The ANDUID is for data-tracking purposes in electronic health records.

◆ GOAL PLANNING

Customized approach to desired outcome development.

ANDUID

▲ Identify Nutrition Intervention Goal(s) 14501

Description of a desired outcome of a nutrition intervention.

- ❑ Identify goal description 14502
- ❑ Identify goal target value 14503
- ❑ Identify goal timeframe 14504
- ❑ Identify goal subject 14505
- ❑ Identify goal setter 14506

◆ PRESCRIPTION PLANNING

Customized approach to care recommendations development.

▲ Nutrition Prescription 10794

The client's tailored recommended intake based on current reference standards and evidenced based nutrition practice guidelines and related to the client's health condition, nutrition diagnosis, and/or client values.

- ❑ Nutrition prescription for oral nutrition 82236
- ❑ Nutrition prescription for enteral nutrition 30095
- ❑ Nutrition prescription for parenteral nutrition 30096
- ❑ Nutrition prescription for intravenous (IV) fluid 30097

◆ FOOD AND/OR NUTRIENT DELIVERY

Individualized approach for food /nutrient provision.

▲ Meals and Snacks 10488

Meals are defined as an eating episode that may or may not occur at a fixed time of the day and include a variety of foods (ie, solid and liquid).Snacks are defined as food eaten between meals

- ❑ Manage composition of oral intake 10828
  - ❑ General healthful diet 10489
  - ❑ Vegetarian diet 30099
  - ❑ Pesco vegetarian diet 30100
  - ❑ Lacto ovo vegetarian diet 30101
  - ❑ Lacto vegetarian diet 30102
  - ❑ Ovo vegetarian diet 30103
  - ❑ Vegan diet 30104
  - ❑ Halal diet 30105
  - ❑ Kosher diet 30106
  - ❑ Mediterranean diet 30107
  - ❑ Texture modified diet 10829

ANDUID

    - ❑ International Dysphagia Diet Standardisation Initiative Framework - Regular Level 7 (Black) food 82180
    - ❑ International Dysphagia Diet Standardisation Initiative Framework - Easy to Chew Level 7 (Black) food 82181
    - ❑ International Dysphagia Diet Standardisation Initiative Framework - Soft and Bite Sized Level 6 (Blue) food 12216
    - ❑ International Dysphagia Diet Standardisation Initiative Framework - Minced and Moist Level 5 (Orange) food 12217
    - ❑ International Dysphagia Diet Standardisation Initiative Framework - Pureed Level 4 (Green) food 12218
    - ❑ International Dysphagia Diet Standardisation Initiative Framework - Extremely Thick Level 4 (Green) drinks 12219
    - ❑ International Dysphagia Diet Standardisation Initiative Framework - Liquidized Level 3 (Yellow) food 12220
    - ❑ International Dysphagia Diet Standardisation Initiative Framework - Moderately Thick Level 3 (Yellow) drinks 12221
    - ❑ International Dysphagia Diet Standardisation Initiative Framework - Mildly Thick Level 2 (Pink) drinks 12222
    - ❑ International Dysphagia Diet Standardisation Initiative Framework - Slightly Thick Level 1 (Grey) drinks 12223
    - ❑ International Dysphagia Diet Standardisation Initiative Framework - Thin Level 0 (White) drinks 82182
    - ❑ Easy to chew diet 10914
    - ❑ Mechanically altered diet 10915
    - ❑ Pureed diet 10916
  - ❑ Energy modified diet 10830
    - ❑ Increased energy diet 10935
    - ❑ Decreased energy diet 10936
  - ❑ Protein modified diet 10831
    - ❑ Consistent protein diet 10896
    - ❑ Increased protein diet 10972
    - ❑ Decreased protein diet 10973

	ANDUID
❑ Decreased casein diet	10999
❑ Decreased gluten diet	11000
❑ Gluten free diet	11027
❑ Amino acid modified diet	10897
❑ Arginine modified diet	10898
❑ Increased arginine diet	10974
❑ Decreased arginine diet	10975
❑ Glutamine modified diet	10899
❑ Increased glutamine diet	10976
❑ Decreased glutamine diet	10977
❑ Histidine modified diet	10900
❑ Increased histidine diet	10978
❑ Decreased histidine diet	10979
❑ Increased homocysteine diet	10980
❑ Isoleucine modified diet	10902
❑ Increased isoleucine diet	10981
❑ Decreased isoleucine diet	10982
❑ Leucine modified diet	10903
❑ Increased leucine diet	10983
❑ Decreased leucine diet	10984
❑ Lysine modified diet	10904
❑ Increased lysine diet	10985
❑ Decreased lysine diet	10986
❑ Methionine modified diet	10905
❑ Increased methionine diet	10987
❑ Decreased methionine diet	10988
❑ Phenylalanine modified diet	10906
❑ Increased phenylalanine diet	11971
❑ Decreased phenylalanine diet	10989
❑ Threonine modified diet	10907
❑ Increased threonine diet	10990
❑ Decreased threonine diet	10991
❑ Tryptophan modified diet	10908
❑ Increased tryptophan diet	10992
❑ Decreased tryptophan diet	10993
❑ Decreased tyramine diet	10994
❑ Tyrosine modified diet	10910
❑ Increased tyrosine diet	10995
❑ Decreased tyrosine diet	10996
❑ Valine modified diet	10911
❑ Increased valine diet	10997
❑ Decreased valine diet	10998
❑ Carbohydrate modified diet	10832
❑ Consistent carbohydrate diet	10860
❑ Increased carbohydrate diet	10930
❑ Increased complex carbohydrate diet	11972
❑ Increased simple carbohydrate diet	11973
❑ Decreased carbohydrate diet	10931
❑ Decreased complex carbohydrate diet	11974

	ANDUID
❑ Decreased simple carbohydrate diet	11975
❑ Galactose modified diet	10861
❑ Increased galactose diet	11976
❑ Decreased galactose diet	10932
❑ Lactose modified diet	10862
❑ Increased lactose diet	11977
❑ Decreased lactose diet	10933
❑ Fructose modified diet	11978
❑ Increased fructose diet	11979
❑ Decreased fructose diet	11980
❑ Carbohydrate counting diet	82183
❑ Fermentable oligosaccharide, disaccharide, monosaccharide and polyols (FODMAP) modified diet	30109
❑ Decreased fermentable oligosaccharide, disaccharide, monosaccharide and polyols (FODMAP) diet	30110
❑ Fermentable oligosaccharide, disaccharide, monosaccharide and polyols (FODMAP) reintroduction diet	30111
❑ Customized low fermentable oligosaccharide, disaccharide, monosaccharide and polyols (FODMAP) diet	30112
❑ Fat modified diet	10833
❑ Increased fat diet	10937
❑ Decreased fat diet	10938
❑ Monounsaturated fat modified diet	10869
❑ Increased monounsaturated fat diet	10939
❑ Decreased monounsaturated fat diet	10940
❑ Polyunsaturated fat modified diet	10870
❑ Increased polyunsaturated fat diet	10941
❑ Increased linoleic acid diet	11981
❑ Decreased polyunsaturated fat diet	10942
❑ Decreased linoleic acid diet	11982
❑ Saturated fat modified diet	10871
❑ Decreased saturated fat diet	10943
❑ Trans fat modified diet	10872
❑ Decreased trans fat modified diet	10944
❑ Omega 3 fatty acid modified diet	11983
❑ Increased omega 3 fatty acid diet	11984
❑ Increased alpha linolenic acid diet	11985

Key: ◆ = NCP Domain; ▲ = NCP Class; ● = NCP Subclass; ☐ = NCP Term

ANDUID

      - ❑ Increased eicosapentaenoic acid diet — 11986
      - ❑ Increased docosahexaenoic acid — 11987
    - ❑ Decreased omega 3 fatty acid diet — 11988
      - ❑ Decreased alpha linolenic acid diet — 11989
      - ❑ Decreased eicosapentaenoic acid diet — 11990
      - ❑ Decreased docosahexaenoic acid diet — 11991
  - ❑ Medium chain triglyceride modified diet — 11992
    - ❑ Increased medium chain triglyceride diet — 11993
    - ❑ Decreased medium chain triglyceride diet — 11994
- ❑ Cholesterol modified diet — 10863
  - ❑ Decreased cholesterol diet — 10934
- ❑ Fiber modified diet — 10834
  - ❑ Increased fiber diet — 10945
  - ❑ Decreased fiber diet — 10946
  - ❑ Soluble fiber modified diet — 10947
    - ❑ Increased soluble fiber diet — 10948
    - ❑ Decreased soluble fiber diet — 10949
  - ❑ Insoluble fiber modified diet — 10950
    - ❑ Increased insoluble fiber diet — 10951
    - ❑ Decreased insoluble fiber diet — 10952
- ❑ Fluid modified diet — 10835
  - ❑ Increased fluid diet — 10874
  - ❑ Fluid restricted diet — 10873
  - ❑ Clear liquid diet — 10876
  - ❑ Full liquid diet — 10877
- ❑ Modification of diet for specific food and/or ingredient — 10836
  - ❑ Beef free diet — 30113
  - ❑ Caffeine free diet — 30114
  - ❑ Cow milk free diet — 30115
  - ❑ Diet with food modified to be low in protein — 12003
  - ❑ Diet modified for egg — 12004
    - ❑ Raw egg free diet — 12005
    - ❑ Egg free diet — 30116
  - ❑ Diet modified for uncooked corn starch — 30117
  - ❑ Fish free diet — 30118
  - ❑ Goat milk free diet — 30119
  - ❑ Lupin free diet — 30120
  - ❑ Mammalian meat free diet — 30121
  - ❑ Mammalian milk free diet — 30122
  - ❑ Peanut free diet — 30123
  - ❑ Pork free diet — 30124

ANDUID

  - ❑ Sesame free diet — 30125
  - ❑ Sheep milk free diet — 30126
  - ❑ Shellfish free diet — 30127
  - ❑ Soy free diet — 30128
  - ❑ Tree nut free diet — 30129
  - ❑ Wheat free diet — 30130
- ❑ Vitamin modified diet — 10837
  - ❑ Vitamin A modified diet — 10923
    - ❑ Increased vitamin A diet — 11013
    - ❑ Decreased vitamin A diet — 11014
  - ❑ Vitamin C modified diet — 10926
    - ❑ Increased vitamin C diet — 11019
    - ❑ Decreased vitamin C diet — 11020
  - ❑ Vitamin D modified diet — 10927
    - ❑ Increased vitamin D diet — 11021
    - ❑ Decreased vitamin D diet — 11022
  - ❑ Vitamin E modified diet — 10928
    - ❑ Increased vitamin E diet — 11023
    - ❑ Decreased vitamin E diet — 11024
  - ❑ Vitamin K modified diet — 10929
    - ❑ Increased vitamin K diet — 11025
    - ❑ Decreased vitamin K diet — 11026
  - ❑ Thiamin modified diet — 10922
    - ❑ Increased thiamin diet — 11011
    - ❑ Decreased thiamin diet — 11012
  - ❑ Riboflavin modified diet — 10921
    - ❑ Increased riboflavin diet — 11009
    - ❑ Decreased riboflavin diet — 11010
  - ❑ Niacin modified diet — 10919
    - ❑ Increased niacin diet — 11005
    - ❑ Decreased niacin diet — 11006
  - ❑ Folic acid modified diet — 10918
    - ❑ Increased folic acid diet — 11003
    - ❑ Decreased folic acid diet — 11004
  - ❑ Vitamin B6 modified diet — 10924
    - ❑ Increased vitamin B6 diet — 11015
    - ❑ Decreased vitamin B6 diet — 11016
  - ❑ Vitamin B12 modified diet — 10925
    - ❑ Increased vitamin B12 diet — 11017
    - ❑ Decreased vitamin B12 diet — 11018
  - ❑ Pantothenic acid modified diet — 10920
    - ❑ Increased pantothenic acid diet — 11007
    - ❑ Decreased pantothenic acid diet — 11008
  - ❑ Biotin modified diet — 10917
    - ❑ Increased biotin diet — 11001
    - ❑ Decreased biotin diet — 11002
- ❑ Mineral modified diet — 10838
  - ❑ Calcium modified diet — 10879
    - ❑ Increased calcium diet — 10953
    - ❑ Decreased calcium diet — 10954
  - ❑ Chloride modified diet — 10880
  - ❑ Iron modified diet — 10886

	ANDUID
❑ Increased iron diet	10960
❑ Decreased iron diet	10961
❑ Magnesium modified diet	10887
❑ Increased magnesium diet	10962
❑ Decreased magnesium diet	10963
❑ Potassium modified diet	10891
❑ Increased potassium diet	10966
❑ Decreased potassium diet	10967
❑ Phosphorus modified diet	10890
❑ Increased phosphorus diet	10964
❑ Decreased phosphorus diet	10965
❑ Sodium modified diet	10893
❑ Increased sodium diet	10968
❑ Decreased sodium diet	10969
❑ Zinc modified diet	10895
❑ Increased zinc diet	10970
❑ Decreased zinc diet	10971
❑ Sulfur modified diet	10894
❑ Fluoride modified diet	10884
❑ Copper modified diet	10883
❑ Increased copper diet	10956
❑ Decreased copper diet	10957
❑ Iodine modified diet	10885
❑ Increased iodine diet	10958
❑ Decreased iodine diet	10959
❑ Selenium modified diet	10892
❑ Manganese modified diet	10888
❑ Chromium modified diet	10881
❑ Increased chromium diet	10955
❑ Molybdenum modified diet	10889
❑ Boron modified diet	10878
❑ Cobalt modified diet	10882
❑ Modification of specific food group	10492
❑ Fruit modified diet	11996
❑ Vegetable modified diet	11997
❑ Starchy vegetable modified diet	11998
❑ Bean and pea modified diet	11999
❑ Grain modified diet	12000
❑ Protein food modified diet	12002
❑ Decreased oxalate diet	30131
❑ Low microbial diet	30132
❑ Advance diet as tolerated	30133
❑ Nil per os (NPO)	30134
❑ Modification of schedule of oral intake	10815
❑ Modification of schedule of intake to limit fasting	11995

▲ Enteral and Parenteral Nutrition Management

Nutrition provided through the GI tract via tube, catheter, or stoma (enteral) or intravenously, centrally or peripherally (parenteral)

	ANDUID
● Enteral Nutrition Management	**10495**
❑ Management of composition of enteral nutrition	10503
❑ Management of concentration of enteral nutrition	10502
❑ Management of delivery rate of enteral nutrition	10500
❑ Management of volume of enteral nutrition	10501
❑ Management of schedule of enteral nutrition	10504
❑ Management of route of enteral nutrition	10792
❑ Insert enteral feeding tube	10497
❑ Management of enteral nutrition site care	10498
❑ Management of flushing of feeding tube	10499
● Parenteral Nutrition/IV Fluid Management	**10505**
❑ Management of composition of parenteral nutrition	10511
❑ Management of concentration of parenteral nutrition	10510
❑ Management of delivery rate of parenteral nutrition	10509
❑ Management of volume of parenteral nutrition	11141
❑ Management of schedule of parenteral nutrition	10512
❑ Management of route of parenteral nutrition	10793
❑ Management of parenteral nutrition site care	10507
❑ Management of intravenous (IV) fluid delivery	10508

▲ Nutrition Supplement Therapy

Foods or nutrients that are not intended as a sole (only) item or a meal or diet, but that are intended to provide additional nutrients

● Medical Food Supplement Therapy	**10514**
❑ Commercial beverage medical food supplement therapy	10515
❑ Commercial food medical food supplement therapy	10516
❑ Modified beverage medical food supplement therapy	10517
❑ Modified food medical food supplement therapy	10518
❑ Purpose of medical food supplement therapy	10519
● Vitamin and Mineral Supplement Therapy	**10520**
❑ Multivitamin mineral supplement therapy	10521
❑ Multitrace element supplement therapy	10522

Key: ◆ = NCP Domain; ▲ = NCP Class; ● = NCP Subclass; ❑ = NCP Term

	ANDUID
❑ Vitamin supplement therapy	10523
❑ Vitamin A supplement therapy	10524
❑ Vitamin C supplement therapy	10525
❑ Vitamin D supplement therapy	10526
❑ Vitamin E supplement therapy	10527
❑ Vitamin K supplement therapy	10528
❑ Thiamin supplement therapy	10529
❑ Riboflavin supplement therapy	10530
❑ Niacin supplement therapy	10531
❑ Folate supplement therapy	10532
❑ Vitamin B6 supplement therapy	10533
❑ Vitamin B12 supplement therapy	10534
❑ Pantothenic acid supplement therapy	10535
❑ Biotin supplement therapy	10536
❑ Mineral supplement therapy	10538
❑ Calcium supplement therapy	10539
❑ Chloride supplement therapy	10540
❑ Iron supplement therapy	10541
❑ Magnesium supplement therapy	10542
❑ Potassium supplement therapy	10543
❑ Phosphorus supplement therapy	10544
❑ Sodium supplement therapy	10545
❑ Zinc supplement therapy	10546
❑ Sulfate supplement therapy	10547
❑ Fluoride supplement therapy	10548
❑ Copper supplement therapy	10549
❑ Iodine supplement therapy	10550
❑ Selenium supplement therapy	10551
❑ Manganese supplement therapy	10552
❑ Chromium supplement therapy	10553
❑ Molybdenum supplement therapy	10554
❑ Boron supplement therapy	10555
❑ Cobalt supplement therapy	10556

● Bioactive Constituent Management **10558**

❑ Plant stanol esters management	10559
❑ Plant sterol esters management	10816
❑ Soy protein management	10561
❑ Psyllium management	10817
❑ Beta glucan management	10563
❑ Food additives management	10564
❑ Alcohol management	10565
❑ Caffeine management	10566

▲ Feeding Assistance Management **10568**

Accommodation or assistance designed to restore the client's ability to eat independently, support adequate nutrient intake, and reduce the incidence of unplanned weight loss and dehydration

❑ Adaptive eating device management	10808
❑ Feeding position management	10570
❑ Meal set up management	10571
❑ Mouth care management	10572
❑ Menu selection assistance	10809

▲ Manage Feeding Environment **10574**

Adjustment of the physical environment, temperature, convenience, and attractiveness of the location where food is served that impact food consumption

	ANDUID
❑ Feeding environment lighting management	10575
❑ Feeding environment odor management	10576
❑ Feeding environment distraction management	10577
❑ Feeding environment table height management	10578
❑ Feeding environment table service management	10849
❑ Feeding environment room temperature management	10580
❑ Feeding environment meal service management	10810
❑ Feeding environment meal location management	10811

▲ Nutrition Related Medication Management **10582**

Modification of a drug or complementary/alternative medicine to optimize client nutritional or health status

❑ Management of nutrition related prescription medication	10839
❑ Management of nutrition related over the counter (OTC) medication	10584
❑ Management of nutrition related complementary and alternative medicine	10799

▲ Infant Feeding Management **14306**

Actions to manage human milk and/or infant formula feeding

❑ Breastmilk feeding management	14143
❑ Management of concentration of breastmilk	14144
❑ Management of human milk fortifier additive in breastmilk	14145
❑ Management of carbohydrate additive in breastmilk	14146
❑ Management of fat additive in breastmilk	14147
❑ Management of protein additive in breastmilk	14148
❑ Management of fiber additive in breastmilk	14149
❑ Management of added infant formula in breastmilk	14150
❑ Management of breastfeeding attempts	14151
❑ Management of volume of breastmilk	14152
❑ Evaluation of breastfeeding plan	14153
❑ Evaluation of breastfeeding	14154

- ❑ Evaluation of breastfeeding behavior 14155
- ❑ Promotion of exclusive breastfeeding 14156
- ❑ Promotion of predominant breastfeeding 14157
- ❑ Promotion of partial breastfeeding 14158

❑ Infant formula management 14159
- ❑ Management of composition of infant formula 14160
- ❑ Management of concentration of infant formula 14161
  - ❑ Management of human milk fortifier additive in infant formula 14162
  - ❑ Management of carbohydrate additive in infant formula 14163
  - ❑ Management of fat additive in infant formula 14164
  - ❑ Management of protein additive in infant formula 14165
  - ❑ Management of fiber additive in infant formula 14166

❑ Management of infant formula feeding attempts 14167

❑ Management of volume of infant formula 14168

❑ Evaluation of infant formula feeding plan 14169

❑ Evaluation of infant formula feeding 14170

❑ Evaluation of infant formula feeding behavior 14171

◆ NUTRITION EDUCATION

Formal process to instruct or train clients in a skill or to impart knowledge to help clients voluntarily manage or modify food, nutrition and physical activity choices and behavior to maintain or improve health

▲ Nutrition Education Content 10587

Instruction or training intended to lead to nutrition related content knowledge

- ❑ Content related nutrition education 13223
- ❑ Education on nutrition's influence on health 10591
- ❑ Physical activity guidance 12012

▲ Nutrition Education Application 10595

Instruction or training leading to nutrition related result interpretation or skills

- ❑ Nutrition related laboratory result interpretation education 10596
- ❑ Nutrition related skill education 10597
- ❑ Technical nutrition education 13222

◆ NUTRITION COUNSELING

A supportive process characterized by a collaborative counselor–client relationship to establish food, nutrition, and physical activity priorities, goals, and individualized action plans that acknowledge and foster responsibility for self-care to treat an existing condition and promote health

ANDUID

▲ Nutrition Counseling Theoretical Basis/Approach 10600

The theories or models used to design and implement an intervention. Theories and theoretical models consist of principles, constructs, and variables, which offer systematic explanations of the human behavior change process. Behavior change theories and models provide a research based rationale for designing and tailoring nutrition interventions to achieve the desired effect. A theoretical framework for curriculum and treatment protocols, it guides determination of:

1. what information clients need at different points in the behavior change process,
2. what tools and strategies may be best applied to facilitate behavior change, and
3. outcome measures to assess effectiveness in interventions or components of interventions.

- ❑ Nutrition counseling based on cognitive behavioral theory approach 10601
- ❑ Nutrition counseling based on health belief model 10602
- ❑ Nutrition counseling based on social learning theory approach 10603
- ❑ Nutrition counseling based on transtheoretical model stages of change approach 10604

▲ Nutrition Counseling Strategies 10606

An evidence based method or plan of action designed to achieve a particular goal. Application of behavior change theories in nutrition practice has provided practitioners with a collection of evidence-based strategies to promote behavior change. Some strategies target change in motivation and intention to change, and others target behavior change. Nutrition and dietetics practitioners selectively apply strategies based on client goals and objectives, and their personal counseling philosophy and skill.

- ❑ Nutrition counseling based on motivational interviewing strategy 10607
- ❑ Nutrition counseling based on goal setting strategy 10608
- ❑ Nutrition counseling based on self monitoring strategy 10609
- ❑ Nutrition counseling based on problem solving strategy 10610
- ❑ Nutrition counseling based on social support strategy 10611
- ❑ Nutrition counseling based on stress management strategy 10612
- ❑ Nutrition counseling based on stimulus control strategy 10613

Key: ◆ = NCP Domain; ▲ = NCP Class; ● = NCP Subclass; ❑ = NCP Term

	ANDUID
❑ Nutrition counseling based on cognitive restructuring strategy	10614
❑ Nutrition counseling based on relapse prevention strategy	10615
❑ Nutrition counseling based on rewards and contingency management strategy	10616

◆ COORDINATION OF NUTRITION CARE BY A NUTRITION PROFESSIONAL

Consultation with, referral to, or coordination of nutrition care with other providers, institutions, or agencies that can assist in treating or managing nutrition-related problems

▲ Collaboration and Referral of Nutrition Care **10840**

Facilitating services with other professionals, institutions, or agencies on behalf of the client prior to discharge from nutrition care

❑ Team meeting involving nutrition professional	10620
❑ Referral by nutrition professional to another nutrition professional with different expertise	10621
❑ Collaboration by nutrition professional with other nutrition professionals	10622
❑ Collaboration by nutrition professional with other providers	10812
❑ Referral by nutrition professional to other providers	10624
❑ Referral by nutrition professional to community agencies and programs	10625

▲ Discharge and Transfer of Nutrition Care to New Setting or Provider **10626**

Discharge planning and transfer of nutrition care from one level or location of care to another

❑ Discharge and transfer of nutrition care to other providers	10813
❑ Discharge and transfer of nutrition care to community agencies and programs	10814
❑ Discharge and transfer of nutrition care from nutrition professional to another nutrition professional	10627

◆ POPULATION BASED NUTRITION ACTION

Interventions designed to improve the nutritional well-being of a population

▲ Population Theoretical Frameworks **12153**

Theories, models, and approaches used to design, implement, and evaluate nutrition interventions at the population level

	ANDUID
❑ Social ecological model	12154
❑ Community organizing	12155
❑ Diffusion of innovations	12156
❑ Social marketing	12157
❑ Organizational change theory	12158
❑ Mass communications	12159
❑ Political action	12160

▲ Population Strategies **12161**

Plans of action that target environmental change, organizational change, and public policy change

❑ Environmental change	12162
❑ Food environment change	12163
❑ Built environment change	12164
❑ Social norm change	12165
❑ Organizational change	12166
❑ Public policy change	12167

▲ Population Settings **12168**

Locations where the population based nutrition intervention is implemented

❑ Residential settings	12169
❑ School settings	12170
❑ Worksite settings	12171
❑ Recreation and sports settings	12172
❑ Food production and provision settings	12173
❑ Service settings	12174
❑ Government settings	12175
❑ Community at large settings	12176

▲ Population Sectors **12177**

Public, private, and nonprofit entities integral to the development and implementation of interventions that impact determinants of the nutritional well-being of the population

❑ Agriculture sector	12178
❑ Education sector	12179
❑ Government sector	12180
❑ Healthcare sector	12181
❑ Food and beverage sector	12182
❑ Business and industry sector	12183
❑ Social welfare sector	12184
❑ Nonprofit sector	12185
❑ Communities, neighborhoods, families sector	12186

◆ NUTRITION INTERVENTION ENCOUNTER CONTEXT

Circumstances for nutrition intervention implementation

▲ Identify Nutrition Intervention Encounter Setting **30136**

Determine the environment where nutrition care is provided (excludes Population settings [P-3])

❑ Ambulatory health setting	30137

	ANDUID
❑ Assisted living setting	30138
❑ Community health care setting	30139
❑ Home health setting	30140
❑ Inpatient care setting	30141
❑ Inpatient rehabilitation environment	30142
❑ Nursing home setting	30143
❑ Outpatient setting	30144
❑ Private practice setting	30145
❑ Skilled nursing setting	30146

▲ Identify Nutrition Intervention Encounter Approach **30147**

Determine the nature of the method for provision of nutrition care

	ANDUID
❑ Individual client direct nutrition intervention encounter	30148
❑ Group client direct nutrition intervention encounter	30149
❑ Telehealth nutrition intervention encounter	30150
❑ Individual client video telehealth nutrition intervention encounter	30151
❑ Group client video telehealth nutrition intervention encounter	30152
❑ Individual client audio only telehealth nutrition intervention encounter	30153
❑ Group client audio only telehealth nutrition intervention encounter	30154
❑ Telehealth nutrition monitoring	30155
❑ Asynchronous nutrition intervention encounter	30156
❑ Provision of written information about nutrition	30157

Identify Nutrition Intervention Goal(s)

Definition

Description of a desired outcome of a nutrition intervention.

Purpose

To communicate specific, measurable, achievable, realistic, time-based (SMART) nutrition goals described and planned for implementation.

Details of Intervention

A typical intervention might be further described with the following details. Nutrition and dietetics practitioners recommend, implement, or order nutrition interventions and the action(s) may be to initiate, modify or discontinue a nutrition intervention(s):

- Identify goal description (based upon nutrition assessment/monitoring and evaluation or nutrition intervention terms)—defined as a summary statement of the desired outcome
- Identify goal target value (based upon nutrition assessment/monitoring and evaluation or nutrition intervention terms)—defined as an indicator from nutrition assessment/monitoring and evaluation and nutrition intervention terms that provides evidence for the goal and desired outcome
- Identify goal timeframe (duration)—defined as the duration of the intervention or date by which the goal is anticipated to be met
- Identify goal subject (individual client, supportive individual, supportive structure)—defined as the individual client, supportive individual (eg, family, caregiver), or supportive structure (eg, social service agencies and faith-based organizations) for whom the goal is planned
- Identify goal setter (individual client, supportive individual, supportive structure; professional, mutually established between individual client and professional)—defined as the party that identified the goal

Identify Nutrition Intervention Goal(s)

Typically Used With the Following

Nutrition Diagnostic Terminology Used in PES Statements	Common Examples
Nutrition Diagnoses	• Inadequate energy intake • Inadequate oral intake • Excessive fat intake • Excessive carbohydrate intake • Inconsistent carbohydrate intake • Growth rate below expected • Food insecurity • Underweight
Etiology	• Lack of access to healthful food choices, eg, current food access, food provided by caregiver • Physiological causes, eg, increased energy needs due to increased activity level, metabolic change, malabsorption, growth, extreme weakness, critical illness • Psychological causes • Neurological causes, eg difficulty chewing, swallowing • Food and nutrition knowledge deficit regarding foods being consumed
Signs and Symptoms	Anthropometric Measurements • Unintentional weight loss • Growth failure • Insufficient maternal body weight gain • Body weight change Nutrition-Focused Physical Findings • Obvious muscle and/or fat wasting • Poor skin turgor (tenting) • Excess subcutaneous fat Food/Nutrition-Related History • Intake less than requirements (insufficient intake) • Intake of fat more than requirements • Reports of food insecurity

Other considerations (eg, client negotiation, client needs and desires, and readiness to change)

- End-of-life issues, ethical considerations, client preferences and values
- Other nutrient intake (oral, enteral nutrition)
- Availability/access to a qualified practitioner for follow-up and monitoring

Identify Nutrition Intervention Goal(s)

Goal Examples

Note: Goals are set using Nutrition Assessment/Monitoring and Evaluation or Nutrition Intervention terms; for individuals and populations; and identified by clients, professionals, or mutually set, so examples are provided to reflect these. The components of each goal are identified in brackets for information only and so that professionals communicate structured and coded components for tracking in electronic health records or reports.

Using a Nutrition Assessment/Monitoring and Evaluation Term

Individual Client Example

[Identify goal description] Increase estimated vegetable serving intake in 24 hours: **[Identify goal setter]** Client identified goal that **[Identify goal subject]** they will **[Identify target value]** eat two vegetable servings with lunch on 5 of 7 days per week **[Identify goal timeframe]** by next encounter in 3 weeks.

Population Example

[Identify goal description] Increase estimated vegetable serving intake in 24 hours: **[Identify goal setter]** Mutually established between individual client and professional that **[Identify goal subject]** client will **[Identify target value]** increase vegetable servings to 4 per day with implementation of new community-supported agriculture incentive program **[Identify goal timeframe]** over the next 6 months.

Using a Nutrition Intervention Term

Individual Client Example

[Identify goal description] Manage rate of enteral nutrition: **[Identify goal setter]** Professional identified goal to increase **[Identify goal subject]** client's **[Identify target value]** enteral nutrition rate from 40 mL/hour to 80 mL/hour of 1 kcal/mL formula **[Identify goal timeframe]** within 48 hours.

Population Example

[Identify goal description] Content-related nutrition education: **[Identify goal setter]** Professional identified goal to provide **[Identify goal subject]** client with **[Identify target value]** content-related education messages on the importance of increasing vegetable servings intake during the implementation of new community supported agriculture incentive program **[Identify goal timeframe]** over the next 6 months.

Note: Items in brackets [Identify goal description] or [Identify goal setter] are provided for education purposes only to illustrate how components are coded in health records. These should not be included when communicating goals.

Nutrition Prescription

Definition

The client's tailored recommended intake based on current reference standards and evidence based nutrition practice guidelines and related to the client's health condition, nutrition diagnosis, and/or client values.

Purpose

To communicate the nutrition professional's intake recommendation based on a nutrition assessment and the nutrition diagnosis.

Details of Intervention

A typical intervention might be further described with the following details.
Nutrition and dietetics practitioners recommend, implement, or order nutrition interventions and the action(s) may be to initiate, modify or discontinue a nutrition intervention(s):

- Nutrition prescription for oral nutrition (ie, energy per day, nutrients [eg, grams, micrograms] per day, foods, texture modification, oral nutrition supplements, values inclusion, and/or eating pattern)—defined as the recommended oral nutrition intake of energy, nutrients, foods, texture modification, oral nutrition supplements, and/or eating pattern; can include the absence of nutrition intake orally (ie, nil per os [NPO]). Examples (not all inclusive): 80 g protein per day, General/healthful diet, Texture modified diet, Increased energy diet, Potassium modified diet, Increased fruits and vegetables, oral nutrition supplement, Lacto ovo vegetarian diet, Halal diet, Nil per os (NPO).
- Nutrition prescription for enteral nutrition (ie, energy per day, nutrients [eg, grams, micrograms] per day, formula composition and volume, method of feeding administration, body position and/or values inclusion)—defined as the recommended intake of energy and/or nutrients for infusion of nutrients distal to the oral cavity via a tube inserted into the gastrointestinal tract; can include the formula, method of feeding administration, and/or body position. Examples (not all inclusive): standard enteral formula with fiber, continuous enteral nutrition feeding, nasoduodenal enteral nutrition feeding administration, prone body position for enteral nutrition administration.
- Nutrition prescription for parenteral nutrition (ie, energy per day, nutrients [eg, grams, micrograms] per day, parenteral solution composition and volume, method of administration and/or values inclusion)—defined as the recommended intake of energy and/or nutrients via a route other than the gastrointestinal tract (ie, intravenous and/or intraperitoneal infusion); can include solution and/or method of administration. Examples (not all inclusive): parenteral nutrition solution, continuous parenteral nutrition administration, central venous parenteral nutrition administration.
- Nutrition prescription for intravenous (IV) fluid (ie, energy per day, nutrients [eg, grams, micrograms] per day, solution, method of administration and/or values inclusion)—defined as the recommended intake of energy and/or nutrients via IV fluids. Examples (not all inclusive): intravenous fluid solution, intravenous fluid administration.

> *Note:* The nutrition prescription can be used as a comparative standard for nutrition assessment and nutrition monitoring and evaluation.

Meals and Snacks

Definition

Meals are defined as an eating episode that may or may not occur at a fixed time of the day and include a variety of foods (ie, solid and liquid). Snacks are defined as food eaten between meals.

Details of Intervention

A typical intervention might be further described with the following details. Nutrition and dietetics practitioners recommend, implement, or order nutrition interventions and the action(s) may be to initiate, modify, or discontinue a nutrition intervention(s):

- Manage composition of oral intake
  - General healthful diet
  - Vegetarian diet
  - Pesco vegetarian diet—defined as a vegetarian diet that includes fish and seafood, eggs, and mammalian milk-based food and excludes all other animal-based protein food and ingredients
  - Lacto ovo vegetarian diet
  - Lacto vegetarian diet
  - Ovo vegetarian diet—defined as a vegetarian diet that includes eggs and excludes other animal-based food and ingredients
  - Vegan diet—defined as a diet that excludes all animal-based foods and animal-based food and ingredients
  - Halal diet—defined as a diet for clients of the Islamic faith and includes only foods considered acceptable. Foods not acceptable include pork, pork products, alcohol as well as other nonapproved food and food ingredients.
  - Kosher diet
  - Mediterranean diet—defined as a diet of minimally processed plant foods with the majority of intake from vegetables, whole grains, fruits, extra virgin olive oil, legumes, nuts, seeds, and herbs, and dairy products (principally yogurt and cheese); moderate intake of fish and seafood; moderate to low intake of poultry; zero to four eggs per week; and low intake of red meat and discretionary foods, such as, sweets and sugar-sweetened beverage
  - Texture modified diet
    - International Dysphagia Diet Standardisation Initiative Framework, Regular Level 7 (Black) food—defined as a diet that includes normal, everyday foods of various textures that are developmentally and age appropriate. Any method may be used to eat these foods and foods may be hard and crunchy or naturally soft. Sample size is not restricted at Level 7, therefore, foods may be of a range of sizes—pediatric: smaller or greater than 8mm pieces; adult: smaller or greater than 15 mm (1.5 cm) pieces. Includes hard, tough, chewy, fibrous, stringy, dry, crispy, crunchy, or crumbly bits. Includes food that contains pips, seeds, pith inside skin, husks, or bones. Includes dual consistency or mixed consistency foods and liquids.*
    - International Dysphagia Diet Standardisation Initiative Framework, Easy to Chew Level 7 (Black) food—defined as a diet that includes normal everyday foods of soft/tender textures that are developmentally and age appropriate. Any method may be used to eat these foods and sample size is not restricted at Level 7; therefore, foods may be of a range of sizes—pediatric: smaller

* Used with permission from the International Dysphagia Diet Standardisation Initiative (IDDSI.org). Please also see the approved synonyms list for the synonyms that can be used for IDDSI concepts.

Meals and Snacks

or greater than 8mm pieces; adults: smaller or greater than 15 mm (1.5 cm) pieces. Does noinclude hard, tough, chewy, fibrous, stringy, crunchy or crumbly bits, pips, seeds, fibrous parts of fruit, husks, or bones. May include dual consistency or mixed consistency foods and liquids

- if also safe for Level 0 and at clinician discretion. If unsafe for Level 0 Thin, liquid portion can be thickened to clinician's recommended thickness level.*
- International Dysphagia Diet Standardisation Initiative Framework, Soft and Bite-Sized Level 6 (Blue) food—defined as a diet that includes foods that can be eaten with a fork, spoon, or chopsticks and can be mashed or broken down with pressure from fork, spoon, or chopsticks. A knife is not required to cut this food but may be used to help load a fork or spoon. Soft, tender, and moist throughout but with no separate thin liquid. Chewing is required before swallowing. Bite-sized pieces as appropriate for size and oral processing skills—pediatric: no larger than 8mm pieces; adults: no larger than 15 mm (1.5 cm) pieces.*
- International Dysphagia Diet Standardisation Initiative Framework, Minced and Moist Level 5 (Orange) food—defined as a diet that includes foods that can be eaten with a fork or spoon and could be eaten with chopsticks in some cases, if the individual has very good hand control. Can be scooped and shaped (eg into a ball shape) on a plate. Soft and moist with no separate thin liquid. Small lumps visible within the food—pediatric: equal to or less than 2 mm width and no longer than 8mm in length; adult: equal to or less than 4mm width and no longer than 15mm in length. Lumps are easy to squash with tongue.*
- International Dysphagia Diet Standardisation Initiative Framework, Pureed Level 4 (Green) food—defined as a diet that includes pureed food that is usually eaten with a spoon (a fork is possible). Cannot be drunk from a cup because it does not flow easily. Cannot be sucked through a straw and does not require chewing. Can be piped, layered, or molded because it retains its shape, but should not require chewing if presented in this form. Shows some very slow movement under gravity but cannot be poured. Falls off spoon in a single spoonful when tilted and continues to hold shape on a plate. No lumps, not sticky, and liquid must not separate from solid.*
- International Dysphagia Diet Standardisation Initiative Framework, Extremely Thick Level 4 (Green) drinks—defined as a diet that includes drinks that are usually eaten with a spoon (a fork is possible). Cannot be drunk from a cup because it does not flow easily. Cannot be sucked through a straw and does not require chewing. Can be piped, layered, or molded because it retains its shape, but should not require chewing if presented in this form. Shows some very slow movement under gravity but cannot be poured. Falls off spoon in a single spoonful when tilted and continues to hold shape on a plate. No lumps, not sticky, and liquid must not separate from solid.*
- International Dysphagia Diet Standardisation Initiative Framework, Liquidized Level 3 (Yellow) food—defined as a diet that includes liquidized foods that can be drunk from a cup. Moderate effort is required to suck through a standard bore or wide bore straw (wide bore straw = 0.275 inch or 6.9 mm). Cannot be piped, layered, or molded on a plate because it will not retain its shape. Cannot be eaten with a fork because it drips slowly in dollops through the prongs. Can be eaten with a spoon. No oral processing or chewing required—can be swallowed directly. Smooth texture with no "bits" (lumps, fibers, bits of shell or skin, husk, particles of gristle or bone).*
- International Dysphagia Diet Standardisation Initiative Framework, Moderately Thick Level 3 (Yellow) drinks—defined as a diet that includes drinks that can be drunk from a cup. Moderate effort is required to suck through a standard bore or wide bore straw (wide bore straw = 0.275 inch or 6.9 mm). Cannot be piped, layered, or molded on a plate because it will not retain its shape. Cannot be eaten with a fork because it drips slowly in dollops through the prongs. Can be eaten

* Used with permission from the International Dysphagia Diet Standardisation Initiative (IDDSI.org). Please also see the approved synonyms list for the synonyms that can be used for IDDSI concepts.

Meals and Snacks

with a spoon. No oral processing or chewing required—can be swallowed directly. Smooth texture with no "bits" (lumps, fibers, bits of shell or skin, husk, particles of gristle or bone).*

- International Dysphagia Diet Standardisation Initiative Framework, Mildly Thick Level 2 (Pink) drinks—defined as a diet that includes drinks that flow off a spoon and are sippable and pour quickly from a spoon but slower than thin drinks. Mild effort is required to drink this thickness through standard bore straw (standard bore straw = 0.209 inch or 5.3 mm diameter).*
- International Dysphagia Diet Standardisation Initiative Framework, Slightly Thick Level 1 (Grey) drinks—defined as a diet that includes drinks that are thicker than water and require a little more effort to drink than thin liquids. It flows through a straw, syringe, teat/nipple. Similar to the thickness of most commercially available anti-regurgitation (AR) infant formulas. IDDSI (International Dysphagia Diet Standardisation Initiative) Flow Test result shows that test liquid flows through a 10 ml slip tip syringe leaving 1 to 4 ml in the syringe after 10 seconds.*
- International Dysphagia Diet Standardisation Initiative Framework, Thin Level 0 (White) drinks—defined as a diet that includes drinks that flow like water with a fast flow and can be drunk through any type of teat/nipple, cup, or straw as appropriate for age and skills. IDDSI (International Dysphagia Diet Standardisation Initiative) Flow Test result shows less than 1 ml of test liquid remaining in the 10 ml slip tip syringe after 10 seconds of flow.*
- Easy to chew diet
- Mechanically altered diet
- Pureed diet

- Energy modified diet
  - Increased energy diet
  - Decreased energy diet
- Protein modified diet
  - Consistent protein diet
  - Increased protein diet
  - Decreased protein diet
  - Decreased casein diet
  - Decreased gluten diet
    - Gluten free diet
  - Amino acid modified diet
    - Arginine modified diet
      - Increased arginine diet
      - Decreased arginine diet
    - Glutamine modified diet
      - Increased glutamine diet
      - Decreased glutamine diet
    - Histidine modified diet
      - Increased histidine diet
      - Decreased histidine diet
    - Increased homocysteine diet

---

* Used with permission from the International Dysphagia Diet Standardisation Initiative (IDDSI.org). Please also see the approved synonyms list for the synonyms that can be used for IDDSI concepts.

- Isoleucine modified diet
  - Increased isoleucine diet
  - Decreased isoleucine diet
- Leucine modified diet
  - Increased leucine diet
  - Decreased leucine diet
- Lysine modified diet
  - Increased lysine diet
  - Decreased lysine diet
- Methionine modified diet
  - Increased methionine diet
  - Decreased methionine diet
- Phenylalanine modified diet
  - Increased phenylalanine diet
  - Decreased phenylalanine diet
- Threonine modified diet
  - Increased threonine diet
  - Decreased threonine diet
- Tryptophan modified diet
  - Increased tryptophan diet
  - Decreased tryptophan diet
- Decreased tyramine diet
- Tyrosine modified diet
  - Increased tyrosine diet
  - Decreased tyrosine diet
- Valine modified diet
  - Increased valine diet
  - Decreased valine diet

- Carbohydrate modified diet
  - Consistent carbohydrate diet
  - Increased carbohydrate diet
    - Increased complex carbohydrate diet
    - Increased simple carbohydrate diet
  - Decreased carbohydrate diet
    - Decreased complex carbohydrate diet
    - Decreased simple carbohydrate diet
  - Galactose modified diet
    - Increased galactose diet
    - Decreased galactose diet
  - Lactose modified diet

Meals and Snacks

        - Increased lactose diet
        - Decreased lactose diet

    - Fructose modified diet
        - Increased fructose diet
        - Decreased fructose diet
    - Carbohydrate counting diet—defined as a diet for a client identifying the grams of carbohydrate to consume per meal and per day
    - Fermentable oligosaccharide, disaccharide, monosaccharide, and polyol (FODMAP)–modified diet—defined as a diet with a lower or higher amount of fermentable oligosaccharide, disaccharide, monosaccharides, and polyols in the diet
        - Low- fermentable oligosaccharide, disaccharide, monosaccharide and polyol (FODMAP) diet—defined as a diet with a reduced amount of fermentable oligo-, di-, monosaccharides and polyol in the diet
        - Fermentable oligosaccharide, disaccharide, monosaccharide and polyol (FODMAP) reintroduction diet—defined as a diet with an overall lower amount of fermentable oligo-, di-, monosaccharides and polyols but with reintroduction of individual FODMAP containing foods to assess tolerance of individual foods
        - Customized low fermentable oligosaccharide, disaccharide, monosaccharide and polyol (FODMAP) diet—defined as a diet with an overall lower amount of fermentable oligo-, di-, monosaccharides and polyols but permits a range of FODMAP containing foods based on the client's diet tolerance
- Fat modified diet
    - Increased fat diet
    - Decreased fat diet
    - Monounsaturated fat modified diet
        - Increased monounsaturated fat diet
        - Decreased monounsaturated fat diet
    - Polyunsaturated fat modified diet
        - Increased polyunsaturated fat diet
            - Increased linoleic acid diet
        - Decreased polyunsaturated fat diet
            - Decreased linoleic acid diet
    - Saturated fat modified diet
        - Decreased saturated fat diet
    - Trans fat modified diet
        - Decreased trans fat modified diet
    - Omega 3 fatty acid modified diet
        - Increased omega 3 fatty acid diet
            - Increased alpha linolenic acid diet
            - Increased eicosapentaenoic acid diet
            - Increased docosahexaenoic acid
        - Decreased omega 3 fatty acid diet
            - Decreased alpha linolenic acid diet

Meals and Snacks

        - Decreased eicosapentaenoic acid diet
        - Decreased docosahexaenoic acid

    - Medium chain triglyceride modified diet
        - Increased medium chain triglyceride diet
        - Decreased medium chain triglyceride diet
- Cholesterol modified diet
    - Decreased cholesterol diet
- Fiber modified diet
    - Increased fiber diet
    - Decreased fiber diet
    - Soluble fiber modified diet
        - Increased soluble fiber diet
        - Decreased soluble fiber diet
    - Insoluble fiber modified diet
        - Increased insoluble fiber diet
        - Decreased insoluble fiber diet
- Fluid modified diet
    - Increased fluid diet
    - Fluid restricted diet
    - Clear liquid diet
    - Full liquid diet
- Modification of diets for specific food and/or ingredient
    - Beef free diet—defined as a diet devoid of beef and beef ingredients
    - Caffeine free diet—defined as a diet devoid of the stimulant caffeine
    - Cow milk free diet—defined as a diet devoid of cow's milk and cow's milk ingredients
    - Diet with foods modified to be low in protein
    - Diet modified for egg
        - Raw egg free diet
        - Egg free diet—defined as a diet devoid of egg and egg ingredients
    - Diet modified for uncooked corn starch
    - Fish free diet—defined as a diet devoid of fish and fish ingredients
    - Goat milk free diet—defined as a diet devoid of goat milk and goat milk ingredients
    - Lupin free diet—defined as a diet devoid of lupins and lupin ingredients
    - Mammalian meat free diet—defined as a diet devoid of all mammalian meat and mammalian meat ingredients
    - Mammalian milk free diet—defined as a diet devoid of mammalian milk and mammalian milk ingredients
    - Peanut free diet—defined as a diet devoid of peanuts and peanut ingredients
    - Pork free diet—defined as a diet devoid of pork and pork ingredients
    - Sesame free diet—defined as a diet devoid of sesame and sesame ingredients
    - Sheep milk free diet—defined as a diet devoid of sheep milk and sheep milk ingredients

Meals and Snacks

- Shellfish free diet—defined as a diet devoid of shellfish and shellfish ingredients
- Soy free diet—defined as a diet devoid of soy and soy ingredients
- Tree nut free diet—defined as a diet devoid of tree nuts and tree nut ingredients
- Wheat free diet

- Vitamin modified diet
  - Vitamin A modified diet
    - Increased vitamin A diet
    - Decreased vitamin A diet
  - Vitamin C modified diet
    - Increased vitamin C diet
    - Decreased vitamin C diet
  - Vitamin D modified diet
    - Increased vitamin D diet
    - Decreased vitamin D diet
  - Vitamin E modified diet
    - Increased vitamin E diet
    - Decreased vitamin E diet
  - Vitamin K modified diet
    - Increased vitamin K diet
    - Decreased vitamin K diet
  - Thiamine modified diet
    - Increased thiamine diet
    - Decreased thiamine diet
  - Riboflavin modified diet
    - Increased riboflavin diet
    - Decreased riboflavin diet
  - Niacin modified diet
    - Increased niacin diet
    - Decreased niacin diet
  - Folic acid modified diet
    - Increased folic acid diet
    - Decreased folic acid diet
  - Vitamin B6 modified diet
    - Increased vitamin B6 diet
    - Decreased vitamin B6 diet
  - Vitamin B12 modified diet
    - Increased vitamin B12 diet
    - Decreased vitamin B12 diet
  - Pantothenic acid modified diet
    - Increased pantothenic acid diet
    - Decreased pantothenic acid diet

Meals and Snacks

    - Biotin modified diet
        - Increased biotin diet
        - Decreased biotin diet
- Mineral modified diet
    - Calcium modified diet
        - Increased calcium diet
        - Decreased calcium diet
    - Chloride modified diet
    - Iron modified diet
        - Increased iron diet
        - Decreased iron diet
    - Magnesium modified diet
        - Increased magnesium diet
        - Decreased magnesium diet
    - Potassium modified diet
        - Increased potassium diet
        - Decreased potassium diet
    - Phosphorus modified diet
        - Increased phosphorus diet
        - Decreased phosphorus diet
    - Sodium modified diet
        - Increased sodium diet
        - Decreased sodium diet
    - Zinc modified diet
        - Increased zinc diet
        - Decreased zinc diet
    - Sulfur modified diet
    - Fluoride modified diet
    - Copper modified diet
        - Increased copper diet
        - Decreased copper diet
    - Iodine modified diet
        - Increased iodine diet
        - Decreased iodine diet
    - Selenium modified diet
    - Manganese modified diet
    - Chromium modified diet
        - Increased chromium diet
    - Molybdenum modified diet
    - Boron modified diet
    - Cobalt modified diet

Meals and Snacks

- Modification of specific food group
    - Fruit modified diet
    - Vegetable modified diet
        - Starchy vegetable modified diet
        - Bean and pea modified diet
    - Grain modified diet
    - Protein food modified diet
- Decreased oxalate diet—defined as a reduction in the oxalate content of the diet compared to the assessed baseline intake of oxalate
- Low microbial diet—defined as a diet that is low in organisms (eg, bacteria, viruses, fungi, parasites) because the organisms might pose a health threat
- Advance diet as tolerated
- Nil per os (ie, NPO)
- Modification of schedule of oral intake (eg, timing of food, number of meals)
- Modification of schedule of intake to limit fasting

Meals and Snacks

Typically Used With the Following

Nutrition Diagnostic Terminology Used in PES Statements	Common Examples
Nutrition Diagnoses	• Increased energy expenditure • Inadequate energy intake • Inadequate oral intake • Excessive fat intake • Excessive carbohydrate intake • Inconsistent carbohydrate intake • Chewing difficulty • Growth rate below expected • Food insecurity • Underweight
Etiology	• Lack of access to healthful food choices, eg, current food access, food provided by caregiver • Physiological causes, eg, increased energy needs due to increased activity level, metabolic change, malabsorption, growth, extreme weakness, critical illness • Psychological causes, eg, disordered eating • Neurological causes, eg difficulty chewing, swallowing • Food and nutrition knowledge deficit regarding foods they are consuming
Signs and Symptoms	Biochemical Data, Medical Tests, and Procedures • Serum cholesterol level • Hemoglobin A1C results Anthropometric Measurements • Body weight change Nutrition-Focused Physical Findings • Dental caries • Diarrhea • Evidence of muscle and/or fat wasting • Hunger Food/Nutrition-Related History • Cultural or religious practices that may impact modified food/nutrition intake • Changes in physical activity • Food and nutrition related knowledge deficit • Limited food and nutrition related skills

Continued on next page

Meals and Snacks

Continued from previous page

Nutrition Diagnostic Terminology Used in PES Statements	Common Examples
Signs and Symptoms (continued)	Client History • Conditions associated with diagnosis or treatment, eg, surgery, trauma, sepsis, diabetes mellitus, inborn errors of metabolism, digestive enzyme deficiency, obesity • Chronic use of medications that increase or decrease nutrient requirements or impair nutrient metabolism

Other considerations (eg, client negotiation, client needs and desires, and readiness to change)

- Adherence skills and abilities
- Economic concerns with purchasing food and/or special food items
- Motivation to change behavior related to diet
- Ability to prepare food
- Availability/access to a qualified practitioner for follow-up and monitoring

Enteral Nutrition Management

Definition

Nutrition provided through the gastrointestinal (GI) tract via tube, catheter, or stoma that delivers nutrients distal to the oral cavity.

Details of Intervention

A typical intervention might be further described with the following details. Nutrition and dietetics practitioners recommend, implement, or order nutrition interventions and the action(s) may be to initiate, modify, or discontinue a nutrition intervention(s):

- Management of composition of enteral nutrition (eg, formula name or description, special additives including supplemental fat, carbohydrate, or protein, fiber)
- Management of concentration of enteral nutrition (eg, calories/kcal/kJ per mL)
- Management of rate of enteral nutrition (eg, mL/hour)
- Management of volume of enteral nutrition (eg, mL/day, mL/feeding)
- Management of schedule of enteral nutrition (eg, number of hours per 24 hours, continuous, intermittent, bolus)
- Management of route of enteral nutrition (eg, nasoentric, oroenteric, percutaneous, or surgical access with gastric, duodenal, or jejunal placement)
- Insert enteral feeding tube
- Management of enteral nutrition site care (eg, change dressings and provide enteral feeding tube site care)
- Management of flushing of feeding tube (eg, type, volume mL/flush, frequency)

Note: Related nutrition interventions, eg, checking gastric residual volume or elevating the head of the bed, are documented using Coordination of Nutrition Care.

Enteral Nutrition Management

Typically Used With the Following

Nutrition Diagnostic Terminology Used in PES Statements	Common Examples
Nutrition Diagnoses	• Swallowing difficulty • Altered GI function • Inadequate oral intake • Increased nutrient needs • Inadequate protein energy intake • Inadequate protein intake • Inadequate enteral nutrition infusion
Etiology	• Altered GI tract function, inability to absorb nutrients • Inability to chew/swallow • Decreased ability to consume sufficient energy, eg, increased nutrient needs due to catabolic illness • Respiratory or other critical illness requiring mechanical ventilation • Disease process or complication of therapy which results in excess fluid loss or retention (eg, heart failure, liver failure, renal failure)
Signs and Symptoms	Anthropometric Measurements • Weight loss • Growth failure • Insufficient maternal weight gain Nutrition Focused Physical Findings • Obvious muscle and/or fat wasting • Poor skin turgor (tenting) • Fluid retention (edema) Food/Nutrition-Related History • Intake < 75% of requirements (insufficient intake) • Existing or expected inadequate intake for 7 to 14 days Client History • Aspiration • Coma

Other considerations (eg, client negotiation, client needs and desires, and readiness to change)

- End-of-life issues, ethical considerations, client rights and family/caregiver issues
- Other nutrient intake (oral, parenteral nutrition), medications containing energy
- Enteral formulary composition and product availability
- Availability/access to a qualified practitioner for follow-up and monitoring
- Economic constraints that limit availability of food/enteral products

Parenteral Nutrition/IV Fluid Management

Definition

Administration of nutrients and fluids intravenously, centrally (delivered into a large-diameter vein, usually the superior vena cava adjacent to the right atrium) or peripherally (delivered into a peripheral vein, usually of the hand or forearm).

Details of Intervention

A typical intervention might be further described with the following details. Nutrition and dietetics practitioners recommend, implement, or order nutrition interventions and the action(s) may be to initiate, modify, or discontinue a nutrition intervention(s):

- Management of composition of parenteral nutrition (formula or description)
- Management of concentration of parenteral nutrition (eg, percent, grams of solute per mL)
- Management of rate of parenteral nutrition (eg, mL/hour)
- Management of volume of parenteral nutrition
- Management of schedule of parenteral nutrition (eg, hours, timing, taper schedule)
- Management of route of parenteral nutrition (eg, peripheral, central, and/or type of catheter)
- Management of parenteral nutrition site care (eg, change dressings and provide line care for parenteral access)
- Management of IV fluid delivery (eg, type; amount mL/day, mL/hr, mL with medications)

Parenteral Nutrition/IV Fluid Management

Typically Used With the Following

Nutrition Diagnostic Terminology Used in PES Statements	Common Examples
Nutrition Diagnoses	• Altered GI function • Inadequate parenteral nutrition infusion • Impaired nutrient utilization
Etiology	• Altered GI tract function, inability to absorb nutrients, or excessive loss of nutrients (eg severe vomiting, diarrhea, high fistula output) • Decreased functional length of GI tract • Bowel obstruction
Signs and Symptoms	Anthropometric Measurements • Unintentional weight loss • Growth failure • Insufficient maternal weight gain Nutrition Focused Physical Findings • Obvious muscle and/or fat wasting • Poor skin turgor (tenting) • Fluid retention (edema, ascites) • Diarrhea • Vomiting Food/Nutrition-Related History • Intake less than requirements (insufficient intake) • Existing or expected inadequate intake for 7 to 14 days Client History • Malabsorption, maldigestion • Emesis • Diffuse peritonitis, intestinal obstruction, paralytic ileus, gastrointestinal ischemia, or perforated viscus, short bowel syndrome

Other considerations (eg, client negotiation, client needs and desires, and readiness to change)

- End-of-life issues, ethical considerations, client rights, and supportive individual issues
- Other nutrient intake (oral, enteral nutrition)
- Parenteral formulary composition and product availability
- Availability/access to a qualified practitioner for follow-up and monitoring
- Economic constraints that limit availability of parenteral products

Medical Food Supplement Therapy

Definition

Commercial or prepared foods or beverages intended to supplement energy, protein, carbohydrate, fiber, and/or fat intake that may also contribute to vitamin and mineral intake.

Details of Intervention

A typical intervention might be further described with the following details. Nutrition and dietetics practitioners recommend, implement, or order nutrition interventions and the action(s) may be to initiate, modify, or discontinue a nutrition intervention(s):

- Commercial beverage medical food supplement therapy
- Commercial food medical food supplement therapy
- Modified beverage medical food supplement therapy
- Modified food medical food supplement therapy
- Purpose of medical food supplement therapy (eg, to supplement energy, protein, carbohydrate, fiber, and/or fat intake)

Medical Food Supplement Therapy

Typically Used With the Following

Nutrition Diagnostic Terminology Used in PES Statements	Common Examples
Nutrition Diagnoses	• Inadequate oral intake • Inadequate fluid intake • Increased nutrient needs • Malnutrition (undernutrition) • Growth rate below expected
Etiology	• Neurologic deficit (stroke) • Difficulty chewing or swallowing • Food allergies or intolerance • Altered GI function • Disease- or treatment-related anorexia (eg, cancer, infection, medication side effects) • Small for gestational age, intrauterine growth restriction, lack of appropriate weight gain, hyperemesis gravidarum • Inborn errors of metabolism
Signs and Symptoms	Anthropometric Measurements • Delayed growth • Unintended weight loss Nutrition Focused Physical Findings • Obvious muscle and/or fat wasting • Poor skin turgor (tenting) Food/Nutrition-Related History • Insufficient usual intake • Insufficient macronutrient and/or micronutrient intake Client History • Diagnosis consistent with elevated nutrient needs • Potential for repletion of nutritional status • Oral/facial trauma

Other considerations (eg, client negotiation, client needs and desires, and readiness to change)

- Appetite sufficient to take medical food supplements
- System constraints that prevent meeting the client's preferences for specific flavors, textures, foods, and the timing of feedings
- Economic concerns and product/food availability
- Ability to procure medical food supplement
- Access to medical food supplement storage

Vitamin and Mineral Supplement Therapy

Definition

A product that is intended to supplement vitamin or mineral intake.

Details of Intervention

A typical intervention might be further described with the following details. Nutrition and dietetics practitioners recommend, implement, or order nutrition interventions and the action(s) may be to initiate, modify, or discontinue a nutrition intervention(s):

- Multivitamin/mineral supplement therapy (yes/no, specify dose, frequency)
- Multi-trace element supplement therapy (yes/no, specify dose, frequency)
- Vitamin supplement therapy:
  - Vitamin A supplement therapy (specify form, µg or RE, frequency)
  - Vitamin C supplement therapy (mg/day, frequency)
  - Vitamin D supplement therapy (specify form, µg or IU, frequency)
  - Vitamin E supplement therapy (specify form, mg or IU, frequency)
  - Vitamin K supplement therapy (µg, frequency)
  - Thiamin supplement therapy (mg, frequency)
  - Riboflavin supplement therapy (mg, frequency)
  - Niacin supplement therapy (specify form, mg, frequency)
  - Folate supplement therapy (specify form, µg, frequency)
  - Vitamin B6 supplement therapy (specify form, mg, frequency)
  - Vitamin B12 supplement therapy (µg, frequency)
  - Pantothenic acid supplement therapy (mg, frequency)
  - Biotin supplement therapy (µg, frequency)
- Mineral supplement therapy:
  - Calcium (specify form, mg, frequency)
  - Chloride supplement therapy (mg, frequency)
  - Iron supplement therapy (specify form, mg, frequency)
  - Magnesium supplement therapy (mg, frequency)
  - Potassium supplement therapy (specify form, g or mg, frequency)
  - Phosphorus supplement therapy (mg, frequency)
  - Sodium supplement therapy (mg or g, frequency)
  - Zinc supplement therapy (mg, frequency)
  - Sulfate supplement therapy (g or mmol, frequency)
  - Fluoride supplement therapy (mg, frequency)
  - Copper supplement therapy (µg or mg, frequency)
  - Iodine supplement therapy (µg, frequency)
  - Selenium supplement therapy (specify form, µg, frequency)
  - Manganese supplement therapy (mg, frequency)
  - Chromium supplement therapy (specify form, µg, frequency)
  - Molybdenum supplement therapy (µg, frequency)
  - Boron supplement therapy (mg, frequency)
  - Cobalt supplement therapy (µg, frequency)

Vitamin and Mineral Supplement Therapy

Typically Used With the Following

Nutrition Diagnostic Terminology Used in PES Statements	Common Examples
Nutrition Diagnoses	• Unbalanced diet pattern • Inadequate vitamin intake • Excessive vitamin intake • Inadequate mineral intake • Excessive mineral intake • Excessive alcohol intake • Altered GI function • Impaired nutrient utilization • Predicted food medication interaction • Food and nutrition related knowledge deficit • Limited food and nutrition related skill
Etiology	• Poor intake of nutrient-dense foods that contain vitamins and minerals • Excessive use of vitamin and mineral supplements • Medical diagnosis or treatment impacting vitamin and mineral requirements or utilization • Malabsorption of vitamins and minerals • Combined ingestion or administration of medication and food that results in undesirable/harmful interaction • Long-term parenteral nutrition dependency
Signs and Symptoms	Biochemical Data, Medical Tests, and Procedures • Laboratory or radiologic indexes of vitamin–mineral depletion Nutrition Focused Physical Findings • Abnormalities consistent with vitamin and mineral deficiency or excess Food/Nutrition-Related History • Nutrient intake analysis reveals vitamin and mineral intake more or less than recommended

Other considerations (eg, client negotiation, client needs and desires, and readiness to change)

- Emerging scientific evidence to support the use of vitamin and mineral supplements in specific populations, medical conditions, and/or medical treatments
- Availability of a qualified practitioner with additional education/training in the use of vitamin and mineral supplements in practice
- Economic considerations and product availability

Bioactive Constituent Management

Definition

Addition or change in provision of bioactive substances (eg, plant stanol and sterol esters, psyllium, food additives, other bioactive substances), alcohol, and caffeine.

Details of Intervention

A typical intervention might be further described with the following details. Nutrition and dietetics practitioners recommend, implement, or order nutrition interventions and the action(s) may be to initiate, modify, or discontinue a nutrition intervention(s):

- Plant stanol esters management (specify g, form, frequency)
- Plant sterol esters management (specify g, form, frequency)
- Soy protein management (specify g, form, frequency)
- Psyllium management (specify g, form, frequency)
- Beta glucan management (specify g, form, frequency)
- Food additives management (those thought to have an impact on a client's health) (specify, eg, amount, form, frequency, pattern)
- Alcohol management (specify, oz/mL/units, form, frequency)
- Caffeine management (specify, eg, mg, oz/mL, form, frequency)

Bioactive Constituent Management

Typically Used With the Following

Nutrition Diagnostic Terminology Used in PES Statements	Common Examples
Nutrition Diagnoses	• Inadequate bioactive substance intake • Excessive bioactive substance intake • Excessive alcohol intake • Predicted food-medication interaction • Food and nutrition related knowledge deficit= • Undesirable food choices • Limited food and nutrition related skill
Etiology	• Food and nutrition related knowledge deficit concerning recommended bioactive substance intake • Lack of or limited access to food that contains a bioactive substance • Contamination, misname, mislabel or lack of labeling, misuse, recent brand change, recent dose increase, recent formulation change of substance consumed • Combined ingestion or administration of medication and food that results in undesirable/harmful interaction • Adverse side effect related to bioactive substance • Limited numeracy skills
Signs and Symptoms	Food/Nutrition-Related History • Nutrient intake analysis reveals bioactive substance intake more or less than recommended • Intake reveals consumption of food additive to which the client is sensitive or intolerant Client History • Medical diagnosis associated with increased bioactive substance need

Other considerations (eg, client negotiation, client needs and desires, and readiness to change)

- Emerging scientific evidence to support the use of bioactive supplements in specific populations, specific medical conditions, and/or with medical treatments
- Availability of a qualified practitioner with additional education/training in the use of bioactive supplements in practice

Feeding Assistance Management

Definition

Accommodation or assistance designed to restore the client's ability to eat independently, support adequate nutrient intake, and reduce the incidence of unplanned weight loss and dehydration.

Details of Intervention

A typical intervention might be further described with the following details. Nutrition and dietetics practitioners recommend, implement, or order nutrition interventions and the action(s) may be to initiate, modify, or discontinue a nutrition intervention(s):

- Adaptive eating device management (equipment or utensils) (eg, specify)
- Feeding position management (eg, specify client position in relationship to eating or degree angle for enteral feeding)
- Meal set up management (eg, specify actions to make food accessible for consumption)
- Mouth care management (eg, specify treatment to promote oral health and hygiene)
- Menu selection assistance (yes/no)
- Other (specify)

Typically Used With the Following

Nutrition Diagnostic Terminology Used in PES Statements	Common Examples
Nutrition Diagnoses	• Inadequate energy intake • Inadequate oral intake • Inadequate enteral nutrition infusion • Unintended weight loss • Self feeding difficulty
Etiology	• Physical disability • Poor food/nutrient intake • Neurological issues, eg, decreased memory, concentration problems
Signs and Symptoms	Anthropometric Measurements • Weight loss Food/Nutrition-Related History • Dropping the utensils or food Client History • Conditions associated with a diagnosis or treatment, eg, cerebral palsy, stroke, dementia • History of aspiration or conditions which increase risk of aspiration • Refusal to use prescribed adaptive eating devices or follow prescribed positioning techniques

Feeding Assistance Management

Other considerations (eg, client negotiation, client needs and desires, and readiness to change)

- Limited acceptance of feeding assistance/feeding devices
- Environment offers limited support to foster adequate intake
- Limited assistance at mealtime
- Limited training in methods of feeding assistance
- Limited available physical therapy, occupational therapy, or speech therapy evaluations
- Limited ability to understand the reasoning behind the recommendations and desire to make personal changes
- Limited assistance when translation of menu items is needed

Manage Feeding Environment

Definition

Adjustment of the physical environment, temperature, convenience, and attractiveness of the location where food is served that impacts food consumption.

Details of Intervention

A typical intervention might be further described with the following details. Nutrition and dietetics practitioners recommend, implement, or order nutrition interventions and the action(s) may be to initiate, modify, or discontinue a nutrition intervention(s):

- Feeding environment lighting management (eg, specify)
- Feeding environment odors management (eg, specify, minimize, or enhance)
- Feeding environment distractions management (eg, specify, minimize)
- Feeding environment table height management (specify)
- Feeding environment table service management (eg, plates, napkins)
- Feeding environment room temperature management
- Feeding environment meal service management (type of service, eg, service at table, buffet)
- Feeding environment meal location management (specify)

Typically Used With the Following

Nutrition Diagnostic Terminology Used in PES Statements	Common Examples
Nutrition Diagnoses	• Inadequate oral intake • Disordered eating pattern • Self feeding difficulty
Etiology	• Dementia • Inability to stick to task/easily distracted by others • Familial, societal, biological/genetic, and/or environmental -related obsessive desire to be thin • Avoidance behavior to strong food aromas • Lack of developmental readiness to perform self-management tasks
Signs and Symptoms	Food/Nutrition-Related History • Changes in appetite attributed to mealtime surroundings • Easily distracted from eating • Food sanitation and safety issues in environment • Available foods not of the client's choosing • Decline in client ability to eat independently • Avoidance of social events at which food is served Client History • Pacing, wandering, changes in affect

Manage Feeding Environment

Other considerations (eg, client negotiation, client needs and desires, and readiness to change)

- Resources available to improve/modify the feeding environment
- Acceptance of feeding environment changes

Nutrition Related Medication Management

Definition

Modification of a drug or nutrition-related complementary/alternative medicine to optimize client nutritional or health status.

Details of Intervention

A typical intervention might be further described with the following details. Nutrition and dietetics practitioners recommend, implement, or order nutrition interventions and the action(s) may be to initiate, modify, or discontinue a nutrition intervention(s):

- Management of nutrition related prescription medication (eg, insulin, appetite stimulants, digestive enzymes) dose, form, schedule, route
- Management of nutrition related over the counter (OTC) medication (eg, antacids, aspirin, laxatives) dose, form, schedule, route
- Management of nutrition related complementary and alternative medicine (eg, peppermint oil, probiotics), dose, form, schedule, route

Nutrition Related Medication Management

Typically Used With the Following

Nutrition Diagnostic Terminology Used in PES Statements	Common Examples
Nutrition Diagnoses	• Altered GI function • Impaired nutrient utilization • Altered nutrition related laboratory values • Food medication interaction • Predicted food medication interaction
Etiology	• Insufficient appetite resulting in inadequate nutrient intake • Frequent hypoglycemia or hyperglycemia • Pancreatic insufficiency • Malabsorption of fat, protein, lactose, or other carbohydrates • Polypharmacy and medication abuse • Combined ingestion or administration of medication and food that results in undesirable/harmful interaction • Reported misuse or lack of use of medication
Signs and Symptoms	Biochemical Data, Medical Tests, and Procedures • Frequent hypoglycemia or hyperglycemia Anthropometric Measurements • Alterations of anthropometric measurements based on medication effect and client conditions, eg, weight gain and corticosteroids Nutrition-Focused Physical Findings • Thin, wasted appearance • Diarrhea Food/Nutrition-Related History • Report of nutrition-related complementary/alternative medicine use Client History • Diabetes with poorly controlled blood glucose • HIV, cancer

Other considerations (eg, client negotiation, client needs and desires, and readiness to change)

- Availability/access to a clinical pharmacist
- Availability of a qualified practitioner with appropriate pharmacology training and/or education

Infant Feeding Management

Definition

Actions to alter human milk and/or infant formula feeding

Details of Intervention

A typical intervention might be further described with the following details. Nutrition and dietetics practitioners recommend, implement, or order nutrition interventions and the action(s) may be to initiate, modify, or discontinue a nutrition intervention(s):

- Breastmilk* feeding management
  - Management of concentration of breastmilk (calories/kcal/kJ per ounce)—defined as actions to alter the energy density of expressed or donor human milk through additives
    - Management of human milk fortifier additive in breastmilk (g/day and mL/day)—defined as actions to alter the quantity of human milk
    - Management of carbohydrate additive in breastmilk (g/day)—defined as actions to alter the quantity of carbohydrate that is added to human milk
    - Management of fat additive in breastmilk (mL/day)—defined as actions to alter the quantity of fat that is added to human milk
    - Management of protein additive in breastmilk (g/day and mL/day)—defined as actions to alter the quantity of protein that is added to human milk
    - Management of fiber additive in breastmilk (g/day and mL/day)—defined as actions to alter the quantity of fiber that is added to human milk
    - Management of added infant formula in breastmilk (g/day and mL/day)—defined as actions to alter the quantity of infant formula that is added to human milk
  - Management of breastfeeding† attempts (number per day)—defined as actions taken to alter the number of breastfeeding attempts in one day
  - Management of volume of breastmilk (eg, in bottle or other route of feeding) (mL/feeding)—defined as actions to alter the volume of human milk provided in each feeding
  - Evaluation of breastfeeding plan—defined as actions to appraise the parent's approach to support infant nourishment via human milk
  - Evaluation of breastfeeding—defined as actions to appraise the parent's breastfeeding of the infant
  - Evaluation of breastfeeding behavior—defined as actions to appraise the behavior of parent and infant while breastfeeding
  - Promotion of exclusive breastfeeding—defined as actions to encourage nourishment of an infant via breastfeeding for the first 6 months of life while permitting oral vitamin and mineral supplements and medicines
  - Promotion of predominant breastfeeding—defined as actions to encourage nourishment of an infant primarily from human milk, including expressed or donor milk, while permitting other liquids, oral vitamin and mineral supplements and medicines
  - Promotion of partial breastfeeding—defined as actions to encourage nourishment of an infant partially from human milk, including expressed or donor milk, with nourishment from other sources

---

* If a synonym for the term "breastmilk" is helpful or needed, an approved alternate is "human milk."

† If a synonym for the term "breastfeeding" is helpful or needed, an approved alternate is "chestfeeding."

Infant Feeding Management

- Infant formula management
  - Management of composition of infant formula (formula name or description)—defined as actions to alter the infant formula provided
  - Management of concentration of infant formula (calories/kcal/kJ per ounce)—defined as actions to alter the energy density of infant formula through additives
    - Management of human milk fortifier additive in infant formula (g/day and mL/day)—defined as actions to alter the quantity of human milk fortifier that is added to infant formula
    - Management of carbohydrate additive in infant formula (g/day)—defined as actions to alter the quantity of carbohydrate that is added to infant formula
    - Management of fat additive in infant formula (mL/day)—defined as actions to alter the quantity of fat that is added to infant formula
    - Management of protein additive in infant formula (g/day and mL/day)—defined as actions to alter the quantity of protein that is added to infant formula
    - Management of fiber additive in infant formula (g/day and mL/day)—defined as actions to alter the quantity of fiber that is added to infant formula
  - Management of infant formula feeding attempts (number per day)—defined as actions taken to alter the number of infant formula feeding attempts in one day
  - Management of volume of infant formula (mL/feeding)—defined as actions to alter the volume of infant formula provided in each feeding
  - Evaluation of infant formula feeding plan—defined as actions to appraise the parent's approach to support infant nourishment via infant formula
  - Evaluation of infant formula feeding—defined as actions to appraise the parent's infant formula feeding of the infant
  - Evaluation of infant formula feeding behavior—defined as actions to appraise the behavior of parent and infant while feeding with infant formula

Infant Feeding Management

Typically Used With the Following

Nutrition Diagnostic Terminology Used in PES Statements	Common Examples
Nutrition Diagnoses	• Inadequate oral intake • Growth rate below expected • Illness related pediatric malnutrition • Non illness related pediatric malnutrition • Food and nutrition related knowledge deficit • Limited food and nutrition related skill
Etiology	• Physiological impairment to feed infant • Diminished ability to feed infant • Diminished ability of infant to feed • Beliefs or attitudes impacting infant feeding • Cultural impact on infant feeding • Social or personal impediment to successful infant feeding
Signs and Symptoms	Anthropometric Measurements • Weight loss or limited weight gain • Growth stunting or failure • Small for gestational age • Preterm birth Biochemical Data, Medical Tests and Procedures • Fewer than six wet diapers per day Nutrition-Focused Physical Findings • Muscle and/or fat wasting • Decreased skin turgor • Evidence of dehydration Food/Nutrition-Related History • Intake less than estimated energy or nutrient requirements Client History • Aspiration • Trauma, significant illness, coma

Other considerations (eg, client negotiation, client needs and desires, and readiness to change)

- Other nutrient intake (oral, parenteral nutrition)
- Medication containing energy
- Availability/access to a qualified practitioner for follow-up and monitoring
- Economic constraints that limit availability of human milk, infant formula, or modifier products

Nutrition Education Content

Definition

Instruction or training intended to lead to nutrition related content knowledge.

Note: This reference sheet only refers to client nutrition education. Please use Nutrition Counseling on pages 483-489 for documentation of the Theoretical Basis/Approach and Strategies used for client behavior change.

Details of Intervention

A typical intervention might be further described with the following details. Nutrition and dietetics practitioners recommend, implement, or order nutrition interventions and the action(s) may be to initiate, modify, or discontinue a nutrition intervention(s):

- Content related nutrition education—defined as instruction intended to lead to nutrition-related knowledge
- Education on nutrition's influence on health—defined as instruction intended to lead to knowledge about the association between nutrition and health and disease status
- Physical activity guidance—defined as instruction intended to lead to physical activity-related knowledge and change

Nutrition Education Content

Typically Used With the Following

<table>
<tr><th>Nutrition Diagnostic Terminology Used in PES Statements</th><th>Common Examples</th></tr>
<tr><td>Nutrition Diagnoses</td><td><ul><li>Predicted food-medication interaction</li><li>Underweight</li><li>Overweight/obesity</li><li>Food and nutrition related knowledge deficit</li><li>Belief finding that hinders food and/or nutrition behavior change</li><li>Attitude finding that hinders food and/or nutrition behavior change</li><li>Self monitoring deficit</li><li>Disordered eating pattern</li><li>Limited adherence to nutrition related recommendations</li><li>Physical inactivity</li><li>Excessive physical activity</li><li>Poor food and/or nutrition quality of life</li><li>Altered nutrition related laboratory values</li><li>Other: Any diagnoses related to inadequate, excessive, or inconsistent intake</li></ul></td></tr>
<tr><td>Etiology</td><td><ul><li>Knowledge deficit related to newly diagnosed medical condition and/or nutrition problem</li><li>Medical or surgical procedure requiring modified diet</li><li>Prior exposure to incorrect information</li></ul></td></tr>
<tr><td>Signs and Symptoms</td><td>Food/Nutrition-Related History<ul><li>Limited ability to explain purpose of the nutrition prescription or rationale for nutrition prescription in relationship to disease/health</li><li>Expresses need for additional information or clarification of education or additional time to learn information</li><li>Limited ability to select appropriate foods or supplements</li><li>Limited ability to choose appropriate timing, volume, or preparation/handling of foods</li><li>Uncertainty of physical activity, type, and frequency</li><li>Limited ability to distinguish legitimate from false information</li></ul>Biochemical Data, Medical Tests and Procedures<ul><li>Laboratory data indicating nutrition education warranted</li></ul></td></tr>
</table>

Nutrition Education Content

Other considerations (eg, client negotiation, client needs and desires, and readiness to change)

- Met with several providers in one day and has limited ability to receive more nutrition education at this time
- Profile reflects complicated situation warranting additional education/instruction
- Being discharged from the hospital
- Caregiver unavailable at time of nutrition education
- Baseline knowledge
- Learning style
- Other education and learning needs, eg, new medication or other treatment administration
- Diminished literacy, including ability to read, write, comprehend information, or language barrier
- Potential for referral to RDN with different expertise
- Promote client-defined health goals and outcomes
- Counseling needed for the unmotivated or precontemplative client

Nutrition Education Application

Definition

Instruction or training intended to lead to nutrition related result interpretation or skills.

Note: This reference sheet only refers to client nutrition education. Please use Nutrition Counseling on pages 483-489 for documentation of the Theoretical Basis/Approach and Strategies used for client behavior change.

Details of Intervention

A typical intervention might be further described with the following details. Nutrition and dietetics practitioners recommend, implement, or order nutrition interventions and the action(s) may be to initiate, modify, or discontinue a nutrition intervention(s):

- Nutrition related laboratory result interpretation education—defined as instruction or training leading to nutrition-related laboratory result interpretation (eg, medical or other results to coincide with nutrition plan, such as such as, distribution of carbohydrates throughout the day based on blood glucose monitoring results)
- Nutrition related skill education—defined as instruction or training leading to nutrition-related skill development (eg, numeracy, glucometer use, home enteral nutrition feeding tube and feeding pump training, cooking and food preparation, physical activity equipment use)
- Technical nutrition education—defined as instruction or training leading to nutrition-related result interpretation or skills (eg, ability to evaluate stool output from ostomy, heart rate during physical activity)

Nutrition Education Application

Typically Used With the Following

Nutrition Diagnostic Terminology Used in PES Statements	Common Examples
Nutrition Diagnoses	• Food and nutrition related knowledge deficit • Belief finding that hinders food and/or nutrition behavior change • Self monitoring deficit • Disordered eating pattern • Physical inactivity • Altered nutrition related laboratory values • Limited food and nutrition related skill • Attitude finding that hinders food and/or nutrition behavior change • Other: Any diagnoses related to inadequate or excessive, or inconsistent intake
Etiology	• Limited understanding of how to interpret nutrition related results • Exposure to incorrect food and nutrition application information • Limited self-management skills
Signs and Symptoms	Food/Nutrition Related History • Expresses desire to apply nutrition information • Food and nutrient intake tracking incomplete Biochemical Data, Medical Tests and Procedures • Laboratory data indicating nutrition education warranted

Other Considerations (eg, client negotiation, client needs and desires, and readiness to change)

- Profile reflects complicated situation warranting additional education/instruction
- Counseling for precontemplative client
- Quality of life may be enhanced with in-depth nutrition education and understanding
- Baseline knowledge
- Lifestyle factors
- Education approaches that enhance skill transfer
- Diminished literacy, including ability to read, write, or comprehend information
- Language barrier

Theoretical Basis/Approach

Definition

The theories or models used to design and implement an intervention. Theories and theoretical models consist of principles, constructs, and variables, which offer systematic explanations of the human behavior change process. Behavior change theories and models provide a research-based rationale for designing and tailoring nutrition interventions to achieve the desired effect. A theoretical framework for curriculum and treatment protocols, it guides determination of: (1) what information clients need at different points in the behavior change process, (2) what tools and strategies may be best applied to facilitate behavior change, and (3) outcome measures to assess effectiveness in interventions or components of interventions.

Application Guidance

One or more of the following theories or theoretical models may influence a practitioner's counseling style or approach. Practitioners are asked to identify those Theories that most influence the intervention being documented. An intervention might also incorporate tools and strategies derived from a variety of behavior change theories and models. The practitioner is also asked to indicate which Strategies they used in a particular intervention session.

Details of Intervention

A typical intervention might be further described with the following details. Nutrition and dietetics practitioners recommend, implement, or order nutrition interventions and the action(s) may be to initiate, modify, or discontinue a nutrition intervention(s).

The following theories and models have proven valuable in providing a theoretical framework for evidence-based individual and interpersonal level nutrition interventions. Other theories may be useful for community level interventions (eg, community organization, diffusion of innovations, communication theory).

- Nutrition counseling based on cognitive behavioral theory approach
- Nutrition counseling based on health belief model
- Nutrition counseling based on social learning theory approach
- Nutrition counseling based on transtheoretical model and stages of change approach

Additional information regarding each of the above theories and models can be found within this reference sheet.

Theoretical Basis/Approach

Typically Used With the Following

Nutrition Diagnostic Terminology Used in PES Statements	Common Examples
Nutrition Diagnoses	• Unbalanced diet pattern • Overweight/obesity • Belief finding that hinders food and/or nutrition behavior change • Not ready for nutrition related behavior change • Self monitoring deficit • Disordered eating pattern • Limited adherence to nutrition-related recommendations • Physical inactivity • Excessive physical activity • Inability to manage self care • Poor food and/or nutrition quality of life • Attitude finding that hinders food and/or nutrition behavior change • Other: Any diagnoses related to inadequate, excessive, or inconsistent intake
Etiology	• New medical diagnosis • Belief finding that hinders food and/or nutrition behavior change • Limited value for behavior change, competing values • Limited efficacy to make changes or to overcome barriers to change • Limited focus/attention to detail, difficulty with time management and/or organization • Perception that time, interpersonal, or financial constraints prevent change • Prior exposure to incorrect or incompatible information • Not ready for nutrition-related behavior change • Limited caretaker or social support for implementing changes • Attitude finding that hinders food and/or nutrition behavior change • High level of fatigue or other side effect of medical condition
Signs and Symptoms (Defining Characteristics)	Food/Nutrition-Related History • Concerns with nutrition and/or physical activity recommendations • Previous challenges changing target behavior • Resistance to change • Sense of lack of control of eating

Continued on next page

Theoretical Basis/Approach

Continued from previous page

Nutrition Diagnostic Terminology Used in PES Statements	Common Examples
Signs and Symptoms (Defining Characteristics, continued)	• Limited ability to apply food- and nutrition-related information/ guidelines • Limited ability to change food- and nutrition-related behavior • Absent or incomplete self-monitoring records • Limited ability to problem solve/self-manage • Irrational thoughts about self and effects of food intake • Unrealistic expectations • Limited flexibility with food selection • Evidence of excessive, inadequate, or inconsistent intake related to needs

Other considerations (eg, client negotiation, client needs and desires, and readiness to change)

- Lifestyle factors
- Language barrier
- Educational level
- Culture
- Socioeconomic status

Strategies

Definition

An evidence-based method or plan of action designed to achieve a particular goal. Application of behavior change theories in nutrition practice has provided practitioners with a collection of evidence-based strategies to promote behavior change. Some strategies target change in motivation and intention to change, and others target behavior change. Nutrition and dietetics practitioners selectively apply strategies based on client goals and objectives, and their personal counseling philosophy and skill.

Application Guidance

An intervention typically incorporates tools and strategies derived from a variety of behavior change theories and models. The practitioner is asked to indicate which Strategies they used in a particular intervention session along with the Theories that most influence the intervention being documented.

Details of Intervention

A typical intervention might be further described with the following details. Nutrition and dietetics practitioners recommend, implement, or order nutrition interventions and the action(s) may be to initiate, modify, or discontinue a nutrition intervention(s).

The following strategies have proven valuable in providing effective nutrition-related (eg nutrition therapy, physical activity) behavior change:

- Nutrition counseling based on motivational interviewing strategy
- Nutrition counseling based on goal setting strategy
- Nutrition counseling based on self monitoring strategy
- Nutrition counseling based on problem solving strategy
- Nutrition counseling based on social support strategy
- Nutrition counseling based on stress management strategy
- Nutrition counseling based on stimulus control strategy
- Nutrition counseling based on cognitive restructuring strategy
- Nutrition counseling based on relapse prevention strategy
- Nutrition counseling based on rewards and contingency management strategy

Additional information regarding each of the above strategies can be found within this reference sheet.

Strategies

Typically Used With the Following

Nutrition Diagnostic Terminology Used in PES Statements	Common Examples
Nutrition Diagnoses	• Unbalanced diet pattern • Overweight/obesity • Belief finding that hinders food and/or nutrition behavior change • Attitude finding that hinders food and/or nutrition behavior change • Not ready for nutrition related behavior change • Self monitoring deficit • Disordered eating pattern • Limited adherence to nutrition-related recommendations • Physical inactivity • Excessive physical activity • Inability to manage self care • Poor food and/or nutrition quality of life • Other: Any diagnoses related to inadequate, excessive, or inconsistent intake
Etiology	• New medical diagnosis • Unsupported beliefs/attitudes about food, nutrition, and nutrition-related topics • Limited value for behavior change, competing values • Limited efficacy to make changes or to overcome barriers to change • Limited focus/attention to detail, difficulty with time management and/or organization • Perception that time, interpersonal, or financial constraints prevent change • Prior exposure to incorrect or incompatible information • Not ready for nutrition-related behavior change • Limited caretaker or social support for implementing changes • High level of fatigue or other side effect of medical condition
Signs and Symptoms (Defining Characteristics)	Food/Nutrition-Related History • Concerns with nutrition and/or physical activity recommendations • Previous challenges when changing target behavior • Resistance to change • Sense of lack of control of eating • Limited ability to apply food- and nutrition-related information/ guidelines

Continued on next page

Strategies

Continued from previous page

Nutrition Diagnostic Terminology Used in PES Statements	Common Examples
Signs and Symptoms (Defining Characteristic, continued)	• Limited ability to change food- and nutrition-related behavior • Absent or incomplete self-monitoring records • Limited ability to problem solve/self-manage • Irrational thoughts about self and effects of food intake • Unrealistic expectations • Limited flexibility with food selection • Evidence of excessive, inadequate, or inconsistent intake related to needs

Other considerations (eg, client negotiation, client needs and desires, and readiness to change)

- Lifestyle factors
- Language barrier
- Educational level
- Culture
- Socioeconomic status

Collaboration and Referral of Nutrition Care

Definition

Facilitating services or interventions with other professionals, institutions, or agencies on behalf of the client prior to discharge from nutrition care.

Details of Intervention

A typical intervention might be further described with the following details. Nutrition and dietetics practitioners recommend, implement, or order nutrition interventions and the action(s) may be to initiate, modify, or discontinue a nutrition intervention(s):

- Team meeting involving nutrition professional (eg, holding a team meeting to develop a comprehensive plan of care)
- Referral by nutrition professional to another nutrition professional with different expertise (eg, a referral for care by other nutrition and dietetics practitioners who provide different expertise)
- Collaboration by nutrition professional with other nutrition professionals (eg, collaboration by nutrition and dietetics practitioner with other nutrition and dietetics practitioners)
- Collaboration by nutrition professional with other providers (eg, collaboration with others such as the physician, dentist, physical therapist, social worker, occupational therapist, speech therapist, nurse, pharmacist, or other specialist dietitian)
- Referral by nutrition professional to other provider (eg, refer to others such as the physician, dentist, physical therapist, social worker, occupational therapist, speech therapist, nurse, pharmacist, or other specialist nutrition and dietetics practitioner)
- Referral by nutrition professional to community agencies and programs (eg, refer to an appropriate agency/program [eg, home delivered meals], assistance programs for women, infants, and children [eg, US Department of Food and Agriculture's Women, Infants & Child Program (WIC)], food assistance programs [eg, food pantry, soup kitchen, food stamps], housing assistance, shelters, rehabilitation, physical and mental disability programs, education training, and employment programs)

Collaboration and Referral of Nutrition Care

Typically Used With the Following

Nutrition Diagnostic Terminology Used in PES Statements	Common Examples
Nutrition Diagnoses	• Inadequate oral intake • Altered nutrition related laboratory values • Underweight • Unintended weight loss • Excessive alcohol intake • Overweight/obesity • Physical inactivity • Food medication interaction • Self feeding difficulty • Food insecurity
Etiology	• Physical ability difference, decreased feeding ability, other changes related to activities of daily living • Mental difference • Growth and development difference • Nutrient drug interactions • Transportation issues • Limited food acceptance • Developmental difference • Economic considerations impacting food/nutrient intake
Signs and Symptoms	Anthropometric Measurements • Body weight loss • Unacceptable growth rates compared to standard growth charts Food/Nutrition-Related History • Inability to procure food • Lack of access to food sources • Lack of food preparation skills Nutrition-Focused Physical Findings • Skin breakdown and poor wound healing Client History • Anorexia nervosa

Other considerations (eg, client negotiation, client needs and desires, and readiness to change)

- Availability of services related to client need (specialty dietitians, clinical pharmacists, speech pathologists, nurse practitioners, etc)
- Anticipated duration of health care encounter/hospital or long-term care discharge
- Resources available for care
- Availability of or access to government medical programs (eg, Medicare/Medicaid, health care exchanges) insurance guidelines and restrictions
- Availability of or access to food assistance program (eg, food assistance program) guidelines and regulations

Discharge and Transfer of Nutrition Care to a New Setting or Provider

Definition

Discharge planning and transfer of nutrition care from one level or location of care to another.

Details of Intervention

A typical intervention might be further described with the following details. Nutrition and dietetics practitioners recommend, implement, or order nutrition interventions and the action(s) may be to initiate, modify, or discontinue a nutrition intervention(s):

- Discharge and transfer of nutrition care to other providers: refer to others such as the physician, dentist, physical therapist, social worker, occupational therapist, speech therapist, nurse, or pharmacist
- Discharge and transfer of nutrition care to community agencies and programs: refer to a community agency/program (eg, home-delivered meals, assistance programs for women, infants and children [eg, US Department of Food and Agriculture's Women, Infants & Child Program (WIC)], food assistance programs [eg, food pantry, soup kitchen, food stamps], housing assistance, shelters, rehabilitation, physical and mental disability programs, education, training and employment programs)
- Discharge and transfer of nutrition care from nutrition professional to another nutrition professional: transfer of nutrition care to another nutrition and dietetics practitioner

Discharge and Transfer of Nutrition Care to a New Setting or Provider

Typically Used With the Following

Nutrition Diagnostic Terminology Used in PES Statements	Common Examples
Nutrition Diagnoses	• Inadequate oral intake • Imbalance of nutrients • Food medication interaction • Underweight • Overweight/obesity • Limited ability to prepare foods for eating • Self feeding difficulty
Etiology	• Long-term insufficient intake mandating home enteral or parenteral nutrition • Growth and development considerations requiring intervention in a new setting
Signs and Symptoms	Biochemical Data, Medical Tests and Procedures • Abnormal lab values Anthropometric Measurements • Less-than-optimal weight status • Continuing weight gain or loss Food/Nutrition-Related History • Less-than-optimal dietary practices • Belief finding that hinders food and/or nutrition behavior change • Attitude finding that hinders food and/or nutrition behavior change Client History • Treatment failure • Readmission

Other considerations (eg, client negotiation, client needs and desires, and readiness to change)

- Availability of discharge planning services, options for care
- Preferences for the level and location of care
- Resources available for care
- Availability of or access to government medical programs (eg Medicare/Medicaid, health exchanges), insurance guidelines and restrictions
- Health literacy
- Ability to implement treatment at home
- Availability of or access to food assistance program (eg, food stamp program) guidelines and regulations

Population Theoretical Frameworks

Definition

Theories, models and approaches used to design, implement and evaluate nutrition interventions at the population level.

Application Guidance

Theories and models are used to analyze and describe a process or occurrence and inform ways to address a problem. Researchers and practitioners draw from theories and models and apply them in systematic approaches relevant to specific situations. Theories, models, and approaches are referred to generally as theoretical frameworks. Theoretical frameworks used to guide change in institutions and society are different from those applied to individual level change. (See Theoretical Bases/Approaches for individual change in the Nutrition Counseling Domain reference sheet on page 484.) The theoretical frameworks listed below are used in assessing, planning, implementing, and evaluating population-based nutrition actions. While the social ecological model provides an overarching model for all intervention approaches, the others provide distinct approaches and concepts to guide and inform the design of population-based interventions. Incorporating theoretical considerations into population based nutrition actions leads to more effective outcomes and is aligned with evidence-based practice. For example, community organizing is used to mobilize action for community gardens and farmers markets, and organizational change theory is used when implementing evidence-based guidelines across systems. Using standard terminology to describe the theoretical foundation for interventions is important for advancing population-based nutrition work.

Details of Intervention

A population based nutrition action is typically described with details regarding the theoretical framework used in its development and implementation. The aim and key concepts of commonly used theories, models, and approaches, and examples of nutrition and dietetic professionals' actions when they are applied are linked to each theoretical framework.

The included theoretical frameworks represent those that are frequently applied in population-based nutrition actions. This is not all inclusive, and nutrition professionals may draw on other theories, models, and approaches as relevant to a particular nutrition problem and its context.

- Social ecological model
- Community organizing
- Diffusion of innovations
- Social marketing
- Organizational change theory
- Mass communications
- Political action

Population Theoretical Frameworks

Typically Used With the Following

Nutrition Diagnostic Terminology Used in PES Statements	Common Examples
Nutrition Diagnoses	• Overweight/obesity • Physical inactivity • Altered nutrition related laboratory values • Unbalanced diet pattern • Limited access to potable water • Other: Any diagnoses related to inadequate, excessive, or inconsistent intake
Etiology	• Food and nutrition related knowledge deficit • Belief finding that hinders food and/or nutrition behavior change • Food insecurity • Availability of shopping facilities • Lack of access to nutrition services • Limited food and nutrition related skill • Attitude finding that hinders food and/or nutrition related behavior change
Signs and Symptoms (Defining Characteristics)	Biochemical Data, Medical Tests and Procedures • Biochemical indicators of at-risk status Anthropometric Measurements • Growth, weight, BMI indicators at risk status Food/Nutrition Related History • Nutrient of food group data indicating inadequate intake or excessive intake • Physical activity, type and frequency • Location, distance to, or rate per population with access to full-service grocery store

Other considerations

- Scope of responsibility of the nutrition and dietetic professional
- Material and economic resources
- Constraints of grants, contracts, and program regulations
- Existing policies and laws
- Opportunities for cross-sectoral collaboration
- Interests, resources, and goals of collaborators

Population Strategies

Definition

Plans of action that target environmental change, organizational change, and public policy change.

Application Guidance

Population strategies are widely used to bring about changes that are external to the individual in order to promote and protect the population's health. The strategies are aimed at the structural aspects of the environment, processes within programs, organizations and systems, and the laws and regulations that are the root causes and contributing factors for many nutrition problems. An aim of these strategies is to create supportive environments that "make the healthy choice the easy choice."

Strategies are classified by the target of change: 1) the environment including food availability and access and the built environment, especially as it affects physical activity opportunities and societal norms; 2) organizational change including the process, procedures, and policies (formal and informal) of programs, organizations, institutions, and systems; and 3) public policy change, including local, state, and national laws and regulations.

Nutrition and dietetic professionals select from these strategies when planning population-based nutrition actions; and when using these strategies they typically work in collaboration with other individuals and organization on cross-sectoral, multi-level, and multi-sector initiatives. The strategy(ies) chosen are guided by the nature of the problem and its determinants. A single initiative can be planned or several strategies may be used simultaneously, resulting in reinforcing, multicomponent programs designed to address different underlying causes of the problem.

Details of Intervention

A population-based nutrition action is typically described by identifying the target of change, and with details regarding the strategy used as identified in the Population Strategies Table on page 506:

- Environmental change
  - Food environment change
  - Built environment change
  - Social norm change
- Organizational change
- Public policy change

Population Strategies

Typically Used With the Following

Nutrition Diagnostic Terminology Used in PES Statements	Common Examples
Nutrition Diagnoses	• Overweight/obesity • Physical inactivity • Altered nutrition related laboratory values • Unbalanced diet pattern • Intake of unsafe food • Other: Any diagnoses related to inadequate, excessive, or inconsistent intake
Etiology	• Food and nutrition related knowledge deficit • Belief finding that hinders food and/or nutrition behavior change • Food insecurity • Availability of shopping facilities • Lack of access to nutrition services • Limited food and nutrition related skill • Attitude finding that hinders food and/or nutrition behavior change
Signs and Symptoms (Defining Characteristics)	Biochemical Data, Medical Tests and Procedures • Biochemical of at-risk status Anthropometric Measurements • Growth, weight, BMI indicators at risk status Food/Nutrition-Related History • Nutrient of food group data indicating inadequate intake or excessive intake • Physical activity, type and frequency • Location, distance to, or rate per population with access to full-service grocery store

Other considerations

- Scope of responsibility of the nutrition and dietetic professional
- Material and economic resources
- Constraints of grants, contracts, and program regulations
- Existing policies and laws
- Opportunities for cross-sectoral collaboration
- Interests, resources, and goals of collaborators

Population Settings

Definition

Locations where the population-based nutrition intervention is implemented.

Application Guidance

The setting specifies the places where the intervention is delivered to most effectively reach and impact the population experiencing the identified nutrition-related problem. A population-based nutrition action may be delivered in more than one setting in a coordinated fashion (eg, school district and community recreation centers). The intervention may involve one or more sites within the setting (eg, one childcare center or all childcare centers in the county or state). The choice of setting has implications for which strategies (see Population Strategies) to employ.

Some of these settings may also be useful in describing and documenting the location for delivery of individual and group nutrition interventions. Nutrition and dietetic professionals, along with collaborators (see Population Sectors on page 502), select from these settings when planning how and where population-based nutrition actions will be implemented in order to have the greatest impact on the problem and its etiology/root causes/determinants. The setting also identifies the target location where data (assessment, monitoring, and evaluation indicators) can be collected to assess progress and determine outcomes.

Details of Intervention

A population based nutrition action is typically described with details regarding the settings where the intervention is implemented. The settings listed in the Population Settings Table below can be used to classify and described the locations utilized:

- Residential settings
- School settings
- Worksite settings
- Recreation and sports settings
- Food production and provisions settings
- Service settings
- Government settings
- Community at large settings

Population Settings

Population Settings Table

Setting	Typical Types Within the Setting	Examples of Population-Based Nutrition Action in the Setting
Residential Settings	• Neighborhood • Residential facility (apartment complex, housing development, public housing, homeless shelter) • Care facility: aged care, assisted living, group home • Prison, correctional institution	• Promotion to increase use of walking and bike paths • Work to increase the number of gardens in homes, at facilities and in the community • Initiative to improve nutritional quality of food and beverage offerings
School Settings	• Early childhood education/preschool • Elementary and secondary school • Training center • College or university	• Policy and process changes to increase availability, visibility, and affordability of healthy foods and beverages on school and college campuses • School program promoting healthy rewards and fundraising options • Implementation of wellness policy for coordinated school health • Curriculum development and capacity building of teachers
Worksite Settings (interventions directed to employees and volunteer staff)	• Workplace • Military establishment	• Establishment of guidelines for activity breaks and healthy meals and refreshments in workplace cafeteria and vending and for all meetings and sponsored events • Initiate breastfeeding friendly workplace
Recreation and Sports Settings	• Sports facility (sports field or arena, community recreation center, YMCA) • Gym/health club • Park, playground, trail • Community group or organization (Boys and Girls Clubs, Parks and Recreation department) • Senior center	• Training for coaches and youth leaders in healthy nutrition for athletic performance; policy on water availability and healthy snacks for athletes; canteen/vending offerings • Partner with YMCA and others to bring more structured and unstructured physical activity into the environment combined with informational outreach activities

Continued on next page

Population Settings

Continued from previous page

Setting	Typical Types Within the Setting	Examples of Population-Based Nutrition Action in the Setting
Food Production and Provision Settings	• Emergency food program: food banks, food shelves/pantries, and soup kitchens • Food service establishment: fast food, restaurants, mobile vendors, catering • Grocery or convenience store • Farms and farmers markets • Community gardens • Food or beverage company (production, processing, and/or distribution)	• Initiative involving local food pantries and regional food banks to place greater emphasis on the nutritional quality of food collected and distributed • Incentive program to encourage offering healthy options and point-of-purchase prompts in retail food outlets and food service facilities • Training of food service personnel on how to prepare, serve, and promote quality, nutritious, appealing meals
Service Settings (interventions directed to clients)	• Childcare facility • Hospital or clinic • Community health center • Business/retail (products and services [other than food] provided to customers) • Service organizations, community-based organizations, fraternal organizations, interest groups • Refugee centers • Faith-based organization (churches, synagogues, mosques) • Government programs (food assistance, social and financial services)	• Initiative with early childhood collaborative to increase capacity and adopt programs for physical activity and healthy eating • Promotion to improve access to breastfeeding-friendly environments • Technical assistance to community organizations that are planning events and celebrations to incorporate physical activity and healthy eating • Vending contracts/procurement policies with nutrition standards requiring healthy food and beverage options for public facilities
Government Settings	• Policy-making body (municipality, county, state, federal) • Administrative agencies (regulatory and planning) • Judicial branch/legal system	• Work with elected officials to formulate wording for policies • Regular monitoring of political issues and action to provide timely input regarding nutrition and health implications of proposed regulations • Event to educate officials and staff on importance of improved nutrition and food access on community health
Community at Large Settings	• Media: print (newspapers, magazines, pamphlets), broadcast (radio/TV), digital (social media, web sites, apps) • Advertising: outdoor billboards, posters	• Community-wide physical activity social marketing initiative • Media campaign on family meals in conjunction with website

Population Settings

Typically Used With the Following

Nutrition Diagnostic Terminology Used in PES Statements	Common Examples
Nutrition Diagnoses	• Overweight/obesity • Physical inactivity • Altered nutrition-related laboratory values • Unbalanced diet pattern • Intake of unsafe food • Other: Any diagnoses related to inadequate, excessive, or inconsistent intake
Etiology	• Food and nutrition related knowledge deficit • Belief finding that hinders food and/or nutrition behavior change • Food insecurity • Availability of shopping facilities • Lack of access to nutrition services • Limited food and nutrition related skill • Attitude finding that hinders food and/or nutrition behavior change
Signs and Symptoms (Defining Characteristics)	Biochemical Data, Medical Tests and Procedures • Biochemical indicators of at-risk status Anthropometric Measurements • Growth, body weight, BMI indicators at risk status Food/Nutrition-Related History • Nutrient of food group data indicating inadequate intake or excessive intake • Physical activity, type and frequency • Location, distance to, or rate per population with access to full-service grocery store

Other considerations

- Scope of responsibility of the nutrition and dietetic professional
- Material and economic resources
- Constraints of grants, contracts, and program regulations
- Existing policies and laws
- Opportunities for cross-sectoral collaboration
- Interests, resources, and goals of collaborators

Population Sectors

Definition

Public, private and non-profit entities integral to the development and implementation of interventions that impact determinants of the nutritional well-being of the population.

Application Guidance

Sectors are unique yet interdependent entities that have differing types of influence on and interest in healthy food and healthy people. Considering a broader range of sectors opens new possibilities for interventions directed to the underlying determinants of population nutrition problems. Each sector has numerous constituencies that are potential collaborators for identifying opportunities and developing, implementing, and evaluating interventions. Through mobilizing cross-sector collaboration, awareness is raised, complementary strengths and combined resources can be applied to problematic aspects of complex nutrition problems, and evidence-based and promising practices can be expanded. Additionally, cross-sector interventions promote solidarity in action and foster transparency and public accountability. For example, food companies, researchers, schools, farmer and producer associations, professional sports teams, government programs, and health care systems have different but coordinated roles in collaborative efforts to address underlying causes of childhood obesity.

The sectors and constituents are frequently involved in collaborative work to tackle problems and their underlying causes and advance population nutrition goals. Cross-sector, multi-level, multi-component programs have been shown to be more effective than single interventions and are commonly used to address challenging nutrition and health issues of the population. Many national and international nutrition intervention efforts attribute success to collaborative and coordinated work that engages multiple sectors.

Other terminology related to the concept of sectors includes stakeholders, partners, players, and affiliates who come together in formal and informal alliances, coalitions, councils, networks, partnerships, or workgroups.

Details of Intervention

A population-based nutrition action is typically described with details regarding who is engaged in collaborative efforts. The sectors and constituents in the Population Sectors Table below can be used to identify potential collaborators and then describe those that participate in the planning, implementation, and/or evaluation of the population-based nutrition action:

- Agriculture sector
- Education sector
- Government sector
- Healthcare sector
- Food and beverage sector
- Business and industry sector
- Social welfare sector
- Nonprofit sector
- Communities, neighborhoods, families sector

Population Sectors

Population Sectors Table

Setting	Examples of Constituents From Which Potential Collaborators Are Identified
Agriculture Sector	• Farmer and grower associations (local and regional) • Commodity organizations/boards • Cooperatives, community-supported agriculture schemes
Education Sector	• Early childhood educators and organizations • Teacher, administrator, school board, school nurse, school nutrition, parent and student associations • School/campus wellness committees • University researchers • Adult education programs
Government Sector (local, state, federal)	• Government food assistance and supplementation programs • Public outreach and education programs • Maternal and child health, aging and refugee health, native and aboriginal health departments • Planning and development agencies • Parks and recreation departments • Public health and social welfare departments • Centers for Disease Control and National Institutes of Health initiatives • Elected officials • Public safety officials and emergency response agencies
Healthcare Sector	• Health promotion and disease management programs • Health professional associations • Health advocacy organizations • Health care systems • Insurance companies
Food and Beverage Industry Sector	• Food manufacturers • Food service supply companies, vending companies • Restaurant chains • Food retailer associations
Business and Industry Sector (excluding food and beverage)	• Pharmaceutical companies • Professional sports teams and leagues • Fitness and apparel companies • Transportation industries • Technology, entertainment, and media industries • Building and construction industries and trade associations

Continued on next page

Population Sectors

Continued from previous page

Setting	Examples of Constituents From Which Potential Collaborators Are Identified
Social Welfare Sector	Food security, shelter, and income subsidy programs
Non-Profit Sector	• Community service organizations • Special interest groups • Charitable organizations and foundations • Food, nutrition, and health advocacy groups • Food policy councils • Nongovernmental organizations
Communities, Neighborhoods, Families Sector	• Community coalitions and community advisory boards • Issue champions • Social clubs and cultural associations • Neighborhood associations

Population Sectors

Typically Used With the Following

Nutrition Diagnostic Terminology Used in PES Statements	Common Examples
Nutrition Diagnoses	• Overweight/obesity • Physical inactivity • Altered nutrition-related laboratory values • Unbalanced diet pattern • Intake of unsafe food • Other: Any diagnoses related to inadequate, excessive, or inconsistent intake
Etiology	• Food and nutrition related knowledge deficit • Belief finding that hinders food and/or nutrition behavior change • Food insecurity • Availability of shopping facilities • Lack of access to nutrition services • Limited food and nutrition related skill • Attitude finding that hinders food and/or nutrition behavior change
Signs and Symptoms (Defining Characteristics)	Biochemical Data, Medical Tests and Procedures • Biochemical indicators of at-risk status Anthropometric Measurements • Growth, body weight, BMI indicators at risk status Food/Nutrition-Related History • Nutrient of food group data indicating inadequate intake or excessive intake • Physical activity, type and frequency • Location, distance to, or rate per population with access to full-service grocery store

Other considerations (eg, client negotiation, client needs and desires, and readiness to change)

- Scope of responsibility of the nutrition and dietetic professional
- Material and economic resources
- Constraints of grants, contracts, and program regulations
- Existing policies and laws
- Opportunities for cross-sectoral collaboration
- Interests, resources, and goals of collaborators

Environmental Change

Population Strategy

Target	Strategy Definitions	Examples of Nutrition and Dietetic Practitioners' Actions
Environmental Change	Actions designed to alter the environment where people live, work, learn and play to promote and support healthful behaviors, prevent disease and disability, and reduce inequities. *Additional information* In simple terms, the aim is to modify the environment to make the healthy choice the easy choice. Environment is subdivided into three areas: the food environment, the built environment, and social norms.	(See following subcategories)
Food Environment Change	Actions to improve the availability, accessibility and quality of food and the places people access food. *Additional information* The food environment includes the continuum from food production, processing and distribution, to places where people access, purchase, and consume food. Food-related facilities and equipment are included here.	• Organize community to increase access to community-supported agriculture schemes • Work with corner stores to improve refrigeration equipment to enable sale of fresh fruits and vegetables • Work with vending companies to improve food choices offered • Implement calorie content signage in cafeterias and fast food outlets • Advocate for pricing changes to influence food choices • Support and improve the nutritional quality of food aid and emergency feeding programs
Built Environment Change	Actions to modify physical features of indoor and outdoor places and spaces to enable and support healthful behaviors, especially to increase opportunities for safe and accessible physical activity for all. *Additional information* The "built" environment refers to structures ("bricks and mortar") and facilities and equipment. (Processes are covered in Organizational Change)	• Work with park and recreation department to update lighting and signage to improve access and safety and increase utilization of walking trails • Work with city planners to increase sidewalks and bike paths, to improve walkability to destinations such as grocery stores, and to incorporate space for physical activity in new housing developments • Work with employee committee to obtain spaces for noon-time exercises classes

Continued on next page

Environmental Change

Continued from previous page

Target	Strategy Definitions	Examples of Nutrition and Dietetic Practitioners' Actions
Social Norm Change	Actions to modify generalized beliefs and values, attitudes and expectations held by segments of the population or the population at large that impact nutrition and health.	• Develop a social marketing campaign to modify expectations regarding portion sizes of food and beverages served • Work with the community to organize support for community gardens and locally-grown food

Mass Communication

Mass Communication

A process in which an entity (person or organization) selects and sends a message through a specialized media or transmitting device to a large group of anonymous and heterogeneous people (target audience or general public) and organizations.

Mass communication draws from many theories that address the processes and mechanisms that allow communication to take place and to impact people, organizations and society.

Aim

To transmit information, frame an issue, and/or shape perceptions to create or change knowledge, attitudes or behaviors of people, societal norms, and/or to modify products and services and structures in the environment.

Key Concepts

- Mass media channels: technological systems and devices that extend communication across time and space. Includes radio, TV, print (books, magazines, pamphlets, billboards, etc) and digital media (email, internet and interactive web sites, blogs, social media, video games)
- Media literacy: ability, of communicator and audience, to access, analyze, evaluate and communicate media messages
- Cultivation of perceptions: through repeated and prolonged exposure to mass media, people's beliefs, values, traditions, behaviors and expectations are shaped
- Mass media campaign: a planned effort that disseminates messages to produce awareness or behavior change among the intended population through channels that reach broad audiences
- Media advocacy: strategic use of mass media to identify and frame issues, increase public awareness and concern, and spur public action
- Framing: taking a leadership role to shape and influence public understanding and discourse about an issue
- Elaboration likelihood model: effectiveness of a message is a function of how people process it and the degree that they engage in elaboration or issue-relevant thinking

Nutrition and Dietetic Practitioner's Actions

- Analyze the communication environment related to the identified nutrition problem, including understanding salient beliefs of the audience, context for decision making, and barriers to behavior change
- Use media analysis to identify competing and reinforcing messages, examine how those messages are framed, and consider how existing coverage of an issue could be improved
- Work with and solicit input of other organizations and community groups to assure the message is relevant and culturally sensitive to the intended audience, expected behaviors are culturally acceptable, and channels are accessible and appropriate
- Determine message, and its framing; and pre-test with the target audience
- Create a comprehensive plan that addresses environmental constraints on the target population as well as individual factors and social and cultural influences
- Develop an exposure strategy to achieve frequent and repeated exposures to the message, through multiple channels
- Select a variety of channels chosen for their ability to reach and engage the target population
- Build in methods for tracking exposure and eliciting feedback

Population Theoretical Frameworks Organizational Change Theory

Numerous theories and models apply to change within organizations. **Two** that are commonly applied in nutrition initiatives are included here.

Oranizational Development (OD)

Organizational development (OD) is any planned and managed process or activity to improve capacity among persons within an organization through continuous diagnoses, action planning, implementation, and evaluation. It involves changing and aligning people with the key goals and challenges facing the organization.

Aim

To expand knowledge, expertise, productivity and effectiveness of people to improve satisfaction, relationships, performance or other desired outcome for the benefit of individuals, groups, work units, or the whole organization.

Key Concepts

- Organizational Climate-The personality of an organization.
- Organizational Culture-The norms, values, and behaviors that are deeply embedded within the members of the organization. The five elements of cultures:
  - Assumptions
  - Values
  - Behavioral norms
  - Behavioral patterns
  - Artifacts
- Organizational Strategies-The organizational development (OD) approach to promote organizational change:
  - Diagnosis
  - Action planning
  - Intervention
  - Evaluation

Nutrition and Dietetic Practitioner's Actions

Nutrition and dietetic practitioner's actions include:

- Analyze changing environmental and organizational trends
- Identify organizational climate and culture enablers and barriers and incorporate them when developing strategies for change
- Recognize where development and realignment of people is necessary to solve current and emerging problems and adapt to changing priorities
- Engage employees in problem solving
- Plan training and team-building and motivational exercises
- Provide training to develop a culturally and linguistically competent nutrition workforce
- Modify position description and performance expectations and adjust recruitment and retention activities
- Use OD concepts to improve the capacity of healthcare professionals to support nutrition needs of clients

Continued on next page

Population Theoretical Frameworks Organizational Change Theory

Continued from previous page

Model for Improvement

The Model for Improvement defines an iterative method for identifying areas for change in a process or system and defining time-specific and measurable goals for improvement, then systematically planning specific actions, implementing them, measuring progress and adjusting the plan as necessary, and finally standardizing and institutionalizing successful innovations and changes.

Models of improvement call for engagement and utilization of a team throughout the steps of the improvement initiative.

Commonly applied in quality improvement programs, updating procedures (eg, evidence-based guidelines), implementing new innovations or technology, and/or in responding to community or customer defined needs and expectations

The PDSA (Plan, Do, Study, Act) Cycle for Learning and Quality Improvement is a widely used application of the model for continuous quality improvement.

Aim

A deliberate and defined method to bring about change in an organization's processes and outcomes to improve internal operations and/or to be responsive to community needs and address population health and nutrition issues.

Key Concepts

Concepts:

- Can be implemented at the program, agency, and/or system levels
- Utilizes a team
- Follows a defined problem solving process, such as the PDSA Cycle

AIM Statement: Preparation step

1. What are we trying to accomplish?
2. How will we know that a change is an improvement?
3. What change can we make that will result in improvement?

The AIM Statement should be clear, specific, measurable and time-bound.

PLAN: Plan a change

1. Identify area, problem or opportunity for improvement
2. Assemble the team
3. Examine the current approach (baseline data, root causes, get input of customers and stakeholders)
4. Identify potential solutions and select best
5. Develop an improvement theory (If..., then...)

DO: Implement the plan

1. Test the change on a small scale
2. Collect data, document successes and problems, examine unintended side effects

Continued on next page

Population Theoretical Frameworks Organizational Change Theory

Continued from previous page

Model for Improvement

Key Concepts (continued)

STUDY: Observe the results

1. Study the results, compare with baseline and intended aim

ACT: Refine the change, as necessary, and implement on large scale

1. Continue testing and adjusting until acceptable level of improvement is achieved
2. Celebrate successes
3. Standardize the improvement
4. Take steps to preserve gains and sustain accomplishments

Nutrition and Dietetic Practitioner's Actions

Nutrition and dietetic practitioner's actions include:

Preparation

- Research and provide evidence for needed changes
- Review best practices and evidence-based approaches
- Determine relevant process and outcome measures
- Secure commitment of resources and administrative approval for effort

Plan

- Specify the area for improvement
- Assemble team, and define roles and responsibilities
- Obtain baseline data and seek input from stakeholders to understand the current approach and opportunities for improvement
- Assess potential solutions and pick solution most likely to accomplish aims
- Prepare detailed plans and timeline for implementation and evaluation

Do

- Oversee or provide guidance to the trial of the new way of doing things
- Collect, chart and display data to determine effectiveness of the test

Study

- Bring expertise to the interpretation of findings and needed action steps
- Report performance with outcome measures and insights for adjustments to plan

Act

- Standardize the improvement and expand implementation, incorporate into procedures and performance expectations
- Communicate accomplishments to internal and external stakeholders and advocate for broader implementation

Organizational Change

Population Stragegy

Organizational Change

Strategy Definitions

Actions designed to alter the operations within a program, organization, institution, or system. Involves durable changes to operating policies, procedures and processes and interactions among constituents.

Additional information: Organizational change can range in scope from actions to establish new or different ways of operating in a single program or site, to comprehensive actions involving many constituents to establish new or different ways of doing complex things throughout a system or across sectors.

Examples of Nutrition and Dietetic Practitioners' Actions

Single organization examples:

- Help worksite establish a healthy eating and activity policy for meetings and events
- Community nutrition staff designs and implements a nutrition module for training community health workers
- Dietitian takes active role as hospital makes changes involving several departments to become certified as a Baby (breastfeeding)-Friendly Hospital

Example of collaboration of two or more organizations:

- Maternal and child health coalition works to implement cross-referrals processes among clinics and community-based programs
- Supplemental food program establishes a system for subsidized purchases at area farmers markets
- A school district and local producers set up a farm to school program

System-wide examples:

- Implementation of electronic medical records, including nutrition terminology, throughout the healthcare system
- Create new system for certification of home care providers that includes food and nutrition knowledge requirements
- BMI screening and follow up implemented in schools and primary healthcare settings across the state
- Country implements evidence-based public health recommendations regarding vitamin/mineral supplementation
- Implement healthy-eating curriculum throughout school system

Political Action

From several theoretical approaches important to advancing political change, two commonly utilized in addressing nutrition issues are included here.They address

1. building advocacy coalitions, and
2. moving to action through the policy window and agenda setting.

Advocacy Coalition Framework

Coalitions form as a result of specific core ideas and beliefs about policy issues and their interests in them. Advocacy coalitions work with policy makers to affect change in policy relevant to the core ideas of the coalition.

Aim

To change policy, and ultimately social or physical conditions, through interactions and coordinated activities among advocacy coalitions, policy makers and political systems.

Key Concepts

Concepts:

- Core beliefs-individuals have core beliefs about problems, their causes and seriousness, and how to solve them. These individuals create coalitions with others sharing the same ideas and beliefs.
- Advocacy coalitions-within a policy area, there can be several different advocacy coalitions representing their own interests. Each coalition will have their own beliefs about issues and solutions, strategies and resources.
- Policy makers-persons responsible for formulating laws, regulations, or rules, or defining policies and practices
- Policy broker-works with both coalitions and policy makers to keep levels of political conflict low and come to reasonable solutions to the problems that the advocacy coalitions are working to change
- Resistance to change-core ideas and beliefs are resistant to change unless major external events or new policy modifies the views of the members of the coalition. New learning can shift views of a coalition

Nutrition and Dietetic Practitioner's Actions

Nutrition and dietetic practitioner's actions include:

- Work with, support, and strengthen alliances with advocacy groups and policy makers that share core ideas or beliefs
- Provide research, information, reports, tools, and education to advocacy coalitions regarding nutrition-related problems, their causes and seriousness, and potential solutions
- Use social or mass media to increase awareness and affect change in public opinion on specific policies that the coalition is trying to change
- Use research and information exchange to change perceptions of opponents
- Prepare and disseminate policy briefs
- Write letters of support or opposition regarding specific policies to policy makers
- Provide public comment or formal testimony at meetings of policy makers and legislative hearings
- Become a recognized and trusted expert for nutrition-related policy issues
- Provide meeting space for coalitions
- Arrange and host policy briefings and dialogues
- Join and actively participate in coalitions that represent food, nutrition and physical activity related issues
- Invite policy makers to visit programs and events
- Recognize policy makers and coalitions for taking action to improve nutrition and health

Continued on next page

Political Action

Continued from previous page

Policy Window and Setting

For issues to get more attention in the policy process, at least two of three streams need to converge at a critical time, known as a policy window. The three streams are problems, policy solutions, and politics/political climate.

Agenda setting is a process in which advocacy groups, decision makers, key stakeholders, constituents, citizens, and the media reciprocally influence one another to get problems on the political agenda.

Aim

To get nutrition-related issues on the political agenda, and to influence the alignment of problem definition, policy solutions, and political climate in the policy window so action can be taken.

Key Concepts

Concepts:

- Problems: social conditions that have been identified by policy makers and advocates, including its status and causes, and potential solutions
- Policy solutions: ideas generated to solve the problem
- Political climate: how the problem is perceived and championed by advocates, and interest groups and policy makers
- The three streams operate independently; the most success comes when all three streams are aligned
- Policy windows- predicable (elections, planning and budget cycles, school years) and unpredictable (dramatic events or crisis [eg, food borne illness outbreak], or natural disasters)
- Agenda setting-to get on an agenda for attention, problems must have an emotional component, a technically feasible solution, be aligned with values and beliefs of decision makers, and have high constituent awareness
- Factors for success-To affect the policy agenda and take advantage of policy windows, advocates must have thorough knowledge of problem and solution, trusted relationships with policy makers, and good reputations

Nutrition and Dietetic Practitioner's Actions

Nutrition and dietetic practitioner's actions include:

- Take an active role in defining nutrition-related problems and potential policy solutions
- Monitor indicators that document the existence, causes and magnitude of the problem
- Initiate special studies to determine the local impact of the issue (health impact assessment)
- Research current and emerging policies, and be prepared to propose viable solution options available
- Frame messages about problems, policies, and political action to align with decision makers' ideologies
- Monitor local, state and national policy issues and advocate to appointed and elected officials before voting occurs
- Draft language for legislation
- Monitor community and stakeholder perceptions and promote constituent feedback and involvement
- Learn how to couple two different streams in order to enact policy change, such as introducing a proposition to city elected officials to solve a problem (eg, sugar-sweetened beverage tax)
- Monitor the political process to recognize a policy window and be prepared to respond
- Influence the political climate by building coalitions, using mass or social media, arranging events, participating in demonstrations, and establishing a rapport with elected officials as the nutrition expert
- Strengthen capacity within the organizational to work on policy change

Public Policy Change

Public Policy Change

Strategy Definitions

Actions related to local, state and federal laws and ordinances and government agency regulations and guidelines that impact factors that contribute to health and nutrition-related outcomes of the population.

Additional information:

This includes actions designed to develop, enact and/or enforce laws and regulations.

Examples of Nutrition and Dietetic Practitioners' Actions

The nutrition and dietetic practitioner takes an active role including:

- Advocating (as appropriate to position)
- Drafting or modifying policies and proposed legislation
- Providing data and testimony
- Organizing community support
- Building coalitions

To effect changes in, for example, restaurant codes, city gardening ordinance, zoning for fast food near schools, taxes on sugar-sweetened beverages, food and menu labeling, supplemental nutrition program regulations, school nutrition and wellness policy, rates for social welfare benefits, and subsidies for rural/remote food access

To advocate for a health-in-all-policies approach

- To reduce inequities in the determinants of health

Identify Nutrition Intervention Encounter Setting

Definition

Determine the environment where nutrition care is provided (excludes Population settings).

Details of Intervention

A typical intervention might be further described with the following details. Nutrition and dietetics practitioners recommend, implement, or order nutrition interventions and the action(s) may be to initiate, modify, or discontinue a nutrition intervention(s):

- Ambulatory health setting
- Assisted living setting
- Community health care setting
- Home health setting
- Inpatient care setting
- Inpatient rehabilitation environment
- Nursing home setting
- Outpatient setting
- Private practice setting
- Skilled nursing setting

Identify Nutrition Intervention Encounter Setting

Typically Used With the Following

Nutrition Diagnostic Terminology Used in PES Statements	Common Examples
Nutrition Diagnoses	• Increased energy expenditure • Inadequate energy intake • Excessive oral intake • Inadequate fiber intake • Inadequate enteral nutrition infusion • Growth rate below expected • Limited access to food • Breastfeeding difficulty • Underweight • Malnutrition
Etiology	• Economic concerns • Physiological causes, eg, increased energy needs due to increased activity level, metabolic change, malabsorption, growth, extreme weakness, critical illness • Fatigue • Limited social support • New need for nutrition knowledge, skills, and/or behavior changes
Signs and Symptoms	Biochemical Data, Medical Tests and Procedures • Hemoglobin A1C results Anthropometric Measures • Body weight change Nutrition-Focused Physical Findings • Diarrhea • Evidence of muscle and/or fat wasting Food/Nutrition-Related History • Cultural or religious practices that do not support food and nutrition goals • Changes in physical activity • Intake of foods inconsistent with goals • Limited food and nutrition related knowledge and/or skills

Continued on next page

Identify Nutrition Intervention Encounter Setting

Continued from previous page

Nutrition Diagnostic Terminology Used in PES Statements	Common Examples
Signs and Symptoms (continued)	Client History • Conditions associated with diagnosis or treatment, eg, surgery, trauma, sepsis, diabetes mellitus, inborn errors of metabolism, digestive enzyme deficiency, obesity • Chronic use of medications that increase or decrease nutrient requirements or impair nutrient metabolism

Other considerations (eg, client negotiations, client needs and desires, and readiness to change)

- Availability of food and/or nutrition related supplies
- Ability to prepare food
- Availability/access to a qualified practitioner for follow-up and monitoring

Identify Nutrition Intervention Encounter Approach

Definition

Determine the nature of the method for provision of nutrition care.

Details of Intervention

A typical intervention might be further described with the following details. Nutrition and dietetics practitioners recommend, implement, or order nutrition interventions and the action(s) may be to initiate, modify, or discontinue a nutrition intervention(s):

- **Individual client: direct nutrition intervention encounter** (and/or including supportive individuals [eg, family or caregiver]) (present/absent)—defined as an intervention where client and professional are in the same physical location for the nutrition intervention; to be used in conjunction with the intervention provided, food and nutrient delivery, education, counseling, coordination of care
- **Group client: direct nutrition intervention encounter** (present/absent)—defined as an intervention where two or more clients and professional are in the same physical location for the nutrition intervention; to be used in conjunction with the intervention provided, food and nutrient delivery, education, counseling, coordination of care, population based nutrition action
- **Telehealth nutrition intervention encounter** (present/absent)—defined as an interactive telecommunication nutrition encounter permitting real-time delivery of nutrition intervention; to be used in conjunction with the intervention provided, food and nutrient delivery, education, counseling, coordination of care
  - **Individual client: video telehealth nutrition intervention encounter** (present/absent)—defined as an interactive audio and video telecommunication encounter permitting real-time communication between the distant site professional and the individual client; to be used in conjunction with the intervention provided, food and nutrient delivery, education, counseling, coordination of care
  - **Group client: video telehealth nutrition intervention encounter** (present/absent)—defined as interactive audio and video telecommunication encounter permitting real-time communication between the distant site professional and two or more clients; to be used in conjunction with the intervention provided, food and nutrient delivery, education, counseling, coordination of care, population based nutrition action
  - **Individual client: audio-only telehealth nutrition intervention encounter** (present/absent)—defined as sound-only telecommunication encounter permitting real-time verbal communication between the distant site professional and the client; to be used in conjunction with the intervention provided, food and nutrient delivery, education, counseling, coordination of care
  - **Group client: audio-only telehealth nutrition intervention encounter** (present/absent)—defined as sound-only communication between the distant site professional and two or more clients; to be used in conjunction with the intervention provided, food and nutrient delivery, education, counseling, coordination of care, population based nutrition action
- **Telehealth nutrition monitoring** (present/absent)—defined as collection and evaluation of data to determine whether goals or expected outcomes are being met
- **Asynchronous nutrition intervention encounter** (present/absent)—defined as a telecommunication-based nutrition encounter where images, data, and/or surveys are transmitted to the professional at a convenient time for assessment offline; to be used in conjunction with the intervention provided, food and nutrient delivery, education, counseling, coordination of care, population based nutrition action
  - **Provision of written information about nutrition** (present/absent)—defined as guidance relevant to nutrition given via email, text, online portal, or other mode of transmission of the written word

Identify Nutrition Intervention Encounter Approach

Typically Used With the Following

Nutrition Diagnostic Terminology Used in PES Statements	Common Examples
Nutrition Diagnoses	• Inadequate oral intake • Excessive oral intake • Inadequate fiber intake • Inadequate enteral nutrition infusion • Growth rate below expected • Food Insecurity • Breastfeeding difficulty • Malnutrition (undernutrition) • Overweight/obesity • Food and nutrition related knowledge deficit • Not ready for nutrition related behavior change • Limited food and nutrition related skill
Etiology	• Economic concerns • Physiological causes, eg, increased energy needs due to increased activity level, metabolic change, malabsorption, growth, extreme weakness, critical illness • Limited food and nutrition knowledge • Limited readiness for nutrition behavior change • Cultural beliefs that may not appear to support nutrition goals • Limited numeracy skills
Signs and Symptoms	Biochemical Data, Medical Tests and Procedures • Hemoglobin A1C results • Vitamin D level Anthropometric Measurements • Weight Nutrition-Focused Physical Findings • Evidence of muscle and/or fat wasting • Cushingoid appearance • Edema

Continued on next page

Identify Nutrition Intervention Encounter Approach

Continued from previous page

Nutrition Diagnostic Terminology Used in PES Statements	Common Examples
Signs and Symptoms (continued)	Food/Nutrition-Related History • Food practices that do not appear to support food and nutrition goals • Changes in physical activity • Intake of foods and/or nutrients inconsistent with goals • Limited food and nutrition related knowledge and/or skills Client History • Conditions associated with diagnosis or treatment, eg, surgery, trauma, sepsis, diabetes mellitus, inborn errors of metabolism, digestive enzyme deficiency, obesity • Chronic use of medications that increase or decrease nutrient requirements or impair nutrient metabolism

Other considerations (eg, client negotiations, client needs and desires, and readiness to change)

- Transportation availability
- Economic concerns
- Home environment

SNAPSHOT
NCP Step 4: Nutrition Monitoring and Evaluation

Definition: The purpose of nutrition monitoring and evaluation is to determine and measure the amount of progress made for the nutrition intervention and whether the goals/expected outcomes are being met.

Determining what to measure for nutrition monitoring and evaluation: During the first interaction, appropriate outcomes/indicators are selected to be monitored and evaluated at the next interaction with the client. During subsequent interactions, these outcomes/indicators are used to demonstrate the amount of progress made and whether the goals or expected outcomes are being met. Factors to consider when selecting indicators are the medical diagnosis, health care outcome goals, nutrition quality management goals, practice setting, client population, and disease state and/or severity.

Please see assessment section for a complete list of Nutrition Monitoring and Evaluation Terms and Reference Sheets.

Terminology for Nutrition Monitoring and Evaluation is organized in eight domains (categories):

Food/Nutrition Related History Outcomes	Food and nutrient intake, food and nutrient administration, medication, complementary/alternative medicine use, knowledge/beliefs, food and supplies availability, physical activity, and nutrition quality of life
Anthropometric Measurement Outcomes	Height, weight, body mass index (BMI), growth pattern indices/percentile ranks, and weight history
Biochemical Data, Medical Tests and Procedure Outcomes	Lab data (eg, electrolytes, glucose) and tests (eg, gastric emptying time, resting metabolic rate)
Physical Finding Outcomes	Findings from a physical exam, interview, or the health record
Assessment, Monitoring, and Evaluation Tools	Tools used for health or disease status or risk assessment, reassessment, and monitoring and evaluation
Etiology Category	Categories to communicate the type of nutrition diagnosis etiology
Comparative Standards	What indicator data are compared against
Progress Evaluation	Evaluation of progress toward a nutrition related goal(s) and resolution of a nutrition diagnosis(es)

Collection and use of nutrition monitoring and evaluation outcome data: This step consists of three actions: monitoring, measuring, and evaluating the changes in nutrition care indicators. Practitioners monitor by providing evidence that the nutrition intervention is or is not changing the client's behavior or status. They measure outcomes by collecting data for outcomes/indicators. Finally, nutrition and dietetics practitioners compare the current findings with previous status, nutrition intervention goals, and/or reference standards (comparative standards) and evaluate the overall impact of the nutrition intervention on the client's nutrition diagnosis(es) and health outcomes. The use of standardized indicators and criteria increases the validity and reliability of outcome data collection and communication. For consistency, nutrition and dietetics practitioners are encouraged to use the labels—new, active, resolved, or discontinued—to communicate the status of each nutrition diagnosis.

Critical Thinking Skills

- Using appropriate reference standards for comparison (Comparative Standards)
- Defining where client is in terms of goals and expected outcomes
- Explaining variance from expected goals and outcomes
- Determining factors that help or hinder progress
- Deciding between discharge or continued care

For more detailed information about the Nutrition Monitoring and Evaluation step, log in as a subscriber to www.nutritioncareprocess.org.

Appendix:
Dietary Reference Intakes Interpretation

Purpose

This section provides guidance to nutrition and dietetics practitioners in countries using the Dietary Reference Intakes (DRIs) on how to appropriately use the DRIs. Because all DRIs are for healthy individuals in a particular life stage and gender group, they may not be applicable reference standards for all scenarios.

Application in the Nutrition Care Process

DRIs can be used to evaluate a "healthy" individual's "usual" intake. Usual intake should reflect long-term average intake over many days; if intake is reported for a small number of days, then the probability of adequacy should be interpreted with caution. However, assessment in the context of the nutrition care process may involve a client whose intake is not "usual" and/or who is not "healthy."

Therefore, when assessing the adequacy of intake for a client, the nutrition and dietetics practitioner will need to use judgment to determine adequacy with special consideration for the following two factors:

- Intake may not be "usual" and/or
- Client may not be "healthy"

Intake May Not Be Usual

The ability and appropriateness of assessing "usual" intake will vary depending on the specific circumstances and may be independent of the care setting.

For example, to evaluate current nutritional status in an acute care setting, it may be necessary to assess current intake (eg, nutrition support for a trauma client) or "usual" intake prior to admission (eg, cystic fibrosis client). Assessing "usual" intake may be appropriate and achievable for the long-term care resident. Additionally, in the ambulatory care setting, "usual" intake will generally be used, but sometimes it may be more appropriate to assess intake since the beginning of an event, such as a new-onset disease diagnosis.

If a client's estimated intake is less than normally recommended for a healthy individual, then the determination of suboptimal nutrient intake(s) based on a comparison with the DRI will need to be carefully evaluated given the specific circumstances.

Client May Not Be Healthy

The DRIs are based on recommendations for apparently healthy individuals. However, when a client has an illness, injury, disease, or other medical condition, he or she may no longer be considered healthy. Therefore, the DRIs may not be the most appropriate reference standard to assess intake adequacy for individuals with altered nutrient requirements due to one or more medical conditions. However, if no other reference standard exists, it may be safe to assume in most situations that a client's intake goal/nutrition prescription should not be below the appropriate DRI (recommended dietary allowance [RDA] or adequate intake [AI]) as long as the potential for altered nutrient requirements is considered.

In summary, although intake data and recommendations are estimates, assessing intake is still worthwhile and may identify nutrients either under- or overconsumed by individuals. To increase dietary assessment accuracy, ensure that dietary data are as complete as possible, portions are correctly specified, and food composition data are accurate. Whenever possible, nutrient intake data should be considered in combination with clinical, biochemical, and anthropometric information; medical diagnosis; clinical status; and other factors to provide a valid assessment of nutritional status based on a totality of the evidence.

What Are the DRIs?

The DRIs are four categories of reference values set when adequate evidence-based information is available about nutrients or food components.

- **Estimated Average Requirement (EAR)**—Mean requirement for a nutrient or the average daily nutrient intake level estimated to meet the requirement of half of the healthy individuals in a particular life stage and gender group.
- **Recommended Dietary Allowance (RDA)**—Recommended intake or the average daily nutrient intake level sufficient to meet the nutrient requirement of 97% to 98% of individuals in a particular life stage and gender group.
- **Adequate Intake (AI)**—*Recommended intake*—A recommended intake level based on observed or experimentally determined approximations or estimates of nutrient intake by a group (or groups) of healthy people that are assumed to be adequate; used when an RDA cannot be determined.
- **Tolerable Upper Intake Level (UL)**—The highest average daily nutrient intake level likely to pose no risk of adverse health effects to almost all individuals in the general population. As intake increases above the UL, the risk of adverse effects increases.

When the DRIs are determined to be appropriate reference standards for assessing intake adequacy, the following must be considered.

DRI	Assessing the intake of healthy individuals in a specific life stage and gender category
RDA	For nutrients with an RDA, estimated usual intakes at or above the RDA have a high probability of adequacy.
EAR	For nutrients with an EAR, estimated usual intakes below the EAR very likely need to be improved (because the probability of adequacy is 50% or less); those between the EAR and the RDA probably need to be improved (because the probability of adequacy is less than 97% to 98%).
AI	For nutrients with an AI, estimated usual intakes at or above the AI can be considered adequate. Although the adequacy of intakes below the AI cannot be determined, they should be improved to meet the AI.
UL	For nutrients with a UL, estimated usual intakes below the UL can be considered to be not at risk for toxicity.

DRI	Assessing the intake of a group
RDA	Do not use to assess intakes of groups.
EAR	For nutrients with an EAR, use the EAR to assess the prevalence of inadequate intakes or the proportion of a population that has estimated usual intakes below median requirements. Choose between two methods-the probability approach or the EAR cut-point method.
AI	For nutrients with an AI, estimated mean intakes at or above this level implies a low prevalence of inadequate intakes. However, when estimated mean intakes of groups are below the AI, it is not possible to make any assumptions about the prevalence of inadequacy.
UL	For nutrients with a UL, estimated usual intakes above the UL are used to estimate the percentage of the population at risk of adverse effects from excessive nutrient intake.

NCPT Approved Synonyms

Throughout the NCPT

Concept	Approved Synonym
Mother (in the context of lactation)	Lactating parent

Nutrition Assessment/Monitoring and Intervention

Terms	Approved Synonym
Breastmilk	Human milk
Glucose, casual	Glucose, random
Breastfeeding	Chestfeeding
Client reported experience measure	Patient reported experience measure (PREM)
Client reported outcome measure	Patient reported outcome (PRO) and/or Patient reported outcome measure (PROM)
Corrected age	Adjusted age

Nutrition Diagnosis

Terms	Approved Synonym
Nutrition diagnosis	Nutrition problem
Breastfeeding difficulty	Chestfeeding difficulty
Predicted breastfeeding difficulty	Predicted chestfeeding difficulty
Food and nutrition related knowledge deficit	Limited food and nutrition related knowledge
Self monitoring deficit	Limited self monitoring
Physical inactivity	Limited physical activity
Unintended weight loss	Involuntary weight loss
Unintended weight gain	Involuntary weight gain
Obesity class III	Morbid obesity

Nutrition Intervention

The nutrition intervention synonyms reflect inclusion of the International Dysphagia Diet Standardisation Initiative (IDDSI) diet modifications and are used with IDDSI's permission.

Terms	Approved Synonym
International Dysphagia Diet Standardisation Initiative Framework—Regular Level 7 (Black) food	International Dysphagia Diet Standardisation Initiative Framework—Regular Level 7 food
	International Dysphagia Diet Standardisation Initiative Framework—RG7 (Regular Level 7) food

Continued on next page

Continued from previous page

Terms	Approved Synonym
International Dysphagia Diet Standardisation Initiative Framework—Easy to Chew Level 7 (Black) food	International Dysphagia Diet Standardisation Initiative Framework—Easy to Chew Level 7 food
	International Dysphagia Diet Standardisation Initiative Framework—EC7 (Easy to Chew Level 7) food
International Dysphagia Diet Standardisation Initiative Framework—Soft and Bite Sized Level 6 (Blue) food	International Dysphagia Diet Standardisation Initiative Framework—Soft and Bite Sized Level 6 food
	International Dysphagia Diet Standardisation Initiative Framework— SB6 (Soft & Bite Sized Level 6) food
International Dysphagia Diet Standardisation Initiative Framework—Minced and Moist Level 5 (Orange) food	International Dysphagia Diet Standardisation Initiative Framework—Minced and Moist Level 5 food
	International Dysphagia Diet Standardisation Initiative Framework—MM5 (Minced & Moist Level 5) food
International Dysphagia Diet Standardisation Initiative Framework—Pureed Level 4 (Green) food	International Dysphagia Diet Standardisation Initiative Framework—Pureed Level 4 food
	International Dysphagia Diet Standardisation Initiative Framework—PU4 (Pureed Level 4) food
International Dysphagia Diet Standardisation Initiative Framework—Extremely Thick Level 4 (Green) drinks	International Dysphagia Diet Standardisation Initiative Framework—Extremely Thick Level 4 drinks
	International Dysphagia Diet Standardisation Initiative Framework—EX4 (Extremely Thick Level 4) drinks
International Dysphagia Diet Standardisation Initiative Framework—Liquidized Level 3 (Yellow) food	International Dysphagia Diet Standardisation Initiative Framework—Liquidized Level 3 food
	International Dysphagia Diet Standardisation Initiative Framework—LQ3 (Liquidized Level 3) food
International Dysphagia Diet Standardisation Initiative Framework—Moderately Thick Level 3 (Yellow) drinks	International Dysphagia Diet Standardisation Initiative Framework - Moderately Thick Level 3 drinks
	International Dysphagia Diet Standardisation Initiative Framework—MO3 (Moderately Thick Level 3) drinks
International Dysphagia Diet Standardisation Initiative Framework—Mildly Thick Level 2 (Pink) drinks	International Dysphagia Diet Standardisation Initiative Framework—Mildly Thick Level 2 drinks
	International Dysphagia Diet Standardisation Initiative Framework—MT2 (Mildly Thick Level 2) drinks
International Dysphagia Diet Standardisation Initiative Framework—Slightly Thick Level 1 (Grey) drinks	International Dysphagia Diet Standardisation Initiative Framework—Slightly Thick Level 1 drinks
	International Dysphagia Diet Standardisation Initiative Framework—ST1 (Slightly Thick Level 1) drinks
International Dysphagia Diet Standardisation Initiative Framework—Thin Level 0 (White) drinks	International Dysphagia Diet Standardisation Initiative Framework—Thin Level 0 drinks
	International Dysphagia Diet Standardisation Initiative Framework—TN0 (Thin Level 0) drinks

Nutrition Diagnosis Etiology Matrix

Below are the etiology categories and their definitions. Etiologies are grouped by the type of cause or contributing risk factor. In two specific instances, Access and Behavior etiologies, these alone may be the cause or contributing risk factor of the nutrition diagnosis or the practitioner may determine a more specific root cause, eg, Belief-Attitudes of the problem.

Etiology Category	Definition
Beliefs–Attitudes Etiologies	Cause or contributing risk factors related to the conviction of the truth of some nutrition-related statement or phenomenon; feelings or emotions toward that truth or phenomenon and activities
Cultural Etiologies	Cause or contributing risk factors related to values, social norms, customs, religious beliefs and/or political systems
Knowledge Etiologies	Cause or contributing risk factors impacting the level of understanding about food, nutrition and health, or nutrition-related information and guidelines
Physical Function Etiologies	Cause or contributing risk factors related to physical ability to engage in specific tasks, may be cognitive in nature
Physiologic–Metabolic Etiologies	Cause or contributing risk factors related to medical/health status that may have a nutritional impact (excludes psychological etiologies—see separate category)
Psychological Etiologies	Cause or contributing risk factors related to a diagnosed or suspected mental health/psychological problem (*Diagnostic and Statistical Manual of Mental Disorders,* DSM)
Social–Personal Etiologies	Cause or contributing risk factors associated with personal and/or social history
Treatment Etiologies	Cause or contributing risk factors related to medical or surgical treatment or other therapies and management or care
Access Etiologies	Cause or contributing risk factors that affect intake and the availability of safe, healthful food, water, and food/nutrition-related supplies. A more specific root cause of Access Etiologies may not be known but may eventually reveal Beliefs-Attitudes, Cultural, Knowledge, Physical Function, Psychological, Social-Personal, or Treatment Etiologies
Behavior Etiologies	Cause or contributing risk factors related to actions which influence achievement of nutrition-related goals. A more specific root cause of Behavior Etiologies may not be known but may eventually reveal Beliefs-Attitudes, Cultural, Knowledge, Physical Function, Psychological, Social-Personal, or Treatment Etiologies.

Etiology	Diagnosis
Category: Beliefs-Attitudes	
Altered body image	Poor food and/or nutrition quality of life
Obsessive desire to be healthy or have a specific body shape	Disordered eating pattern
Food preference	Limited food acceptance, Excessive fat intake, Intake of types of fats inconsistent with needs, Unbalanced diet pattern
Limited acceptance need to change	Not ready for nutrition related behavior change
Disbelief in science-based food and nutrition information	Belief finding that hinders food and/or nutrition behavior change
End-of-life care if client or supportive individuals do not desire nutrition support	Enteral nutrition composition inconsistent with needs, Enteral nutrition administration inconsistent with needs, Parenteral nutrition composition inconsistent with needs, Parenteral nutrition administration inconsistent with needs
Cultural, societal, biological/genetic, and/or environmental related to fear of body weight gain	Disordered eating pattern
Food faddism	Imbalance of nutrients, Excessive protein intake, Intake of types of proteins inconsistent with needs, Excessive intake of calcium, Excessive intake of chloride, Excessive intake of iron, Excessive intake of magnesium, Excessive intake of potassium, Excessive intake of phosphorus, Excessive intake of sodium, Excessive intake of zinc, Excessive intake of sulfate, Excessive intake of fluoride, Excessive intake of copper, Excessive intake of iodine, Excessive intake of selenium, Excessive intake of manganese, Excessive intake of chromium, Excessive intake of molybdenum, Excessive intake of boron, Excessive intake of cobalt
Limited food acceptance due to food aversion	Inadequate oral intake, Limited food acceptance
Belief finding that hinders food and/or nutrition behavior change	Excessive energy intake, Inadequate oral intake, Excessive oral intake, Limited food acceptance, Excessive alcohol intake, Imbalance of nutrients, Excessive fat intake, Intake of types of fats inconsistent with needs, Excessive protein intake, Intake of types of proteins inconsistent with needs, Intake types of amino acids inconsistent with needs, Excessive fiber intake, Excessive intake of calcium, Excessive intake of chloride, Excessive intake of iron, Excessive intake of magnesium, Excessive intake of potassium, Excessive intake of phosphorus, Excessive intake of sodium, Excessive intake of zinc, Excessive intake of sulfate, Excessive intake of fluoride, Excessive intake of copper, Excessive intake of iodine, Excessive intake of selenium, Excessive intake of manganese, Excessive intake of chromium, Excessive intake of molybdenum, Excessive intake of boron, Excessive intake of cobalt, Unbalanced diet pattern, Predicted breastfeeding difficulty, Underweight, Growth rate below expected, Food and

Etiology	Diagnosis
Category: Beliefs-Attitudes	
Belief finding that hinders food and/or nutrition behavior change (continued)	nutrition related knowledge deficit, Not ready for nutrition related behavior change, Limited adherence to nutrition related recommendations, Limited food and nutrition related skill, Physical inactivity, Excessive physical activity, Food insecurity, Limited access to potable water
Irritability	Breastfeeding difficulty
Limited self efficacy for making change or demoralization from previous challenges associated with change	Food and nutrition related knowledge deficit, Not ready for nutrition related behavior change, Limited adherence to nutrition related recommendations, Poor food and/or nutrition quality of life
Limited confidence in ability to change	Limited adherence to nutrition related recommendations, Belief finding that hinders food and/or nutrition behavior change
Limited value for behavior change or competing values	Excessive energy intake, Excessive oral intake, Excessive alcohol intake, Excessive fat intake, Intake of types of fats inconsistent with needs, Self monitoring deficit, Limited adherence to nutrition related recommendations, Physical inactivity, Inability to manage self care
Limited motivation and/or readiness to apply or support systems change	Belief finding that hinders food and/or nutrition behavior change, Unbalanced diet pattern, Limited food acceptance
Perceived negative impact of current or previous medical nutrition therapy (MNT)	Poor food and/or nutrition quality of life
Not ready for nutrition related behavior change	Overweight, adult or pediatric, Obesity, adult or pediatric, Obesity, pediatric, Obesity Class I, Obesity Class II, Obesity Class III, Unintended weight gain, Excessive growth rate, Self monitoring deficit, Belief finding that hinders food and/or nutrition behavior change, Inability to manage self care, Poor food and/or nutrition quality of life
Perception of inadequate milk supply	Breastfeeding difficulty, Predicted breastfeeding difficulty
Perception that lack of or limited resources (eg, time, financial, or interpersonal) prevent:	
• Selection/food choices consistent with recommendations	Unbalanced diet pattern
• Changes	Not ready for nutrition related behavior change, Limited adherence to nutrition related recommendations
• Sufficient level of activity	Physical inactivity

Etiology	Diagnosis
• Self monitoring	Self monitoring deficit, Inability to manage self care
Category: Beliefs-Attitudes	
Limited interest/motivation/ prioritization:	
• Learning information/ applying skill	Food and nutrition related knowledge deficit, Not ready for nutrition related behavior change, Limited adherence to nutrition related recommendations, Unbalanced diet pattern, Limited food acceptance, Limited food and nutrition related skill, Inability to manage self care
• Reducing energy intake	Excessive energy intake
• Reducing intake	Excessive oral intake
• Modify protein or amino acid intake	Intake of types of proteins inconsistent with needs, Intake types of amino acids inconsistent with needs
• Tracking progress	Self monitoring deficit
• Unwillingness to purchase or consume fiber-containing foods	Inadequate fiber intake
• Body weight regulation/ preoccupation	Disordered eating pattern
Limited emotional ability	Limited food and nutrition related skill
Limited self-efficacy for applying skill	Limited food and nutrition related skill
Beliefs and/or attitudes leading to inadequate intake and/or limited physical activity	Sarcopenia
Perceived risk of a disease	Belief finding that hinders food and/or nutrition behavior change
Perceived benefits of adopting a food and/or nutrition behavior	Belief finding that hinders food and/or nutrition behavior change
Perceived barriers to adopting a food and/or nutrition behavior (eg, personal, social, cultural, environmental, economic)	Belief finding that hinders food and/or nutrition behavior change
Perceived cues to action to adopt a food and/or nutrition behavior, such as internal cues (eg, experiencing signs or symptoms of illness) or external cues (eg, recommendation of a health care provider, access to food and/or nutrition information)	Belief finding that hinders food and/or nutrition behavior change
Perceived control about adopting the food and/or nutrition behavior (eg, beliefs about what makes it easier or harder to adopt the behavior)	Belief finding that hinders food and/or nutrition behavior change

Etiology	Diagnosis
Category: Beliefs-Attitudes	
Perceived norms about the approval or disapproval of the client's food and/or nutrition behavior by supportive individuals (eg, family, caregivers) and/or supportive structures (eg, social service agencies, faith-based organizations) [injunctive norm]	Belief finding that hinders food and/or nutrition behavior change
Limited emotional ability	Limited food and nutrition related skill
Limited self-efficacy for applying skill	Limited food and nutrition related skill
Beliefs and/or attitudes leading to inadequate intake and/or limited physical activity	Sarcopenia
Perceived risk of a disease	Belief finding that hinders food and/or nutrition behavior change
Perceived benefits of adopting a food and/or nutrition behavior	Belief finding that hinders food and/or nutrition behavior change
Perceived barriers to adopting a food and/or nutrition behavior (eg, personal, social, cultural, environmental, economic)	Belief finding that hinders food and/or nutrition behavior change
Perceived cues to action to adopt a food and/or nutrition behavior, such as internal cues (eg, experiencing signs or symptoms of illness) or external cues (eg, recommendation of a health care provider, access to food and/or nutrition information)	Belief finding that hinders food and/or nutrition behavior change
Perceived control about adopting the food and/or nutrition behavior (eg, beliefs about what makes it easier or harder to adopt the behavior)	Belief finding that hinders food and/or nutrition behavior change
Perceived norms about the approval or disapproval of the client's food and/or nutrition behavior by supportive individuals (eg, family, caregivers) and/or supportive structures (eg, social service agencies, faith-based organizations) [injunctive norm]	Belief finding that hinders food and/or nutrition behavior change
Belief that supportive individuals (eg, family, caregivers) and/or supportive structures (eg, social service agencies, faith-based organizations) do or do not adopt the food and/or nutrition behavior [descriptive norm]	Belief finding that hinders food and/or nutrition behavior change

Etiology	Diagnosis
Category: Beliefs-Attitudes	
Craving for nonfood item	Belief finding that hinders food and/or nutrition behavior change
Emotional response to adopting the food and/or nutrition behavior (how the client feels about the behavior, such as feeling anger, sadness, fear, ambivalence)	Attitude finding that hinders food and/or nutrition behavior change
Beliefs about the outcome of adopting the food and/or nutrition behavior (what the client perceives as the plusses or minuses of the behavioral outcome, such as weight loss or weight gain)	Attitude finding that hinders food and/or nutrition behavior change
Attitude finding that hinders food and/or nutrition behavior change	Unbalanced diet pattern, Limited food acceptance
Category: Cultural	
Culture of overeating	Predicted excessive energy intake
Practices that affect nutrient intake	Predicted inadequate nutrient intake
Cultural beliefs that may affect ability to and receptivity to:	
• Access to food, fluid, nutrients	Inadequate energy intake, Inadequate oral intake, Inadequate fluid intake, Moderate starvation related malnutrition (undernutrition), Severe starvation related malnutrition (undernutrition), Inadequate protein–energy intake, Inadequate protein intake, Inadequate carbohydrate intake, Inadequate intake of vitamin A, Inadequate intake of vitamin C, Inadequate intake of vitamin D, Inadequate intake of vitamin E, Inadequate intake of vitamin K, Inadequate intake of thiamin, Inadequate intake of riboflavin, Inadequate intake of niacin, Inadequate intake of folate, Inadequate intake of vitamin B6, Inadequate intake of vitamin B12, Inadequate intake of pantothenic acid, Inadequate intake of biotin, Inadequate intake of calcium, Inadequate intake of chloride, Inadequate intake of iron, Inadequate intake of magnesium, Inadequate intake of potassium, Inadequate intake of phosphorus, Inadequate intake of sodium, Inadequate intake of zinc, Inadequate intake of sulfate, Inadequate intake of fluoride, Inadequate intake of copper, Inadequate intake of iodine, Inadequate intake of selenium, Inadequate intake of manganese, Inadequate intake of chromium, Inadequate intake of molybdenum, Inadequate intake of boron, Inadequate intake of cobalt, Unintended weight loss, Food insecurity, Limited access to potable water
• Make food choices consistent with reference intake standards, guidelines, and/or nutrition prescription for oral nutrition	Inadequate fat intake

Etiology	Diagnosis
Category: Cultural	
• Breastfeed	Breastfeeding difficulty, Predicted breastfeeding difficulty
• Learn information/apply skill	Food and nutrition related knowledge deficit, Unbalanced diet pattern, Limited food acceptance, Limited food and nutrition related skill
• Manage self care	Inability to manage self care
• Reduce carbohydrate intake	Excessive carbohydrate intake
• Regulate types of protein or amino acids consumed	Intake of types of proteins inconsistent with needs, Intake types of amino acids inconsistent with needs
• Regulate timing of carbohydrate consumption	Inconsistent carbohydrate intake
• Regulate types of carbohydrate consumed	Intake of types of carbohydrate inconsistent with needs
• Track personal progress	Self monitoring deficit
• Perform skill	Limited food and nutrition related skill
Category: Knowledge	
Food and nutrition knowledge deficit	Inadequate energy intake, Excessive energy intake, Excessive oral intake, Inadequate fluid intake, Excessive fluid intake, Inadequate bioactive substance intake, Excessive bioactive substance intake, Excessive alcohol intake, Moderate starvation related malnutrition (undernutrition), Severe starvation related malnutrition (undernutrition), Moderate acute disease or injury related malnutrition (undernutrition), Severe acute disease or injury related malnutrition (undernutrition), Inadequate protein–energy intake, Imbalance of nutrients, Excessive fat intake, Inadequate protein intake, Excessive protein intake, Inadequate carbohydrate intake, Inadequate fiber intake, Excessive intake of calcium, Excessive intake of chloride, Excessive intake of iron, Excessive intake of magnesium, Excessive intake of potassium, Excessive intake of phosphorus, Excessive intake of sodium, Excessive intake of zinc, Excessive intake of sulfate, Excessive intake of fluoride, Excessive intake of copper, Excessive intake of iodine, Excessive intake of selenium, Excessive intake of manganese, Excessive intake of chromium, Excessive intake of molybdenum, Excessive intake of boron, Excessive intake of cobalt, Predicted breastfeeding difficulty, Sarcopenia, Overweight, adult or pediatric, Obesity, adult or pediatric, Obesity, pediatric, Obesity Class I, Obesity Class II, Obesity Class III, Excessive growth rate, Self monitoring deficit, Inability to manage self care, Limited ability to prepare food for eating, Poor food and/or nutrition quality of life, Food insecurity, Limited access to nutrition related supplies, Limited access to potable water
Food and nutrition knowledge deficit concerning:	
Sufficient oral food/beverage intake	Inadequate oral intake

Etiology	Diagnosis
Category: Knowledge	
Consumption of an appropriate variety of foods	Excessive intake of calcium, Excessive intake of chloride, Excessive intake of iron, Excessive intake of magnesium, Excessive intake of potassium, Excessive intake of phosphorus, Excessive intake of sodium, Excessive intake of zinc, Excessive intake of sulfate, Excessive intake of fluoride, Excessive intake of copper, Excessive intake of iodine, Excessive intake of selenium, Excessive intake of manganese, Excessive intake of chromium, Excessive intake of molybdenum, Excessive intake of boron, Excessive intake of cobalt
• Potentially unsafe food	Intake of unsafe food
• Proper infant feeding, food/feeding preparation and storage	Intake of unsafe food
• Adequate energy intake	Underweight
• Appropriate amount or types of dietary protein or amino acids	Mild non illness related pediatric malnutrition (undernutrition), Moderate non illness related pediatric malnutrition (undernutrition), Severe non illness related pediatric malnutrition (undernutrition), Inadequate protein–energy intake, Inadequate protein intake, Intake of types of proteins inconsistent with needs, Intake types of amino acids inconsistent with needs
• Appropriate amount or type of dietary fat	Inadequate protein–energy intake, Inadequate fat intake, Excessive fat intake, Intake of types of fats inconsistent with needs
• Appropriate amount and types of dietary carbohydrate	Excessive carbohydrate intake, Intake of types of carbohydrate inconsistent with needs
• Appropriate timing of carbohydrate intake	Inconsistent carbohydrate intake
• Physiological causes requiring careful timing and consistency in the amount of carbohydrate	Inconsistent carbohydrate intake
• Physiological causes altering carbohydrate digestion or metabolism	Intake of types of carbohydrate inconsistent with needs
• Physiological causes requiring use of modified carbohydrate intake	Excessive carbohydrate intake
• Desirable quantities of fiber	Inadequate fiber intake, Excessive fiber intake
• Correct enteral formula needed	Inadequate enteral nutrition infusion
• Food and supplemental sources of vitamins	Inadequate intake of vitamin A, Inadequate intake of vitamin C, Inadequate intake of vitamin D, Inadequate intake of vitamin E, Inadequate intake of vitamin K, Inadequate intake of thiamin, Inadequate intake of riboflavin, Inadequate intake of niacin, Inadequate intake of folate, Inadequate intake of vitamin B6, Inadequate intake of vitamin B12, Inadequate intake of pantothenic acid, Inadequate intake of biotin, Excessive intake of vitamin A, Excessive intake of vitamin C, Excessive intake

Etiology	Diagnosis
Category: Knowledge	
• Food and supplemental sources of vitamins (continued)	of vitamin D, Excessive intake of vitamin E, Excessive intake of vitamin K, Excessive intake of thiamin, Excessive intake of riboflavin, Excessive intake of niacin, Excessive intake of folate, Excessive intake of vitamin B6, Excessive intake of vitamin B12, Excessive intake of pantothenic acid, Excessive intake of biotin
• Food and supplemental sources of minerals	Inadequate intake of calcium, Inadequate intake of chloride, Inadequate intake of iron, Inadequate intake of magnesium, Inadequate intake of potassium, Inadequate intake of phosphorus, Inadequate intake of sodium, Inadequate intake of zinc, Inadequate intake of sulfate, Inadequate intake of fluoride, Inadequate intake of copper, Inadequate intake of iodine, Inadequate intake of selenium, Inadequate intake of manganese, Inadequate intake of chromium, Inadequate intake of molybdenum, Inadequate intake of boron, Inadequate intake of cobalt
• Recommended dose of vitamin and mineral supplements	Imbalance of nutrients
• Management of diagnosis requiring mineral restriction	Excessive intake of calcium, Excessive intake of chloride, Excessive intake of iron, Excessive intake of magnesium, Excessive intake of potassium, Excessive intake of phosphorus, Excessive intake of sodium, Excessive intake of zinc, Excessive intake of sulfate, Excessive intake of fluoride, Excessive intake of copper, Excessive intake of iodine, Excessive intake of selenium, Excessive intake of manganese, Excessive intake of chromium, Excessive intake of molybdenum, Excessive intake of boron, Excessive intake of cobalt
• Management of diagnosed genetic disorder altering mineral homeostasis	Excessive intake of calcium, Excessive intake of chloride, Excessive intake of iron, Excessive intake of magnesium, Excessive intake of potassium, Excessive intake of phosphorus, Excessive intake of sodium, Excessive intake of zinc, Excessive intake of sulfate, Excessive intake of fluoride, Excessive intake of copper, Excessive intake of iodine, Excessive intake of selenium, Excessive intake of manganese, Excessive intake of chromium, Excessive intake of molybdenum, Excessive intake of boron, Excessive intake of cobalt
• Correct amount of enteral/parenteral formula	Excessive energy intake, Excessive parenteral nutrition infusion
• Correct parenteral nutrition components or administration	Inadequate parenteral nutrition infusion, Parenteral nutrition composition inconsistent with needs, Parenteral nutrition administration inconsistent with needs
• Appropriate/correct access for delivering EN/PN	Inadequate enteral nutrition infusion, Inadequate parenteral nutrition infusion, Parenteral nutrition administration inconsistent with needs
• Health benefits of physical activity	Physical inactivity
• How to make nutrition related changes	Limited adherence to nutrition related recommendations
• Food drug interactions	Food medication interaction, Predicted food medication interaction

Etiology	Diagnosis
Category: Knowledge	
• On the part of the caregiver	Excessive enteral nutrition infusion, Excessive parenteral nutrition infusion, Enteral nutrition composition inconsistent with needs, Enteral nutrition administration inconsistent with needs, Parenteral nutrition composition inconsistent with needs, Parenteral nutrition administration inconsistent with needs
• Consumption of high-dose nutrient supplements	Imbalance of nutrients
• Infant/child hunger cues	Food and nutrition related knowledge deficit, Limited food and nutrition related skill
Limited prior exposure or exposure to misinformation, disinformation, and/or contradictory nutrition related information	Food and nutrition related knowledge deficit, Belief finding that hinders food and/or nutrition behavior change, Self monitoring deficit, Unbalanced diet pattern, Limited food and nutrition related skill, Inability to manage self care
Limited prior exposure to accurate information regarding physical activity	Physical inactivity
Limited adjustment for lifestyle changes or restricted mobility and decreased metabolism	Excessive energy intake
Limited literacy	Food and nutrition related knowledge deficit, Limited food and nutrition related skill, Belief finding that hinders food and/or nutrition behavior change
Limited numeracy	Food and nutrition related knowledge deficit, Limited food and nutrition related skill, Belief finding that hinders food and/or nutrition behavior change
Limited access to sources of reliable food and nutrition information	Food and nutrition related knowledge deficit
Limited prior application of skill	Limited food and nutrition related skill
New skill requirement due to recent medical diagnosis or change in health or disease status	Limited food and nutrition related skill, Limited ability to prepare food for eating
New skill requirement due to change in life-course stage or responsibility for self or others	Limited food and nutrition related skill
Category: Physical Function	
Irritability	Breastfeeding difficulty
Inability to physically: • Bend elbow at wrist • Grasp cups and utensils • Sit with hips square and back straight • Support neck and/or control head and neck • Coordinate hand movement to mouth	Self feeding difficulty

Etiology	Diagnosis
Category: Physical Function	
Limited physical ability	Limited food and nutrition related skill, Sarcopenia
Limited self feeding ability	Unintended weight loss
Diminished ability to shop	Food insecurity, Limited access to nutrition related supplies, Limited access to potable water, Sarcopenia
Limited physical strength or range of motion	Self feeding difficulty, Sarcopenia
Limited physical activity	Sarcopenia, Overweight, adult or pediatric, Obesity, adult or pediatric, Obesity, pediatric, Obesity Class I, Obesity Class II, Obesity Class III, Excessive growth rate
Change in physical activity anticipated	Predicted inadequate energy intake, Predicted excessive energy intake
Voluntary or involuntary physical activity/movement	Increased energy expenditure
Category: Physiologic-Metabolic	
Age-related demands	Inadequate protein intake, Growth rate below expected
Alteration in gastrointestinal tract:	
• Decreased functional length of GI tract	Increased nutrient needs, Moderate starvation related malnutrition (undernutrition), Severe starvation related malnutrition (undernutrition), Moderate chronic disease or condition related malnutrition (undernutrition), Severe chronic disease or condition related malnutrition, Moderate acute disease or injury related malnutrition (undernutrition), Severe acute disease or injury related malnutrition (undernutrition), Mild illness related pediatric malnutrition (undernutrition), Moderate illness related pediatric malnutrition, Severe illness related pediatric malnutrition, Altered GI function, Growth rate below expected
• Alteration in gastrointestinal (GI) anatomical structure	Increased nutrient needs, Moderate starvation related malnutrition (undernutrition), Severe starvation related malnutrition (undernutrition), Moderate chronic disease or condition related malnutrition (undernutrition), Severe chronic disease or condition related malnutrition,Moderate acute disease or injury related malnutrition (undernutrition), Severe acute disease or injury related malnutrition (undernutrition), Mild illness related pediatric malnutrition (undernutrition), Moderate illness related pediatric malnutrition (undernutrition), Severe illness related pediatric malnutrition (undernutrition), Altered GI function, Inadequate fat intake, Growth rate below expected
• Alteration in GI function	Limited food acceptance, Inadequate bioactive substance intake, Excessive bioactive substance intake, Increased nutrient needs, Moderate starvation related malnutrition (undernutrition), Severe starvation related malnutrition (undernutrition), Moderate chronic disease or condition related malnutrition (undernutrition), Severe chronic disease or condition related malnutrition, Moderate acute disease or injury related malnu-

Etiology	Diagnosis
Category: Physiologic-Metabolic	
• Alteration in GI function (continued)	trition (undernutrition), Severe acute disease or injury related malnutrition (undernutrition), Mild illness related pediatric malnutrition (undernutrition), Moderate illness related pediatric malnutrition (undernutrition), Severe illness related pediatric malnutrition (undernutrition), Inadequate fat intake, Altered GI function, Sarcopenia, Growth rate below expected
• Change in GI tract motility	Altered GI function
• Change in GI related organ function	Increased nutrient needs, Altered GI function, Growth rate below expected
• Compromised endocrine function	Impaired nutrient utilization, Growth rate below expected
• Change in GI related organ function	Increased nutrient needs, Altered GI function, Growth rate below expected
• Compromised endocrine function	Impaired nutrient utilization, Growth rate below expected
Altered cholesterol metabolism/ regulation	Decreased nutrient needs
Breast tissue with lactating capability or nipple abnormality	Breastfeeding difficulty, Predicted breastfeeding difficulty
Changes in taste, appetite	Excessive fat intake, Intake of types of fats inconsistent with needs
Conditions leading to excess fluid loss	Inadequate fluid intake
Craniofacial malformations	Difficulty chewing
Decreased energy needs	Overweight, adult or pediatric, Obesity, adult or pediatric, Obesity, pediatric, Obesity Class I, Obesity Class II, Obesity Class III, Excessive growth rate
Decreased ability to consume sufficient energy, nutrients	Inadequate energy intake, Inadequate oral intake, Inadequate protein–energy intake, Inadequate protein intake, Inadequate intake of vitamin A, Inadequate intake of vitamin C, Inadequate intake of vitamin D, Inadequate intake of vitamin E, Inadequate intake of vitamin K, Inadequate intake of thiamin, Inadequate intake of riboflavin, Inadequate intake of niacin, Inadequate intake of folate, Inadequate intake of vitamin B6, Inadequate intake of vitamin B12, Inadequate intake of pantothenic acid, Inadequate intake of biotin, Inadequate intake of calcium, Inadequate intake of chloride, Inadequate intake of iron, Inadequate intake of magnesium, Inadequate intake of potassium, Inadequate intake of phosphorus, Inadequate intake of sodium, Inadequate intake of zinc, Inadequate intake of sulfate, Inadequate intake of fluoride, Inadequate intake of copper, Inadequate intake of iodine, Inadequate intake of selenium, Inadequate intake of manganese, Inadequate intake of chromium, Inadequate intake of molybdenum, Inadequate intake of boron, Inadequate intake of cobalt, Sarcopenia, Unintended weight loss, Growth rate below expected

Etiology	Diagnosis
Category: Physiologic-Metabolic	
Decreased nutrient needs related to low activity levels due to chronic disease or organ failure	Excessive enteral nutrition infusion, Excessive parenteral nutrition infusion, Excessive intake of vitamin A, Excessive intake of vitamin C, Excessive intake of vitamin D, Excessive intake of vitamin E, Excessive intake of vitamin K, Excessive intake of thiamin, Excessive intake of riboflavin, Excessive intake of niacin, Excessive intake of folate, Excessive intake of vitamin B6, Excessive intake of vitamin B12, Excessive intake of pantothenic acid, Excessive intake of biotin
Decreased total fat need or recommendation	Excessive fat intake
Altered fatty acid need or recommendation	Intake of types of fats inconsistent with needs
Developmental delay	Limited food acceptance
Difficulty chewing or swallowing high-fiber foods	Inadequate fiber intake
Difficulty latching on	Breastfeeding difficulty
Excessive energy intake	Overweight, adult or pediatric, Obesity, adult or pediatric, Obesity, pediatric, Obesity Class I, Obesity Class II, Obesity Class III, Excessive growth rate
Food allergies and aversions impeding food choices consistent with guidelines	Unbalanced diet pattern, Limited food acceptance
Food intolerances	Decreased nutrient needs, Limited food acceptance, Unbalanced diet pattern
Genetic predisposition to overweight/obesity	Predicted excessive energy intake
Heart failure	Decreased nutrient needs
Illness causing unexpected body weight gain because of head trauma, immobility, paralysis or related condition	Unintended weight gain
Limited cognitive ability, including learning disabilities, neurological or sensory impairment, and dementia	Inadequate fluid intake, Moderate starvation related malnutrition (undernutrition), Severe starvation related malnutrition (undernutrition), Food and nutrition related knowledge deficit, Not ready for nutrition related behavior change, Self monitoring deficit, Limited food and nutrition related skill, Inability to manage self care, Limited ability toprepare food for eating, Self feeding difficulty, Food insecurity
Inadequate energy intake	Sarcopenia, Underweight, Moderate chronic disease or condition related malnutrition (undernutrition), Severe chronic disease or condition related malnutrition, Moderate acute disease or injury related malnutrition (undernutrition), Severe acute disease or injury related malnutrition (undernutrition)
Inadequate milk supply	Breastfeeding difficulty

Etiology	Diagnosis
Category: Physiologic-Metabolic	
Increased energy needs	Underweight
Injury, condition, physical disability or limitation that reduces physical activity or activities of daily living	Physical inactivity, Sarcopenia Mild illness related pediatric malnutrition (undernutrition), Moderate illness related pediatric malnutrition (undernutrition), Severe illness related pediatric malnutrition (undernutrition), Limited ability to prepare food for eating
Intolerance of enteral nutrition (EN)/parenteral nutrition (PN)	Inadequate enteral nutrition infusion, Inadequate parenteral nutrition infusion, Mild non illness related pediatric malnutrition (undernutrition), Moderate non illness related pediatric malnutrition (undernutrition), Severe non illness related pediatric malnutrition (undernutrition), Mild illness related pediatric malnutrition (undernutrition), Moderate illness related pediatric malnutrition (undernutrition), Severe illness related pediatric malnutrition (undernutrition)
Kidney, liver, cardiac, endocrine, neurologic, and/or pulmonary dysfunction	Limited food acceptance, Excessive fluid intake, Difficulty chewing, Altered nutrition related laboratory values, Growth rate below expected
Limited developmental readiness to perform self management tasks	Inability to manage self care
Lethargy, sleepiness	Breastfeeding difficulty
Limited vision	Self feeding difficulty
Limited food acceptance	Inadequate oral intake, Growth rate below expected
Liver dysfunction	Decreased nutrient needs, Excessive protein intake, Intake of types of proteins inconsistent with needs, Intake types of amino acids inconsistent with needs
Loss of appetite awareness	Excessive oral intake
Malnutrition/malabsorption	Increased nutrient needs, Breastfeeding difficulty, Predicted breastfeeding difficulty, Growth rate below expected
Mastitis and/or painful breast tissue with lactating capability, nipples	Breastfeeding difficulty, Predicted breastfeeding difficulty
Mechanical issues such as inflammation, surgery, stricture, or oral, pharyngeal and esophageal tumors, mechanical ventilation	Swallowing difficulty, Difficulty chewing
Inborn errors of metabolism	Intake of types of proteins inconsistent with needs, Intake types of amino acids inconsistent with needs, Altered nutrition related laboratory values, Mild illness related pediatric malnutrition (undernutrition), Moderate illness related pediatric malnutrition (undernutrition), Severe illness related pediatric malnutrition (undernutrition)
Metabolic abnormality	Excessive protein intake, Intake of types of proteins inconsistent with needs, Intake types of amino acids inconsistent with needs, Mild illness related pediatric malnutrition (undernutrition), Moderate illness related pediatric malnutrition (undernutrition), Severe illness related pediatric malnutrition (undernutrition)

Etiology	Diagnosis
Category: Physiologic-Metabolic	
Metabolic disorders	Impaired nutrient utilization, Intake types of amino acids inconsistent with needs, Mild illness related pediatric malnutrition (undernutrition), Moderate illness related pediatric malnutrition (undernutrition), Severe illness related pediatric malnutrition (undernutrition)
Motor causes related to neurological or muscular disorders	Swallowing difficulty
Oral pain	Breastfeeding difficulty
Other organ dysfunction that leads to biochemical changes	Altered nutrition related laboratory values
Partial or complete edentulism	Difficulty chewing
Physical disability	Limited ability to prepare food for eating, Food insecurity, Limited access to potable water
Physiological causes that put emphasis on food, body weight, or shape	Disordered eating pattern
Physiologic causes requiring modified amount or timing of carbohydrate intake	Excessive carbohydrate intake, Intake of types of carbohydrate inconsistent with needs, Inconsistent carbohydrate intake
Physiological causes that put emphasis on food, body weight, or shape	Disordered eating pattern
Physiologic causes requiring modified amount or timing of carbohydrate intake	Excessive carbohydrate intake, Intake of types of carbohydrate inconsistent with needs, Inconsistent carbohydrate intake
Physiological causes increasing nutrient needs due to:	
• Accelerated growth or anabolism	Increased energy expenditure, Inadequate enteral nutrition infusion, Inadequate parenteral nutrition infusion, Increased nutrient needs, Inadequate intake of calcium, Inadequate intake of chloride, Inadequate intake of iron, Inadequate intake of magnesium, Inadequate intake of potassium, Inadequate intake of phosphorus, Inadequate intake of sodium, Inadequate intake of zinc, Inadequate intake of sulfate, Inadequate intake of fluoride, Inadequate intake of copper, Inadequate intake of iodine, Inadequate intake of selenium, Inadequate intake of manganese, Inadequate intake of chromium, Inadequate intake of molybdenum, Inadequate intake of boron, Inadequate intake of cobalt, Growth rate below expected
• Altered absorption or metabolism	Inadequate fluid intake, Increased nutrient needs, Inadequate protein intake, Inadequate carbohydrate intake, Inadequate intake of vitamin A, Inadequate intake of vitamin C, Inadequate intake of vitamin D, Inadequate intake of vitamin E, Inadequate intake of vitamin K, Inadequate intake of thiamin, Inadequate intake of riboflavin, Inadequate intake of niacin, Inadequate intake of folate, Inadequate intake of vitamin B6, Inadequate

Etiology	Diagnosis
Category: Physiologic-Metabolic	
• Altered absorption or metabolism (continued)	intake of vitamin B12, Inadequate intake of pantothenic acid, Inadequate intake of biotin, Inadequate intake of calcium, Inadequate intake of chloride, Inadequate intake of iron, Inadequate intake of magnesium, Inadequate intake of potassium, Inadequate intake of phosphorus, Inadequate intake of sodium, Inadequate intake of zinc, Inadequate intake of sulfate, Inadequate intake of fluoride, Inadequate intake of copper, Inadequate intake of iodine, Inadequate intake of selenium, Inadequate intake of manganese, Inadequate intake of chromium, Inadequate intake of molybdenum, Inadequate intake of boron, Inadequate intake of cobalt, Predicted inadequate nutrient intake, Moderate chronic disease or condition related malnutrition (undernutrition), Severe chronic disease or condition related malnutrition, Mild illness related pediatric malnutrition (undernutrition), Moderate illness related pediatric malnutrition (undernutrition), Severe illness related pediatric malnutrition (undernutrition), Inadequate protein–energy intake, Unintended weight loss, Growth rate below expected
• Disease/condition	Inadequate enteral nutrition infusion, Inadequate parenteral nutrition infusion, Inadequate fluid intake, Increased nutrient needs, Moderate chronic disease or condition related malnutrition (undernutrition), Severe chronic disease or condition related malnutrition, Mild illness related pediatric malnutrition (undernutrition), Moderate illness related pediatric malnutrition (undernutrition), Severe illness related pediatric malnutrition (undernutrition), Inadequate protein–energy intake, Inadequate protein intake, Intake of types of proteins inconsistent with needs, Intake types of amino acids inconsistent with needs, Inadequate intake of vitamin A, Inadequate intake of vitamin C, Inadequate intake of vitamin D, Inadequate intake of vitamin E, Inadequate intake of vitamin K, Inadequate intake of thiamin, Inadequate intake of riboflavin, Inadequate intake of niacin, Inadequate intake of folate, Inadequate intake of vitamin B6, Inadequate intake of vitamin B12, Inadequate intake of pantothenic acid, Inadequate intake of biotin, Sarcopenia, Unintended weight loss, Growth rate below expected
Maintenance of body temperature	Increased energy expenditure, Inadequate fluid intake, Growth rate below expected
Prolonged catabolic illness	Inadequate energy intake, Inadequate oral intake, Inadequate fluid intake, Moderate chronic disease or condition related malnutrition (undernutrition), Severe chronic disease or condition related malnutrition,Mild illness related pediatric malnutrition (undernutrition), Moderate illness related pediatric malnutrition (undernutrition), Severe illness related pediatric malnutrition (undernutrition),Inadequate protein–energy intake, Inadequate protein intake, Inadequate intake of vitamin A, Inadequate intake of vitamin C, Inadequate intake of vitamin D, Inadequate intake of vitamin E, Inadequate intake of vitamin K, Inadequate intake of thiamin, Inadequate intake of riboflavin, Inadequate intake

Etiology	Diagnosis
Category: Physiologic-Metabolic	
Prolonged catabolic illness (continued)	of niacin, Inadequate intake of folate, Inadequate intake of vitamin B6, Inadequate intake of vitamin B12, Inadequate intake of pantothenic acid, Inadequate intake of biotin, Inadequate intake of calcium, Inadequate intake of chloride, Inadequate intake of iron, Inadequate intake of magnesium, Inadequate intake of potassium, Inadequate intake of phosphorus, Inadequate intake of sodium, Inadequate intake of zinc, Inadequate intake of sulfate, Inadequate intake of fluoride, Inadequate intake of copper, Inadequate intake of iodine, Inadequate intake of selenium, Inadequate intake of manganese, Inadequate intake of chromium, Inadequate intake of molybdenum, Inadequate intake of boron, Inadequate intake of cobalt, Sarcopenia, Unintended weight loss, Growth rate below expected
Altered metabolism	Predicted excessive energy intake, Predicted excessive nutrient intake
Poor sucking ability	Breastfeeding difficulty, Predicted breastfeeding difficulty, Growth rate below expected
Prematurity	Altered nutrition related laboratory values, Growth rate below expected, Mild illness related pediatric malnutrition (undernutrition), Moderate illness related pediatric malnutrition (undernutrition), Severe illness related pediatric malnutrition (undernutrition),
Renal dysfunction	Decreased nutrient needs, Excessive protein intake, Intake of types of proteins inconsistent with needs, Intake types of amino acids inconsistent with needs
Small for gestational age, intrauterine growth retardation/restriction and/or Lack of or limited progress/appropriate body weight gain per day	Underweight, Growth rate below expected
Soft tissue disease (primary or oral manifestations of a systemic disease)	Difficulty chewing, Moderate starvation related malnutrition (undernutrition), Severe starvation related malnutrition (undernutrition),
Swallowing difficulty, and altered suck and breathing patterns in infants	Swallowing difficulty, Breastfeeding difficulty, Predicted breastfeeding difficulty
Xerostomia	Difficulty chewing
Recent medical diagnosis or change in health or disease status	Food and nutrition related knowledge deficit
Loss of muscle mass, decreased strength, and/or decreased physical performance related to aging, hormonal balance, and/or inflammation	Sarcopenia
Alcohol or drug addiction	Excessive alcohol intake, Impaired nutrient utilization

Etiology	Diagnosis
Category: Psychological	
Addictive personality	Excessive physical activity
Mental illness, confusion, or altered awareness	Intake of unsafe food, Excessive oral intake
Personality characteristics or temperament associated with eating disorders	Disordered eating pattern
Psychological causes that put emphasis on food, body weight, or shape	Disordered eating pattern
Psychological causes such as depression and disordered eating	Inadequate energy intake, Inadequate oral intake, Inadequate fluid intake, Excessive fluid intake, Moderate starvation related malnutrition (undernutrition), Severe starvation related malnutrition (undernutrition), Non illness related pediatric malnutrition (undernutrition), Mild illness related pediatric malnutrition (undernutrition), Moderate illness related pediatric malnutrition (undernutrition), Severe illness related pediatric malnutrition (undernutrition), Inadequate protein–energy intake, Inadequate fat intake, Inadequate protein intake, Inadequate carbohydrate intake, Excessive carbohydrate intake, Intake of types of carbohydrate inconsistent with needs, Inconsistent carbohydrate intake, Inadequate fiber intake, Inadequate intake of vitamin A, Inadequate intake of vitamin C, Inadequate intake of vitamin D, Inadequate intake of vitamin E, Inadequate intake of vitamin K, Inadequate intake of thiamin, Inadequate intake of riboflavin, Inadequate intake of niacin, Inadequate intake of folate, Inadequate intake of vitamin B6, Inadequate intake of vitamin B12, Inadequate intake of pantothenic acid, Inadequate intake of biotin, Excessive intake of vitamin A, Excessive intake of vitamin C, Excessive intake of vitamin D, Excessive intake of vitamin E, Excessive intake of vitamin K, Excessive intake of thiamin, Excessive intake of riboflavin, Excessive intake of niacin, Excessive intake of folate, Excessive intake of vitamin B6, Excessive intake of vitamin B12, Excessive intake of pantothenic acid, Excessive intake of biotin, Inadequate intake of calcium, Inadequate intake of chloride, Inadequate intake of iron, Inadequate intake of magnesium, Inadequate intake of potassium, Inadequate intake of phosphorus, Inadequate intake of sodium, Inadequate intake of zinc, Inadequate intake of sulfate, Inadequate intake of fluoride, Inadequate intake of copper, Inadequate intake of iodine, Inadequate intake of selenium, Inadequate intake of manganese, Inadequate intake of chromium, Inadequate intake of molybdenum, Inadequate intake of boron, Inadequate intake of cobalt, Unintended weight loss, Growth rate below expected, Unbalanced diet pattern, Excessive physical activity, Food insecurity, Limited access to nutrition related supplies
Limited psychological ability	Limited food and nutrition related skill
Psychological factors leading to inadequate intake and/or limited physical activity	Sarcopenia

Etiology	Diagnosis
Category: Social-Personal	
Limited psychological ability	Limited food and nutrition related skill
Psychological factors leading to inadequate intake and/or limited physical activity	Sarcopenia
Limited role models	Breastfeeding difficulty, Physical inactivity
Limited social support for implementing changes	Breastfeeding difficulty, Predicted breastfeeding difficulty, Mild non illness related pediatric malnutrition (undernutrition), Moderate non illness related pediatric malnutrition (undernutrition), Severe non illness related pediatric malnutrition (undernutrition), Not ready for nutrition related behavior change, Self monitoring deficit, Limited adherence to nutrition related recommendations, Limited food and nutrition related skill, Physical inactivity, Inability to manage self care, Poor food and/or nutrition quality of life
Family or social history of overeating	Predicted excessive energy intake
Increased psychological/life stress	Predicted breastfeeding difficulty, Overweight, adult or pediatric, Obesity, adult or pediatric, Obesity, pediatric, Obesity Class I, Obesity Class II, Obesity Class III, Predicted inadequate energy intake, Predicted excessive energy intake
Traumatic event(s) that causes a physical or psychological stress reaction	Disordered eating pattern
Change in living situation	Predicted inadequate energy intake, Predicted excessive energy intake, Predicted inadequate nutrient intake, Predicted breastfeeding difficulty
Living in a geographic location with danger for environmental emergency	Predicted inadequate nutrient intake
Change in life-course stage or responsibility for self or others	Food and nutrition related knowledge deficit
Social-Personal factors leading to inadequate intake and/or limited physical activity	Sarcopenia
Category: Treatment	
Accidental vitamin and/or mineral overdose from oral, enteral or parenteral sources	Excessive intake of vitamin A, Excessive intake of vitamin C, Excessive intake of vitamin D, Excessive intake of vitamin E, Excessive intake of vitamin K, Excessive intake of thiamin, Excessive intake of riboflavin, Excessive intake of niacin, Excessive intake of folate, Excessive intake of vitamin B6, Excessive intake of vitamin B12, Excessive intake of pantothenic acid, Excessive intake of biotin, Excessive intake of calcium, Excessive intake of chloride, Excessive intake of iron, Excessive intake of magnesium, Excessive intake of potassium, Excessive intake of phosphorus, Excessive intake of sodium, Excessive intake of zinc, Excessive intake of sulfate, Excessive intake of fluoride, Excessive intake of copper, Excessive intake of iodine,

Etiology	Diagnosis
Category: Treatment	
Accidental vitamin and/or mineral overdose from oral, enteral or parenteral sources (continued)	Excessive intake of selenium, Excessive intake of manganese, Excessive intake of chromium, Excessive intake of molybdenum, Excessive intake of boron, Excessive intake of cobalt
Calories/kcal/kJ unaccounted for from intravenous (IV) infusion and/or medications	Excessive energy intake
Changes in taste, appetite	Excessive fat intake, Intake of types of fats inconsistent with needs
Changes in GI tract motility	Altered GI function, Unbalanced diet pattern
Chronic use of medications known to cause body weight gain, such as use of certain antidepressants, antipsychotics, corticosteroids, certain HIV medications	Unintended weight gain, Excessive growth rate
Difficulty chewing or swallowing high-fiber foods	Inadequate fiber intake
Excessive energy intake	Overweight, adult or pediatric, Obesity, adult or pediatric, Obesity, pediatric, Obesity Class I, Obesity Class II, Obesity Class III
Food intolerances	Decreased nutrient needs
High level of fatigue or other side effect of therapy	Unbalanced diet pattern, Limited ability to prepare food for eating
Improvement in client status, allowing return to total or partial oral diet; changes in the course of disease resulting in changes in nutrient requirements	Enteral nutrition composition inconsistent with needs, Enteral nutrition administration inconsistent with needs, Parenteral nutrition composition inconsistent with needs, Parenteral nutrition administration inconsistent with needs
Inadequate energy intake	Sarcopenia, Underweight
Infusion volume not reached or schedule for infusion interrupted	Inadequate enteral nutrition infusion, Inadequate parenteral nutrition infusion
Insufficient electrolyte replacement when initiating feeding (PN/EN, including oral)	Imbalance of nutrients
Lack of or limited, compromised, or incorrect access for delivering EN/PN	Inadequate enteral nutrition infusion, Inadequate parenteral nutrition infusion
Mechanical issues such as inflammation, surgery, stricture, or oral, pharyngeal and esophageal tumors, mechanical ventilation	Swallowing difficulty, Difficulty chewing
Medications that increase appetite	Excessive energy intake, Excessive oral intake,
Medications that increase nutrient needs	Increased nutrient needs

Etiology	Diagnosis
Category: Treatment	
Medications that affect nutrient metabolism	Impaired nutrient utilization
Medications that increase fluid needs or decrease thirst	Inadequate fluid intake
Misused specialized protein products	Intake of types of proteins inconsistent with needs
Misused specialized amino acid products	Intake types of amino acids inconsistent with needs
Misdiagnosis of lactose intolerance/lactase deficiency	Inadequate intake of calcium, Inadequate intake of magnesium, Inadequate intake of potassium, Inadequate intake of phosphorus
Nutrient/nutrient interaction and/or drug/nutrient interaction	Inadequate enteral nutrition infusion, Inadequate parenteral nutrition infusion, Inadequate intake of vitamin A, Inadequate intake of vitamin C, Inadequate intake of vitamin D, Inadequate intake of vitamin E, Inadequate intake of vitamin K, Inadequate intake of thiamin, Inadequate intake of riboflavin, Inadequate intake of niacin, Inadequate intake of folate, Inadequate intake of vitamin B6, Inadequate intake of vitamin B12, Inadequate intake of pantothenic acid, Inadequate intake of biotin, Excessive intake of vitamin A, Excessive intake of vitamin C, Excessive intake of vitamin D, Excessive intake of vitamin E, Excessive intake of vitamin K, Excessive intake of thiamin, Excessive intake of riboflavin, Excessive intake of niacin, Excessive intake of folate, Excessive intake of vitamin B6, Excessive intake of vitamin B12, Excessive intake of pantothenic acid, Excessive intake of biotin, Inadequate intake of calcium, Inadequate intake of chloride, Inadequate intake of iron, Inadequate intake of magnesium, Inadequate intake of potassium, Inadequate intake of phosphorus, Inadequate intake of sodium, Inadequate intake of zinc, Inadequate intake of sulfate, Inadequate intake of fluoride, Inadequate intake of copper, Inadequate intake of iodine, Inadequate intake of selenium, Inadequate intake of manganese, Inadequate intake of chromium, Inadequate intake of molybdenum, Inadequate intake of boron, Inadequate intake of cobalt, Excessive intake of calcium, Excessive intake of chloride, Excessive intake of iron, Excessive intake of magnesium, Excessive intake of potassium, Excessive intake of phosphorus, Excessive intake of sodium, Excessive intake of zinc, Excessive intake of sulfate, Excessive intake of fluoride, Excessive intake of copper, Excessive intake of iodine, Excessive intake of selenium, Excessive intake of manganese, Excessive intake of chromium, Excessive intake of molybdenum, Excessive intake of boron, Excessive intake of cobalt, Food Medication Interaction, Predicted food medication interaction
Overfeeding of parenteral/enteral nutrition (PN/EN)	Excessive energy intake

Etiology	Diagnosis
Category: Treatment	
Planned procedure, therapy or medication predicted to increase energy expenditure or nutrient need	Predicted inadequate energy intake, Predicted inadequate nutrient intake, Sarcopenia
Planned therapy or medication predicted to reduce energy/nutrient need or metabolic rate/metabolism	Predicted excessive energy intake, Predicted excessive nutrient intake
Planned procedure, therapy or medication predicted to hinder breastfeeding	Predicted breastfeeding difficulty
Planned procedure, therapy or medication predicted to decrease ability to consume sufficient energy or nutrients	Predicted inadequate energy intake, Predicted inadequate nutrient intake, Sarcopenia
Prolonged adherence to a low-fiber or low-residue diet	Inadequate fiber intake
Prolonged hospitalization	Sarcopenia Unintended weight loss
Renal dysfunction	Decreased nutrient needs, Excessive protein intake, Intake of types of proteins inconsistent with needs, Intake types of amino acids inconsistent with needs
Limited training availability	Limited food and nutrition related skill
Impacting physical activity level	Sarcopenia, Limited ability to prepare food for eating
Category: Access	
Access to foods and supplements in excess of needs	Excessive intake of vitamin A, Excessive intake of vitamin C, Excessive intake of vitamin D, Excessive intake of vitamin E, Excessive intake of vitamin K, Excessive intake of thiamin, Excessive intake of riboflavin, Excessive intake of niacin, Excessive intake of folate, Excessive intake of vitamin B6, Excessive intake of vitamin B12, Excessive intake of pantothenic acid, Excessive intake of biotin
Caregiver intentionally or unintentionally not providing access to food or nutrition related supplies	Food insecurity, Limited access to nutrition related supplies, Limited access to potable water
Community and geographical constraints	Inadequate intake of vitamin A, Inadequate intake of vitamin C, Inadequate intake of vitamin D, Inadequate intake of vitamin E, Inadequate intake of vitamin K, Inadequate intake of thiamin, Inadequate intake of riboflavin, Inadequate intake of niacin, Inadequate intake of folate, Inadequate intake of vitamin B6, Inadequate intake of vitamin B12, Inadequate intake of pantothenic acid, Inadequate intake of biotin, Food insecurity, Limited access to nutrition related supplies, Limited access to potable water

Etiology	Diagnosis
Category: Access	
Environmental causes (eg, inadequately tested nutrient bioavailability of fortified foods, beverages, and supplements; marketing of fortified foods, beverages, supplements as a substitute for natural food source of nutrient(s))	Inadequate intake of vitamin A, Inadequate intake of vitamin C, Inadequate intake of vitamin D, Inadequate intake of vitamin E, Inadequate intake of vitamin K, Inadequate intake of thiamin, Inadequate intake of riboflavin, Inadequate intake of niacin, Inadequate intake of folate, Inadequate intake of vitamin B6, Inadequate intake of vitamin B12, Inadequate intake of pantothenic acid, Inadequate intake of biotin, Inadequate intake of calcium, Inadequate intake of chloride, Inadequate intake of iron, Inadequate intake of magnesium, Inadequate intake of potassium, Inadequate intake of phosphorus, Inadequate intake of sodium, Inadequate intake of zinc, Inadequate intake of sulfate, Inadequate intake of fluoride, Inadequate intake of copper, Inadequate intake of iodine, Inadequate intake of selenium, Inadequate intake of manganese, Inadequate intake of chromium, Inadequate intake of molybdenum, Inadequate intake of boron, Inadequate intake of cobalt
Exposure to contaminated water or food (eg, community outbreak of illness documented by surveillance and/or response agency)	Intake of unsafe food, Food insecurity, Limited access to potable water
Reluctance to participate in federal food programs such as women and children food program, school breakfast and/or lunch program, supplemental food resources	Food insecurity, Limited access to potable water
Financial constraints that may prevent sufficient level of activity (eg, to address cost of equipment or shoes or club membership to gain access)	Physical inactivity
Limited access to:	
• Adaptive foods or eating devices conducive for self feeding	Self feeding difficulty
• Available and safe physical activity environment and/or equipment	Physical inactivity
• Fluid	Inadequate fluid intake, Inadequate fiber intake,
• Fortified foods and beverages	Inadequate intake of calcium, Inadequate intake of chloride, Inadequate intake of iron, Inadequate intake of magnesium, Inadequate intake of potassium, Inadequate intake of phosphorus, Inadequate intake of sodium, Inadequate intake of zinc, Inadequate intake of sulfate, Inadequate intake of fluoride, Inadequate intake of copper, Inadequate intake of iodine, Inadequate intake of selenium, Inadequate intake of manganese, Inadequate intake of chromium, Inadequate intake of molybdenum, Inadequate intake of boron, Inadequate intake of cobalt

Etiology	Diagnosis
Category: Access	
• Specialized protein products	Excessive protein intake
• Food or artificial nutrition	Inadequate energy intake, Inadequate oral intake, Moderate starvation related malnutrition (undernutrition), Severe starvation related malnutrition (undernutrition), Mild non illness related pediatric malnutrition (undernutrition), Moderate non illness related pediatric malnutrition (undernutrition), Severe non illness related pediatric malnutrition (undernutrition), Inadequate protein energy intake, Inadequate fat intake, Inadequate protein intake, Intake of types of proteins inconsistent with needs, Intake of types of amino acids inconsistent with needs, Inadequate carbohydrate intake, Inadequate intake of vitamin A, Inadequate intake of vitamin C, Inadequate intake of vitamin D, Inadequate intake of vitamin E, Inadequate intake of vitamin K, Inadequate intake of thiamin, Inadequate intake of riboflavin, Inadequate intake of niacin, Inadequate intake of folate, Inadequate intake of vitamin B6, Inadequate intake of vitamin B12, Inadequate intake of pantothenic acid, Inadequate intake of biotin, Inadequate intake of calcium, Inadequate intake of chloride, Inadequate intake of iron, Inadequate intake of magnesium, Inadequate intake of potassium, Inadequate intake of phosphorus, Inadequate intake of sodium, Inadequate intake of zinc, Inadequate intake of sulfate, Inadequate intake of fluoride, Inadequate intake of copper, Inadequate intake of iodine, Inadequate intake of selenium, Inadequate intake of manganese, Inadequate intake of chromium, Inadequate intake of molybdenum, Inadequate intake of boron, Inadequate intake of cobalt, Underweight, Unintended weight loss, Growth rate below expected, Poor food and/or nutrition quality of life
• Fiber-containing foods	Inadequate fiber intake
• Food that contains a bioactive substance	Inadequate bioactive substance intake
• Sufficient quantity and/or variety of culturally appropriate healthful food	Excessive energy intake, Excessive oral intake, Excessive fat intake, Intake of types of fats inconsistent with needs, Unbalanced diet pattern, Food insecurity
• Sufficient quantity of potable water	Limited access to potable water
• Safe and/or clear and accurately labeled food supply	Excessive bioactive substance intake Intake of unsafe food
• Food storage equipment/ facilities	Intake of unsafe food
• Self management tools or decision guides or other nutrition related supplies	Inability to manage self care, Limited access to nutrition related supplies
• Resources	Food and nutrition related skill, Food insecurity

Etiology	Diagnosis
Category: Access	
Limited participation in community supplemental food programs such as food pantries, emergency kitchens, or shelters, with a sufficient variety of culturally appropriate healthful foods or nutrition related supplies	Food insecurity, Unbalanced diet pattern, Limited access to nutrition related supplies, Limited access to potable water
Schools lacking nutrition/wellness policies or application of policies ensuring convenient, appetizing, competitively priced culturally appropriate healthful foods and/or water at meals, snacks, and school sponsored activities	Food insecurity, Limited access to potable water
Factors leading to inadequate intake and/or limited physical activity	Sarcopenia
Limited health care coverage	Food insecurity
Disruption of food production, processing, and/or distribution network	Food insecurity
Limited food outlet options or one that has abundance of food outlets lacking nutrient rich foods	Food insecurity, Unbalanced diet pattern
Category: Behavior	
Addictive behavior	Excessive physical activity
Consumption of high-dose nutrient supplements	Imbalance of nutrients
Eating behavior serves a purpose other than nourishment	Unbalanced diet pattern, Limited food acceptance
Excessive energy intake	Overweight, adult or pediatric, Obesity, adult or pediatric, Obesity, pediatric, Obesity Class I, Obesity Class II, Obesity Class III
Excessive physical activity	Underweight
Food and nutrition adherence limitations	Excessive carbohydrate intake, Intake of types of carbohydrate inconsistent with needs, Inconsistent carbohydrate intake
Food or activity behavior-related difficulty	Poor food and/or nutrition quality of life
Food preparation or eating patterns that involve only high-fiber foods to the exclusion of other nutrient-dense foods	Excessive fiber intake

Etiology	Diagnosis
Category: Behavior	
Disordered eating pattern	Excessive physical activity, Underweight, Overweight, adult or pediatric, Obesity, adult or pediatric, Obesity, pediatric, Obesity Class I, Obesity Class II, Obesity Class III, Mild non illness related pediatric malnutrition (undernutrition), Moderate non illness related pediatric malnutrition (undernutrition), Severe non illness related pediatric malnutrition (undernutrition), Mild illness related pediatric malnutrition (undernutrition), Moderate illness related pediatric malnutrition (undernutrition), Severe illness related pediatric malnutrition (undernutrition)
Feeding via bottle or other route that may affect breastfeeding	Breastfeeding difficulty, Predicted breastfeeding difficulty
Frequent intake of foods containing bioactive substances	Excessive bioactive substance intake
Limited food acceptance due to behavioral issues	Inadequate oral intake, Growth rate below expected
Inability to limit or refuse offered foods	Excessive oral intake
Inadequate energy intake	Underweight
Limited focus and attention to detail, difficulty with time management and/or organization	Self monitoring deficit
Lifestyle change that reduces physical activity or activities of daily living	Physical inactivity
Limited physical activity	Sarcopenia
Over consumption of a limited variety of foods	Excessive intake of calcium, Excessive intake of chloride, Excessive intake of iron, Excessive intake of magnesium, Excessive intake of potassium, Excessive intake of phosphorus, Excessive intake of sodium, Excessive intake of zinc, Excessive intake of sulfate, Excessive intake of fluoride, Excessive intake of copper, Excessive intake of iodine, Excessive intake of selenium, Excessive intake of manganese, Excessive intake of chromium, Excessive intake of molybdenum, Excessive intake of boron, Excessive intake of cobalt
Poor food planning, purchasing and preparation practices	Excessive oral intake, Inadequate fiber intake, Food insecurity
Reluctance or avoidance of self feeding	Self feeding difficulty